BEFORE PROZAC

Before Prozac

The Troubled History of Mood Disorders in Psychiatry

Edward Shorter

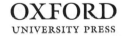

UNIVERSITY PRESS

2009

OXFORD
UNIVERSITY PRESS

Oxford University Press, Inc., publishes works that further
Oxford University's objective of excellence
in research, scholarship, and education.

Oxford   New York
Auckland   Cape Town   Dar es Salaam   Hong Kong   Karachi
Kuala Lumpur   Madrid   Melbourne   Mexico City   Nairobi
New Delhi   Shanghai   Taipei   Toronto

With offices in
Argentina   Austria   Brazil   Chile   Czech Republic   France   Greece
Guatemala   Hungary   Italy   Japan   Poland   Portugal   Singapore
South Korea   Switzerland   Thailand   Turkey   Ukraine   Vietnam

Copyright © 2009 by Oxford University Press, Inc.

Published by Oxford University Press, Inc.
198 Madison Avenue, New York, New York 10016
www.oup.com

Oxford is a registered trademark of Oxford University Press

Library of Congress Cataloging-in-Publication Data
Shorter, Edward.
Before Prozac: the troubled history of mood disorders in psychiatry / Edward Shorter.
p. ; cm.
Includes bibliographical references and index.
ISBN: 978-0-19-536874-1
1. Affective disorders—Chemotherapy—United States—History. 2. Psychotropic
drugs—United States—History. 3. Psychopharmacology—United States—History.
4. Serotonin uptake inhibitors—Therapeutic use—History. 5. Psychotropic drugs
industry—United States—History. 6. Pharmaceutical policy—United
States—History. I. Title.
[DNLM: 1. United States. Food and Drug Administration. 2. Psychopharmacology—
history—United States. 3. Drug Approval—history—United States. 4. Government
Agencies—history—United States. 5. History, 20th Century—United States. 6. Mood
Disorders—drug therapy—United States. 7. Psychotropic Drugs—history—United States.
QV 11 AA1 S559b 2008.]
RC537.S52 2008
616.85'27061—dc22

                                                                      2008008082

9 8 7 6 5 4 3 2 1

Printed in the United States of America
on acid-free paper

To my teachers

PREFACE

When I lecture to my students, I tell them that medicine has two arms. One is diagnosis, and I hold out my left arm and wiggle it. The other is treatment, and I extend my right arm and wave it a bit. Psychiatry, as part of medicine, also has two arms, and events with them over the last 50 years have gone seriously awry. As the discipline pulled itself out of the swamp of psychoanalysis in the middle third of the twentieth century, one might have expected to see progress, as achievement was built upon achievement, and the wall of knowledge rose higher. This is approximately what happens in the other medical disciplines.

This increment of knowledge has not happened in psychiatry, at least not in the diagnosis and treatment of mood disorders, the bulk of the discipline's clinical burden. Instead, knowledge has been forgotten, with the result that in the early twenty-first century psychiatry is not demonstrably further down the road on which it found itself in the mid-1950s. This is not only a scandal for the responsible advancement of knowledge, it is a disaster for public health, as patients in the grips of often terrible illnesses cannot count on the certainty of state-of-the-art diagnosis and treatment, simply because the state of the art has been duly forgotten, or trampled in the latest surge of herd behavior that seems to characterize psychiatrists more than clinicians in other disciplines. How something that wasn't supposed to happen actually occurred is the subject of this book.

As someone trained as a historian, I have learned much from a small and scattered group of psychiatrists—thoughtful scientists and distinguished clinicians—whom I regard, doubtless somewhat self-inflatedly, as my teachers. They are Thomas Ban, Tom Bolwig, Bernard Carroll, Max Fink, David Healy, Conrad Swartz, and Michael Alan Taylor. That I have not learned all they have to teach is doubtless owing to my own inadequacies as a student, for not all of them will agree with every-thing that is in this book. But I am terribly grateful to them for years of intellectual companionship and camaraderie.

In addition, I must thank Tom Ban and David Healy for giving each chapter a critical reading.

It is, I realize, tedious for readers to see the interlibrary loan service at the author's local university acknowledged. Yet I must mention mine for coping uncomplainingly with a volume of requests that ranged from the excessive to the hallucinatory.

In the years it has taken to research and write this book, I have a special debt to researchers Susan Bélanger, Heather Dichter, and Ellen Tulchinsky, as well as my longtime secretary Andrea Clark, now hap-pily retired and away from the office with its shouts and screams.

My literary agent and dear friend Bev Slopen has, as always, been terribly helpful. Marion Osmun at Oxford University Press is a won-derful editor, and I feel privileged to have worked with her.

Edward Shorter
Toronto
February 2008

CONTENTS

Main Drug Classes Discussed in *Before Prozac*[1]

Drug Class	Generic Drug Name	Trade Name (Drug Company and Year Introduced)[2]
Amphetamines *(includes some phenylethylamine [PEA] derivatives)* *Use: antidepressant; stimulant; antihyperactivity*	amphetamine sulfate	*Benzedrine Sulfate* (Smith, Kline & French marketed 1935)
	bupropion, a PEA derivative	*Wellbutrin* (Burroughs-Wellcome introduced 1986)
	dextroamphetamine	*Dexedrine Sulfate* (Smith, Kline & French marketed 1944)
	methamphetamine	*Desoxyn* (Abbott Laboratories marketed 1943)
	methylphenidate (amphetamine-related in structure)	*Ritalin* (Ciba launched in 1954 in Switzerland, in 1956 in United States)
	pipradrol	*Meratran* (Merrell marketed 1955); considered a stimulant
Antihistamines *Use: antipanic; antidepressant. (See also phenothiazines)*	chlorpheniramine	*Chlor-Trimeton* (Schering Labs marketed 1949)
	diphenhydramine	*Benadryl* (Parke Davis marketed 1946)
Barbiturates *Use: sedative; hypnotic; anticonvulsant*	allobarbital	*Dial* (Ciba patented and marketed 1912)
	amobarbital	*Sodium Amytal* (Lilly patented and marketed 1924)
	barbital (also diemal malonal barbitone)	*Veronal* (Merck and Bayer marketed in 1903 in Germany; also brought out as *Medinal* by Schering, 1903)
	butabarbital	*Butisol Sodium* (Lilly patented, and McNeil Laboratories marketed in 1932)
	phenobarbital	*Luminal* (Bayer marketed in 1911 in Germany)
	secobarbital sodium	*Seconal* (Lilly synthesized in 1934; marketed in 1936)
	talbutal	*Lotusate* (synthesized in 1925; Winthrop marketed in 1955)

(continued)

Main Drug Classes *(continued)*

Drug Class	Generic Drug Name	Trade Name (Drug Company and Year Introduced)[2]
Benzodiazepines *Use: anxiolytic; hypnotic; anticonvulsant; muscle relaxant*	alprazolam	*Xanax* (Upjohn launched 1981; later, also antipanic)
	chlordiazepoxide	*Librium* (Hoffmann-La Roche introduced 1960)
	clonazepam	*Rivotril* (Hoffmann-La Roche marketed in 1973 in France; and as *Clonopin* [*Klonopin*] in 1975 in United States)
	clorazepate	*Tranxene* (Abbott marketed in 1968 in France, in 1972 in United States)
	diazepam	*Valium* (Hoffmann-La Roche marketed in Italy in 1962, in United States in 1963)
	flurazepam	*Dalmane* (Hoffmann-La Roche launched 1970)
	lorazepam	*Ativan* (Wyeth marketed in 1977 in United States; brought out previously as *Temesta* in Europe in 1972; used also for catatonia)
	oxazepam	*Serax* (Wyeth marketed 1965)
	prazepam	*Verstran* (Warner-Lambert marketed 1977)
	triazolam	*Halcion* (Upjohn launched in 1979 in United Kingdom, in 1982 in United States)
Bicyclic and Tetracyclic Antidepressants *Use: antidepressant*	maprotiline	*Ludiomil* (Ciba introduced in 1973 in Germany, in United States in 1981)
	nomifensine	*Alival* (Hoechst introduced in 1976 in Germany; also brought out at as *Merital* in 1985 in United States); withdrawn 1986
	trazodone	*Trittico* (Angelini developed and marketed in 1972 in Italy; brought out by Mead Johnson as *Desyrel* in 1982 in United States; later used as hypnotic)

Drug Class	Generic Drug Name	Trade Name (Drug Company and Year Introduced)[2]
Carbamates *Use: antineurotic;* *sedative; anxiolytic*	emylcamate	*Striatran* (synthesized 1912 and marketed by Merck in 1960)
	ethinamate	*Valmid*, later *Valamin* (Lilly marketed 1955)
	hydroxyphenamate	*Listica* (Armour launched 1961)
	meprobamate	*Miltown* (Carter Products, later called Carter-Wallace, marketed in 1955, and licensed to Wyeth as *Equanil*)
	methylparfynol (methylpentynol; meparfynol*)*	*Dormison* (Schering launched in 1951; a cogener brought out as *N-Oblivon* in 1955)
Diphenylmethane *Use: antineurotic;* *antidepressant;* *anxiolytic*	azacyclonal	*Frenquel* (Merrell introduced 1955; also used as antipsychotic)
	benactyzine	*Suavitil* (Merck marketed 1957; also used as antiphobic)
	hydroxyzine	*Atarax* (Union Chimique Belge synthesized in 1956; Pfizer marketed in 1956 in the United States)
Lithium Salts *Use: antimanic;* *antidepressant*	lithium carbonate	*Lithium* (efficacy reestablished 1949; marketed in United States by Rowell; Smith, Kline & French; and Pfizer, 1970)
Monoamine Oxidase Inhibitors (MAOIs) *Use: antidepressant*	iproniazid	*Marsilid* (Hoffmann-La Roche marketed in 1951 for tuberculosis; in 1957 for depression)
	isocarboxazid	*Marplan* (Hoffmann-La Roche marketed 1959)
	nialamide	*Niamid* (Pfizer launched 1959)
	phenelzine	*Nardil* (Warner-Chilcott marketed 1959)
	pheniprazine	*Catron* (Lakeside introduced 1959)
	tranylcypromine	*Parnate* (Smith, Kline & French introduced in 1960 in United Kingdom, in 1961 in United States)

(continued)

Main Drug Classes *(continued)*

Drug Class	Generic Drug Name	Trade Name (Drug Company and Year Introduced)[2]
Phenothiazines *Use: antipsychotic; anxiolytic*	chlorpromazine	*Largactil* (Rhône-Poulenc synthesized in 1950 and introduced in 1953 worldwide; also brought out as *Thorazine* by Smith, Kline & French in 1954 in United States [entered clinical trials in 1952])
	levomepromazine (later methotrimeprazine)	*Nozinan* (Rhône-Poulenc synthesized in 1958, marketed in France in 1963; also brought out as *Levoprome* by Lederle in 1966 in United States as sedative/analgesic, later antimelancholic)
	mepazine	*Pacatal* (Promonta synthesized in 1952 in Germany; Warner-Chilcott marketed in 1957 in United States)
	prochlorperazine	*Compazine* (Rhône-Poulenc developed; Smith, Kline & French marketed in United States, 1956)
	promazine	*Sparine* (Rhône-Poulenc patented in 1950; Wyeth Laboratories introduced in 1956)
	promethazine	*Phenergan* (Rhône-Poulenc synthesized in 1944; marketed in 1951 in United States)
	thioridazine	*Mellaril* (Sandoz synthesized in 1958; introduced in 1959 in United States)
Propanediol *Use: tranquilizer; muscle relaxant; antineurotic*	mephenesin	*Tolserol* (synthesized in 1908; Squibb marketed 1954)
Reserpine *Use: antipsychotic*	reserpine, derived from *Rauwolfia serpentina*	*Serpasil* (Ciba introduced for hypertension in 1953; Riker Labs brought out a mixture of alkaloids from the plant as "Raudwidrine" for "mood elevation," 1954)

Drug Class	Generic Drug Name	Trade Name (Drug Company and Year Introduced)[2]
Selective Serotonin Reuptake Inhibitors (SSRIs) *Use: antidepressant; anxiolytic*	citalopram	*Cipramil* (Lundbeck patented in 1977, launched in 1989 in Denmark; also brought out as *Celexa* by Forest Laboratories in 1998 in United States)
	fluoxetine	*Prozac* (Lilly patented in 1975, marketed in Belgium in 1986, in United States in 1988)
	fluvoxamine	*Floxyfral* (Philips-Duphar, subsidiary of Solvay, patented in 1975; launched in Switzerland in 1983; brought out as *Faverin* in United Kingdom in 1987; and as *Luvox* in United States 1995 for obsessive-compulsive disorder)
	indalpine	*Upstène* (Fournier Frères-Pharmuka patented in 1977; launched in 1983 in France; withdrawn in 1985)
	paroxetine	*Paxil* (Ferrosan developed in 1974; SmithKline Beecham introduced in 1993 in United States; also brought out as *Seroxat* in United Kingdom)
	sertraline	*Zoloft* (Pfizer patented in 1981; introduced in 1992)
	zimelidine (zimeldine)	*Zelmid* (Astra-Hässle synthesized in 1969; launched in 1981 in Europe; withdrawn in 1983)
Tricyclic Antidepressants (TCAs) *Use: antidepressant* (continued)	amitriptyline	*Elavil* (Merck marketed 1961)
	amoxapine	*Asendin* (Lederle launched 1980, antidepressant with neuroleptic properties)
	clomipramine	*Anafranil* (Geigy launched 1967 in France; in United States in 1990, for obsessive-compulsive disorder)
	desipramine	*Pertofrane* (Geigy marketed in 1963 in United Kingdom, in 1964 in United States)

(continued)

Drug Class	Generic Drug Name	Trade Name (Drug Company and Year Introduced)[2]
Tricyclic Antidepressants (TCAs) *Use: antidepressant* (continued)	dothiepin (dosulepin)	*Prothioden* (Knoll launched in 1969 in United Kingdom)
	doxepin	*Sinequan* (Pfizer introduced in United States in 1969; uses: anxiolytic, antidepressant
	imipramine	*Tofranil* (Geigy marketed in 1957 in Switzerland and in 1959 in United States)
	nortriptyline	*Aventyl* (Merck developed; Lilly introduced in 1963 in United Kingdom, 1965 in United States)
	protriptyline	*Concordin* (Merck marketed in 1966 in United Kingdom; also brought out as *Vivactil* in 1967 in United States)
	tianeptine	*Stablon* (synthesized in 1970; Servier marketed in 1983 in France)

[1] Please refer to the book's glossary for a more extensive listing of the medications identified or discussed in the text.

[2] Unless otherwise noted, the year refers to when the drug was first introduced in the United States.

Before Prozac

1
Introduction

Most of the antidepressants today don't work very well. This is in contrast to the 1950s and '60s, when some truly effective medications for mood disorders were available. Similarly, many of the diagnoses of mood disorder today really don't make a lot of sense; they don't "cut Nature at the joints," as one says. This is unlike 40 years ago, when some sensible diagnoses of depression and anxiety were current, diagnoses that corresponded to what people actually had.

How did this happen?

Medicine is supposed to make progress, to go forward in scientific terms so that each successive generation knows more and does better than previous generations. This hasn't occurred by and large in psychiatry, at least not in the diagnosis and treatment of depression and anxiety, where knowledge has probably been subtracted rather than added. There is such a thing as real psychiatric illness, and effective treatments for it do exist. But today we're seeing medicines that don't work for ill-defined diagnoses of dubious validity. This has caused a crisis in psychiatry.

The usual villains of this piece are the wicked drug companies. And indeed the pharmaceutical industry has not always clung to the high road of science, especially when their commercial interests are threatened. But this is well known, and really a minor note in the story. Instead, the spotlight of blame for the crisis now afflicting psychiatry falls upon two players that normally come off with accolades: the regulatory agencies, particularly the United States Food and Drug Administration (FDA), and the academic psychiatrists who produce the classification of diseases known by the opaque acronym *DSM*, or *Diagnostic and*

Statistical Manual of Mental Disorders of the American Psychiatric Association. *DSM* is the official list of diagnoses that dictates how each psychiatric researcher or practitioner, and each health insurance provider, especially in North America, identifies a psychiatric illness or condition. In the rather ineffective drug treatments for depression known as the selective serotonin reuptake inhibitors (SSRIs)—the Prozac-style drugs—and in the triumph of such diagnoses as "major depression" that exist more in the shadowland of artifact than in the world of Nature—academic psychiatry has a lot to answer for.

The history of psychopharmacology, that is, of the study of the effect of drugs on behavior and mental activity, is littered with burnt-out volcanoes. Ever since the early twentieth century, when the first major psychoactive drug class—the barbiturates—made its appearance, medications have been picked up and laid aside. A drug class will come into popularity, enjoy wide currency, and then vanish. Why has it vanished? Lost efficacy perhaps or some deadly new side effect discovered? Not really. The drugs that worked in the 1940s would still be as effective and as safe if they were routinely prescribed now. One major reason for their vanishing act is the expiration, usually after 20 years (in the United States), of their patent protection, after which their manufacturer ceases to promote them. As pharma sales reps are the main source of drug information for prescribing physicians, an end of such promotion means the end of a drug's public exposure. Thus, it is not at all implausible that there are a number of effective drugs in psychiatry's history that, like burnt-out volcanoes, have simply been forgotten. And in their place are medications that are not necessarily better. Indeed, as far as medications for mood disorders are concerned, it may be illusory to think of progress in clinical psychopharmacology, as opposed to the underlying neuroscience of mood disorders where there have been clear advances in research. If anything, drug efficacy seems to have decreased, while the volume of side effects has stayed the same.

The same is true of the diagnosis of mood disorders, or affective disorders as they are also called. Here, too, progress has proven illusory. The diagnoses that flourished in the middle third of the twentieth century did a better job of cutting Nature at the joints than many of the diagnoses we have today, which are artifacts born of political compromises and sustained by pharmaceutical promotion rather than scientifically accurate descriptions of what is actually wrong with someone. Thus we have been losing ground in this area as well.

How can there not be progress in pharmaceuticals? We spend billions of dollars a year on research in this field. Is this money thrown out the window? One problem comes at the regulatory level: Pharmaceutical companies are willing enough to produce innovative drugs, but they must get them approved by the FDA. Today, the FDA makes things easy. Rather than insisting that a new drug be superior to existing drugs, the agency permits the companies to test new products only against placebo. If you can beat sugar pills in your drug trial, you get your drug licensed. The FDA is not interested in whether your drug represents progress or will cause a therapeutic loss by sweeping from the shelves competing drugs that may be superior but that have lost patent protection.

That is the situation today. Yet in the past the drug-approval process was quite different: In the 1960s, the FDA did a lot of muscle flexing, taking on the star drugs of big companies as an exercise in empire building. There is no doubt that today, the FDA towers punishingly over the pharmaceutical industry: For a drug company, challenging the FDA bureaucrats is a good way of going out of business. Yet in establishing this menacing reputation during the 1960s, the FDA broke a number of eggs in the psychiatric pharmacopeia of that time, and some of them were useful drugs, today forgotten.

Is this merely an exercise in nostalgia? All that existed in the 1950s, together with Bobby Darin, was wonderful? Everything today, including Britney Spears, a pile of overblown hype? Not at all. History doesn't have a lot of uses in the practice of medicine. You can be a quite successful nephrologist and not know the first thing about the history of your field. But psychiatry today offers a barren tundra of remedies and diagnoses. There is little in the industry pipeline of new drugs. And we have a nosological system, or system of classifying diseases, that does not tell us which patients will respond to which drugs. Here, knowing about the past can be genuinely helpful, in recalling much forgotten but useful knowledge about diagnoses that do seem to correspond to natural disease entities. Similarly, we have wrongly cast drugs aside because of a staggering overestimation of their side effects and an underestimation of their clinical benefits—misestimates subtly encouraged by the manufacturers of competing drugs.

Psychiatrists are more subject to herd behavior than physicians in other medical specialties, where a genuine knowledge of disease mechanisms helps ward off therapeutic fads. Nephrologists might say, "No, we reject moonbeam treatments because we don't see how they could possibly affect the nephron." Psychiatrists have no real way of warding off moonbeam treatments, of proving them wrong, because they know little about how the brain affects the mind. So they rush in hordes back and forth across the stage, animated by the principle that if everybody else is prescribing this or that psychiatric med, it must be right. Looking at the past offers a means of checking this herd behavior, by demonstrating its very ridiculousness and absence of scientific method.

I am not advocating therapeutic antiquarianism. Every drug and diagnosis in psychiatry's past was not necessarily virtuous. One thinks of "hysteria" and the toxic salts of the element bromine, the "bromides." The future of today's psychiatry does not lie in resurrecting the past but in respecting the scientific method, in abandoning diagnoses fashioned by consensus, and in doing away with ineffective therapies dictated by the corporate bottom line. It does not necessarily lie in reviving the first drug set of the 1950s. Yet mental therapeutics today seems bereft of ideas. As we wait for science to percolate, maybe we can derive some practical benefit from looking backward and gaining a humbling reminder that knowledge can be lost, and therapeutics fail to progress—or worse.

A Word About Evidence

Confronting the history of psychopharmacology means facing, right up front, the question of evidence. How do we know whether one drug is more effective than another? Today, only the evidence of randomly controlled clinical trials, called RCTs, is acceptable. It is the gold standard of evidence, meaning trials that are sufficiently "powered" (enroll enough patients) to produce clinically significant results. These are placebo-controlled trials in which patients are randomly allocated to drug or placebo (rather than allocated on the basis of who is most likely to respond); such trials are also "double blind," meaning that investigators and patients alike are unaware of which group of participants is taking the drug or placebo. Such trials were not conducted before the 1970s.

In the long decades before the advent of proper RCTs, what are we to use for evidence? Some psychopharmacologists oriented to the gold standard may say, "Why don't you give it up? The history of drugs is impossible under these circumstances." But I don't think that it is impossible. Other kinds of evidence exist that may not give us the same scientifically exact measurements as modern RCTs but that nonetheless offer rough ballpark estimates of drugs that were or were not effective.

One kind of evidence derives from small "open" trials, conducted usually by physicians in their own practices, in which they gave a drug to many of their patients and then described the results. There was no control group, save the doctor's own recollection of how similar patients have done on other drugs in the past. Physicians chronicled the results of such trials in the medical press, and the medicine of the day accepted the results as valid guidelines. There is no reason why the conclusions of such small open trials would be completely misleading, even though the trials did not control for the effects of such influences as medical suggestion from the physicians themselves who, convinced of the drug's effectiveness, might psychologically convey its benefits to their patients. (Such suggestive effects occur in today's RCTs as well—for example, when patients break the blind and realize they must be on placebo because they are not experiencing the side effects of which they were warned.)

A second kind of evidence is the wisdom of accumulated medical experience. William Wardell and Louis Lasagna, senior psychopharmacologists at the University of Rochester, observed in a book they wrote together in 1975 that "anecdotal" drug testing is not really uncontrolled. "The control consists of what the observer believes would have occurred in the absence of the drug."[1] This is a question that experience answers. On another occasion Lasagna, the dean of American pharmacology, observed,

> There may be a good deal of clinical experience suggesting that your hypothetical drug does work. I am not willing to throw out a lot of naturalistic experience on the basis of one or two negative double-blind trials. I have seen too many negative double-blind trials. . . . There are a number of drugs for which we don't have double-blind control placebo tests, for instance, digitalis, antiepileptic drugs, antibiotics, and anti-Parkinsonian drugs. In these cases, the medical profession and the academic experts have decided, "I have enough feeling for this drug on the basis of what I have seen in ordinary 'uncontrolled' clinical experience to conclude that it is O.K.[2]

Thus, many wise observers regarded the accumulation of clinical experience with respect, all the more so when this accumulation is passed on across the generations. In other words, doctors know if a drug clearly works; they don't need an RCT to demonstrate it. We don't need RCTs to show that penicillin works in pneumococcal pneumonia, or that electroconvulsive therapy is effective in catatonia. It just works!

Yet one can take the wisdom of accumulated clinical experience only so far. After all, at one point there was a medical consensus that bleeding was an effective remedy and that enemas were the quickest route to restored health. But in those days, the mid-nineteenth century and before, medical knowledge was based upon rote learning from tradition—precepts about humors passed down since the days of Hippocrates. Late in the nineteenth century, medicine started to become data-oriented, and doctrines about humors gave way to statistical procedures for determining which accumulated wisdom was valid, and which was not. Today, this is called "evidence-based medicine," but the basic concept of establishing truth with quantitative evidence has been with us for a century or more.

Thus, modern medicine has an intellectual reflex that traditional medicine lacked: assessing supposed verities with a constantly critical eye on weeding out untruths. We have, alas, plenty of evidence that this does not always happen, for example in the persistence of unnecessary tonsillectomies for upper respiratory infections. Nonetheless, the demand for ongoing scrutiny has been for a century part of the culture of medicine: It is taught in the first year of medical school, and not all physicians forget it. On the whole, therefore, the accumulated medical experiences of today have been subjected to a winnowing that did not occur in the long centuries of medicine's past. It is a winnowing in which everything is always more or less up for grabs, and in which useless and dangerous remedies fail to retain the kind of traction they once had.

The point is that when senior clinicians with decades of experience behind them arrive at a judgment, it might at least be weighed reflectively and not instantly cast aside as failing the RCT gold standard of evidence. Congress wrote this respect for clinical experience into an early draft of the Kefauver-Harris legislation of 1962, the law that greatly expanded the power of the Food and Drug Administration. William Goodrich, FDA general counsel at the time, said later, "We put in a provision that clinical experience adequately documented would be considered along with adequate and well-controlled studies" in evaluating the efficacy of drugs. But the provision was dropped in the final legislation.[3]

Regardless, in medical practice today, it is the accumulated wisdom of clinical experience, not controlled trials in the literature, that tends to give a drug its reputation. The mood agent trazodone, launched in the United States in the 1980s under the trade name Desyrel, was abandoned not necessarily because someone had done an RCT proving it useless but because word somehow got out in collegial conversations. And the word in that case was correct: Trazodone *was* ineffective as an antidepressant. It turned out, however, to be terrific as a hypnotic (sleeping medication), with relatively few side effects and little addictiveness. And this, too, was word that got out in corridor conversations rather than in articles in influential journals.

One must cautiously delimit this argument. The wisdom of collective experience would not, for example, apply to most medical and surgical procedures, in which compensation may be based on whether one does the procedure or not. Nor would it apply to areas of high-liability risk, such as obstetrics, in which omitting a procedure could fuel a lawsuit. But we may be on safer ground in psychopharmacology, in which something would always be prescribed. The question is what is prescribed? Here physicians' defensive medicine plays less of a role, and consensus may be taken more at face value. I am not saying it is absolute proof of a drug's effectiveness that a number of doctors believe it—again, such herd mentality isn't reliable evidence. Yet it entitles us briefly to suspend disbelief and ask, what other evidence is available? As for the deification of randomly controlled trials, we've learned in recent years that their value can be undermined all too easily: One recalls that it was thanks to such trials—to their manipulation and, as recently publicized, to the obfuscation in some studies of negative results—that one of the least effective drug classes in the history of psychopharmacology lurched onto the stage, the Prozac-style drugs, the so-called selective serotonin reuptake inhibitors.

But let's not get ahead of our story.

What's Coming

The first third of this story pivots about the introduction in the 1950s of a new wave of truly effective drugs for depression and anxiety, which I call "the first drug set." In order to appreciate the significance of this innovation, we have to go back a step and look at drugs available before the 1950s.

The second part of the book turns to the hitherto unknown story of the FDA's power flexing against the pharmaceutical industry by taking down a good deal of the first drug set and other medications, such as the first of the benzodiazepine drugs that were launched in the early 1960s. It was an influence grab that had little to do with science and much to do with the imperatives of inside-the-Beltway empire building in Washington, D.C. We spend three chapters on this subject, because it resulted in cutting the psychopharmacopoeia nearly in half, and in reifying the concept of "antidepressant" as the main drug class for patients who were not out-and-out psychotic. The first of these chapters treats the smackdown of a now forgotten drug called meprobamate, trade named Miltown and Equanil, the first blockbuster drug in psychiatry. Then we look at the FDA's assault upon the "benzos," Librium and Valium. Finally, in this Food and Drug triplet, an obscurely titled but enormously influential bureaucratic sweep of the pharmaceutical table comes up called. . . . No, I can't even bear to reveal at this point what it was called. But it is discussed in Chapter 6.

The story ends with the triumph of the SSRIs for depression, a victory to which the FDA had pointed the way by outlawing, restricting, or stigmatizing so much of the competition. Academic psychiatry played a crucial role here by making "major depression" the only kind of depression on the table. The whole original concept of two depressions, melancholia and nonmelancholia, as different from each other as chalk and cheese, became clouded as the term *major depression* was coined in 1975 and reached a worldwide audience in 1980 in the influential third edition of the *Diagnostic and Statistical Manual*, or *DSM-III*, of the American Psychiatric Association.

In the last chapter, we see how the rise of the SSRIs fit hand in glove with this new unitary concept of depression: a single drug class for a single depression, as opposed to the many agents that had thrived before for a complexly layered notion of mood disorders. This Prozac-style drug class went on to drive all the competing drug classes, many of them more effective, from the stage. Thus the story ends in the triumph of a manifestly less effective class of drugs for a kind of illness, major depression, that was, essentially, a political artifact born of academic infighting. This is not supposed to happen.

2

Before Psychopharmacology

The psychopharmacologic era is said to have begun in the 1950s, with the advent in 1952 of the first antipsychotic drug, chlorpromazine. No question it was an extraordinary time of pharmaceutical discovery, but in fact, effective treatments existed long before then. Merely, they have been forgotten, or crucified by the drug cops. It helps us to avoid over-valuing later contributions to recall that the cupboard has never been entirely bare.

"Some Griefs Are Medicinable"[1]

What does a world without psychopharmacology look like?

In 1913, Mr. X, a 25-year-old employee of the London branch of a Swiss bank, came to see Dr. Frederick Parkes-Weber, an internist with an office on chic Harley Street, in London's West End. Parkes-Weber con-sulted to the elite, and his practice consisted heavily of well-to-do people with complaints that were often nervous rather than organic. "Nothing special in past history," wrote Parkes-Weber in Mr. X's chart, "except that he was disappointed in love 2 or 3 years ago. Has been wasting dur-ing last 12 months and looks very thin." Mr. X's mother was said to be "highly nervous." Parkes-Weber performed a physical exam but found nothing. "No actual delusions. He is said to think a girl is in love, when she is pleasant to him, and is angry when he finds out that she is not."

Parkes-Weber wrote the patient's employer that Mr. X was suffer-ing from a "physical 'run down' condition, secondary to a condition of psychical depression, bordering on insanity." Mr. X was often invited to the home of a colleague. "He will sit in a chair or on a sofa when visiting B [the colleague] for an hour without (hardly) opening his mouth. The only thing he cares to talk of is his unfortunate love affair . . . Typical of his psychic depression is the tendency to lividity of his nose, with his emaciated face—I suppose he has cold hands and tendency to cyanosis too."

What to do? Parkes-Weber had numerous treatments for this "psychical depression" available, but he proposed the one he thought most effective: a course of treatment in a "water-cure institute" at Bendorf on the Rhine in Germany. But the treatment failed, and in July 1914 Mr. X was sent back to Switzerland.[2]

In 1913 Parkes-Weber had customary remedies for mood disorders, such as the water-cure resorts that had come into existence during the nineteenth century. He was also beginning to profit from modern treatments, such as opium injections, which had become practical with the introduction of the syringe in the 1850s, and aspirin, launched by the German pharmaceutical house Bayer in 1899. Parkes-Weber often prescribed aspirin for nervousness.

Parkes-Weber lived in a world without psychopharmacology—that is, without the understanding that drugs might have differential responsiveness in different mental diseases, with some drugs working in some conditions but not others. If we had to assign a birth hour to psychopharmacology as a discipline, it would probably be a meeting at Neuchâtel and the nearby cantonal mental hospital in Perreux, Switzerland, on June 21–22, 1930, when the Swiss Psychiatric Society discussed "pharmacology and psychiatry."[3] Before then, the concept of differential responsiveness was poorly understood, and treatment of psychiatric conditions was something of a hit-or-miss proposition, although people agreed that you did not prescribe the sedative valerian for madness, or send fully psychotic patients to spas.

And yet, over the centuries, physicians have always been able to propose something for mood disorders. Sometimes the remedy proposed was ineffectual by our standards. Early in the eighteenth century, for example, "spleen," "vapors," and "hyp" were fashionable psychiatric diagnoses. What did physicians prescribe for these? According to Doctor James Adair, who consulted at the general hospital in the spa town of Bath whither the fashionable of London retreated, relief was sought in a "pearl cordial" (a drink containing powdered pearl).[4] As English physician George Cheyne counseled novelist Samuel Richardson, who had a history of depression, in 1738, "I am heartily sorry that a sound head which belongs to so honest a heart is so troublesome. Nothing can possibly cure you durably but vomits frequently repeated at least as often as the symptoms exasperate." Half a dram of the emetic ipecac once a week, Cheyne said, should put the novelist back in form.[5]

But often the remedies offered worked. Just as psychiatry today has physical treatments for mood disorders, such as electroconvulsive therapy (ECT) and magnetic stimulation therapy, so did the medicine of yore. Convinced that the emotional life of women was dominated by their sexual organs, around 1870 Berlin gynecologist Louis Mayer cured an episode of melancholia involving constant crying in a 57-year-old female patient by applying a pessary: "It relieved her physical problems and many severe disorders of mood. . . . Previously, a quite inexplicable anxiety had overcome her, sending the most terrible thoughts day and night through her head, giving her no rest, robbing her of sleep, leaving her indifferent toward her children, husband and the entire world. She felt an urge to free herself of these tortures through suicide." But after the pessary, the relief was magical: "The application of a Mayer Ring improved her quite considerably."[6]

The Earliest Effective Drugs

In terms of medication, there have always been drugs to soothe the mind and tame the agitated spirit. Alkaloids, widely found in nature, especially in plants in the Solanaceae family, have always served as sedatives. Belladonna, or deadly nightshade (*Atropa belladonna*), contains anticholinergic alkaloids such as atropine, hyoscyamine, and scopolamine that act against the neurotransmitter acetylcholine. The pure alkaloid hyoscyamine was isolated in 1871 "from the inert mass of resin, fixed oil and extractives that had held it captive," as Henry Wetherill at the Pennsylvania Hospital for the Insane put it; it came into wide use in asylums and in family practice.[7] Hyoscyamine and scopolamine served in many drug cocktails in the past, such as the "green medicine" beloved by English family doctors before the Second World War. "It very often worked," reminisced one physician.[8] The mandrake plant (*Mandragora officinarum*), also a Solanaceae, offers another source of these alkaloids, and mandrake has been known in medicine since the Middle Ages.[9]

In the late 1930s and '40s a highly effective set of drugs was introduced for psychiatric diseases, illnesses now so rare they have been forgotten. In 1938 Conrad Arnold Elvehjem isolated nicotinic acid as the crucial vitamin deficiency in pellagra, a finding that eventually emptied the mental asylums of the U.S. South (and parts of Italy) of poor people whose niacin-deficient diets had condemned them to the psychosis and dementia of the disease. Pellagra is now found mainly in the history books.[10]

Neurosyphilis, or the syphilitic infiltration of the central nervous system, once called "general paralysis of the insane," had been partially treatable ever since Julius von Wagner-Jauregg devised his malarial fever cure in 1917. Neurosyphilis came to a definitive end when Philadelphia dermatologist John H. Stokes led a team that discovered in 1944 the effectiveness of penicillin for it.[11] Syphilis of the nervous system, which once had populated the men's wards of asylums with its psychiatric manifestations such as mania, became a clinical curiosity.

Wernicke-Korsakoff syndrome is a brain inflammation to which chronic alcoholics are subject, resulting in memory loss and a variety of other psychiatric and neurological symptoms. Asylums were once filled with alcoholic, middle-aged men suffering "Korsakoff psychosis" or "Wernicke's disease." In 1947 Hugh Edward De Wardener, on the basis of his experiences with a rice-only diet in a Japanese prison camp, figured out that Wernicke's encephalopathy was due to thiamine deficiency.[12] Thiamine treatments almost wiped out "Wernicke's." So these are drugs that really do work in psychiatry.

What else?

Alcohol is another substance with medicinal purposes and in the past was often used to alleviate certain mood symptoms.

Let me just insert here, before we proceed with alcohol, a point of clarification about "mood" and related terms: I tend not to speak in this book simply of "depression" but distinguish, when the sources permit, between melancholic and nonmelancholic mood disorders. Melancholia (also called endogenous depression) is a well-defined mood disorder characterized by high-serum cortisol, slowing of mind and muscle, and severe feelings of self-worthlessness; it can deteriorate into psychosis, meaning loss of contact with reality in the form of delusions and hallucinations. By contrast, nonmelancholia may include low mood or mild depression, anxiety, tension, and general unhappiness; it is a heterogeneous group of illnesses that nineteenth-century Austrian psychiatrist Richard von Krafft-Ebing called *psychoneurosis*, which later became a favorite term of the Freudians. Collectively, melancholia, non-melancholia, mania, and sometimes anxiety are all called *mood disorders*, or *affective disorders*.

Alcohol is not a specific for melancholia, but it does have a soothing effect in nonmelancholic illness and has been prescribed in medicine since time out of mind. It is interesting that the substance, so stigmatized today in American medicine, has served such a therapeutic role in the past. In low spirits in the elderly, counseled London family physician Adolphus Bridger in 1892, give port and brandy. "Full-bodied Burgundy, high class claret, port, the better white French, German, and Italian wines, stout or good brandy, may with a clear conscience and great hopefulness, be recommended to the aged. A suitable form of alcohol will often do more to restore nervous health in old age than any medicine."[13] Europeans have not lost sight of these virtues: "Alcohol has done more good than bad to mankind," said Swedish psychopharmacologist and Nobel Prize winner Arvid Carlsson in 1996. "I am convinced of that. There is so much that has come out of the increased interaction between individuals because of alcohol."[14] Thus, hyoscyamine, scopolamine, and ethanol (the chemical name for beverage alcohol), all worthy drugs, have always been available in the psychopharmacopoeia. Yet none are specific for any particular mood disorder.

There were, however, several treatments, aside from the endless tonics, infusions of valerian, and sea baths, that do seem to have had an elective effect in mood disorders. Today they are regarded as narcotics, but that does not make them less effective.

Opium, the milky juice of the unripe poppy plant *Papaver somniferum*—native to Asia Minor—has been known medically since the ancient Greeks (it is dried to a brownish gummy mass, which is then powdered to form pharmacy-type opium).[15] There is an age-old medical tradition of prescribing opium for melancholia and mania, reinforced in the seventeenth century by British physician Thomas Sydenham's standardizing of opium together with alcohol in "laudanum," or opium tincture.[16] To be sure, what was termed mania and melancholia in past times does not always correlate with our concepts of these illnesses, yet both terms were not just synonyms for "madness" but possessed a core of symptoms that has remained constant.

The systematic "opium cure" of anxious-melancholic moods was initiated with the Engelken family in eighteenth-century Germany, who founded beginning in 1746 two private psychiatric clinics in villages near Bremen. The generations of Engelken physicians kept their methods secret until Hermann Engelken published a memoir about them in 1844.[17] The cure consisted of doses of 2–3 grains of opium, titrating up to 8–10 and even to 16 grains, in intervals of 10 hours. (An apothecary "grain" is 64 mg.) The Engelken clinic in Rockwinkel bei Bremen used up to 40 pounds of opium a year.[18]

The Engelken opium cure became famous throughout Europe. Its popularity was much accelerated by the above-mentioned invention of the syringe in the 1850s, so that opium could be injected. In his 1879 textbook, Krafft-Ebing—at the time professor of psychiatry in Graz, Austria—recommended opium injections as well as suppositories. "Opium is of incalculable value in cases of beginning melancholia," he wrote. "It treats the psychic hyperesthesia and shows itself to be of special value in compulsive thoughts and precordial anxiety."[19] (*Precordial* refers to anxious pains in the chest.)

In 1977, German psychiatrist Günter Elsässer looked back upon the earlier days. "You have to keep in mind that at the beginning of the Thirties there were very few treatments available in psychiatry. There was the malarial treatment of neurosyphilis, the opium cure for depression, very limited medications for the convulsive disorders, and above and beyond that, only work therapy and morphine-scopolamine injections for agitation."[20] Thus, the opium cure belonged to the few treatments that worked.

The opium cure started to go out of fashion in psychiatry as the problem of addiction and street abuse of morphine swelled in the twentieth century. For all the benefits that opiates brought when appropriately prescribed by a physician, they were also capable of wreaking great damage. Morphine could easily convert those who had started injecting it on medical advice into lifelong addicts. So it is not that opiates were problem-free drugs, but rather that they represent the first specific for melancholic illness and might even today deserve a second look.

Indeed, in the real world of psychiatric practice, they *are* getting a second inspection. In the 1990s a New England psychiatrist was "treating a woman with severe, refractory depression and dissociative disorder. We tried everything. . . . Really aggressive approach but to no avail." Then the psychiatrist came across a reference in the literature to codeine, an alkaloid of opium, in the treatment of depression:

> The pharmacy easily prepared either codeine or placebo in
> identical capsules. We randomized it and in a double blind

fashion gave her either active drug or placebo for a week or so. Bottom line: after three months the results in this randomized, double blind, n = 1 ABAB design showed highly consistent efficacy with the codeine, as demonstrated by a strong drop in the HAMD [the Hamilton Depression Scale] and some dissociative scale. As a result, she was placed on a low dose of codeine (15 mg a day) and in three-year follow up did great and never increased the dose![21]

Thus an anecdotal report from the trenches: Psychiatry's oldest drug still remains among its most effective.

Likewise, the sedative and hypnotic uses of cannabis, derived from the flowering tops of the hemp plant, go back to Antiquity.[22] Cannabis was neglected for ages, then underwent a nineteenth-century revival. At Ticehurst House Asylum in England, *Cannabis indica*, a variety of the genus *Cannabis*, was routinely given to patients having melancholia and mania, with apparently good results.[23] In the 1860s a private psychiatric hospital near Halle in Germany used a half grain of the extract or ten drops of the tincture per day, obtaining in "very severe hallucinations of terrifying content and in chronic insomnia . . . always a calming effect."[24] At a meeting in Switzerland in 1916, Max Cloetta, professor of pharmacology in Zurich, noted with interest the uses of potassium bromide in melancholia, but asked if hashish, a form of cannabis, could not also be employed.[25]

Cannabis actually became in Europe a marketed drug. In the 1930s a commercial hypnotic consisting of barbital, a barbiturate, and *Cannabis indica* was marketed in England as Indonad.[26] In Germany it was available as Indonal-Bürger.[27] So there is no doubt that cannabis was on the radar of psychological medicine in the prepsychopharmacologic era before the 1950s.

Finally, among the narcotic drugs used for mood disorders in past times was cocaine, obtained from the leaves of South American *Erythroxylon coca*, the medical applications of which were discovered in Vienna late in the nineteenth century by Sigmund Freud.[28] Cocaine became hugely popular in America in those years and was used in all kinds of patent medicines, soft drinks (e.g. Coca-Cola), and pharmaceutical preparations. Historian David Musto calls the Parke Davis Company "an exceptionally enthusiastic producer of cocaine, even sold coca-leaf cigarettes and coca cheroots to accompany their other products . . . such as a liqueurlike alcohol mixture called Coca Cordial, tablets, hypodermic injections, ointments and sprays."[29] Boston psychiatrist Leo Alexander later called cocaine, "the first really great wave of psychopharmacology in this country." He noted that Sigmund Freud had initiated it. "In a way, the poor man is now seeking vengeance . . . by having flooded this country with psychoanalysis."[30]

Was there anything to this cocaine hype? Cocaine is another of the narcotic drugs to which restless minds have later returned in search of active pharmacological principles in the treatment of mood disorders. As a young man in the early 1960s, Norbert Matussek of the Max Planck Institute for Psychiatry in Munich had studied at pharmacologist Bernard Brodie's lab at the National Heart Institute, part of the National Institutes of Health in Bethesda, Maryland. Once back in Munich, "applying the knowledge I had gained at the NIH, I began to unravel the mysteries of the release and uptake of NE [the neurotransmitter norepinephrine]." Matussek discovered that cocaine inhibited the reuptake of norepinephrine, making it an interesting candidate as an antidepressant, because other antidepressants had a similar action. Moreover, unlike other drugs under study, cocaine caused the release of norepinephrine from the neurons into the synapse, thus increasing even more the amount of the neurotransmitter available to the brain (a supposedly good effect). "In view of this we hypothesized that cocaine should be a better antidepressant than the ones in clinical use." Yet this insight was never acted on because of the prevailing fears of addiction from even tiny amounts of cocaine. Matussek did, however, try some cocaine on himself yet felt nothing, "probably because I took it orally."[31]

Cocaine had been known to South American Indians to be psychoactive since time out of mind. Cannabis and opium have been understood for ages in Western society as psychoactive. It is curious that the earliest drugs in psychiatry are among the most interesting.

Barbiturates

In the late nineteenth century, a slew of new treatments started to become available thanks mainly to the magic of the German chemical industry. In 1857, the salts of bromine—for "hysteria" and epilepsy—hit the market. In 1869 the psychiatric uses of chloral hydrate, a minor sedative, were discovered. In 1882 paraldehyde, a major sedative for asylum patients, was introduced into medicine.[32] All were key sedatives of the day but are now largely forgotten because the great wheel of therapeutics has turned further, with the possible exception of chloral hydrate (which remains used as a sedative almost without side effects).

Then in 1903 the psychoactive drug scene was transformed with the arrival of the first barbiturates, drugs that are a combination of uric acid and malonic acid.[33] Unlike paraldehyde, which you would probably not want to take in your home before bedtime if you were feeling a bit nervous (it smelled awful, for one thing), the barbiturates were more palatable drugs for the family medicine chest. In the March 1903 issue of *Contemporary Therapeutics*, Emil Fischer, professor of chemistry in Berlin, and Josef von Mering, professor of internal medicine at Halle University, announced the discovery of "a new class of hypnotics."[34] The initial drug in this class was generically named barbital (barbitone in the United Kingdom), and jointly marketed by Merck and Bayer as Veronal, and by Schering Labs as Medinal. Both names quickly became household words, and Veronal in particular found a place in homes across the Western world.

The advantage of the barbiturates over the other drugs was their safety and lack of side effects, certainly compared to the bromides—rich in side effects of acne, headache, stomach upset, and dizziness—which the barbiturates began to displace in the 1930s. Also, the barbiturates had a longer half-life than paraldehyde, permitting patients to sleep through the night. "That was the real goal," said Benjamin Wiesel, head of psychiatry at Hartford Hospital in Connecticut "There wasn't any concept at that time of changing a patient's thinking."[35]

In 1911 Bayer brought out phenobarbital (Luminal), which even today is in use as an anticonvulsant. Barbital and phenobarbital have a long duration of action, which made them suitable as sedatives for anxious and agitated individuals, and phenobarbital especially, with its heavy phenyl (six-carbon ring) side chain, became the prototype for the long-duration barbiturate sedatives. As hypnotics, both barbital and phenobarbital also enjoyed wide currency, although people complained of feeling drugged the following morning. Lighter drugs then became popular as sleeping medicines, such as amobarbital (Sodium Amytal), patented by Eli Lilly in 1924, and butabarbital, which Lilly patented in 1932 and McNeil Labs marketed as Butisol. In fact, there was much unhappiness in state hospitals when Lilly stopped manufacturing blue "Amytal" placebo capsules. Said psychopharmacologist Louis Lasagna much later, "Amytal had been used for years as a sedative drug during the day or at night. Then it was found, just empirically, that a fair number of patients were quite happy just getting a blue capsule that looks like Amytal."[36] Amytal also developed a niche reputation for "narcoanalysis" and later for the "Amytal interview," meaning that it was used to encourage patients to talk freely in the hopes of uncovering buried material from the "unconscious."[37] Such was the value attached to this drug's supposed truth-revealing effects that the New York courts would ask psychiatrists at Bellevue Hospital to inject murder defendants with Amytal to see if they were faking mental illness. The injections were involuntary.[38]

The uptake of the barbiturates was enormous, far surpassing that of any psychoactive drug class ever previously marketed. Their great popularity ensured that many manufacturers sprang into the market. More than sixty different versions were available by 1944, and over 1,200 were theoretically possible on the basis of the structure of the molecule.[39] "The British patient, just back from the Black Forest or from Lausanne," mocked one tony London general practitioner in 1934, "proudly takes a carton of the latest isomer of Veronal out of her pocket or vanity bag and says, 'You will not have seen this new drug, doctor.' And she is quite frequently correct."[40]

In those years, the diagnosis of depression was conferred grudgingly, and it was for "nerves," "tension," and the like that the barbiturates flourished—and for insomnia, because helping patients sleep often opens the door to recovery. Yet London novelist Virginia Woolf took Veronal for periodic depression,[41] and Amytal in particular had a solid reputation in the relief of mood disorders. In 1930 William Bleckwenn at the University of Wisconsin—the originator of narcotherapy—said of Amytal that in "manic-depressive psychosis," manic episodes could be immediately broken up and "the patient is asleep in about five minutes." As for the depressed phase, "the favorable response takes the form of a greater willingness to eat. . . . They are more active, more talkative, have less constrained and less awkward attitudes, and certainly the course of their depressions [is] materially shortened." In the depression of midlife, Amytal had "striking" results: some "complete recoveries in from two to four weeks."[42]

Eric Lindemann at the University of Iowa followed these results up in 1931 in a paper that laid the foundation for Amytal as some kind of truth drug (which it is not). Lindemann said, "Depressed patients told about subjective reasons for their feelings of guilt" and became more willing to divulge.[43] The University of Iowa was already becoming a psychiatric powerhouse in those days, and Lindemann became known as the pioneering trialist of Amytal.[44] (Later, while at Harvard, he became famous in 1944 for his psychological analysis of trauma following the terrible fire in November 1942 at the Cocoanut Grove nightclub in Boston.)[45]

It was actually after the Second World War that the barbiturates enjoyed their greatest popularity, right up to the advent of the "tranquilizers" such as meprobamate, launched in 1955. The tricyclic antidepressants and the benzodiazepines of the late 1950s and early '60s then truly tipped the barbiturates into a terminal decline. In the United States, 231,000 pounds of "barbituric acid and derivatives" were consumed in 1936, 852,000 pounds in 1960, the high point. As one scholar observed, "The 1960 figure . . . would be enough raw material to make approximately 6 billion one-grain barbiturate capsules or tablets, or about 33 for every man, woman, and child in the United States."[46] This represents an almost fourfold increase in barbiturate consumption over the 1930s.

Especially popular were barbiturate combos, a barbiturate such as phenobarbital plus some other agent such as aspirin. It was really via these combos that the barbiturates worked their way by the 1950s into almost every corner of American therapeutics: Phenobarbital plus hyoscyamine and atropine were the A. H. Robins Company's combo Donnatal for irritable bowel syndrome; phenobarbital plus thiamine became Smith, Kline & French's Eskaphen B Elixir for whatever complaints baby might have (plus the bonus: "Patients who 'know all about sleeping tablets' don't know you are prescribing a barbiturate").[47] In Spain in the 1980s, two-thirds of the total consumption of sedative-hypnotic drugs were in these barbiturate (and benzodiazepine) combos. Said one authority, "For most of these drugs the main indication is not anxiety, insomnia or nervousness, but pain, and less frequently digestive symptoms, cardiovascular conditions and non-specific problems of old age."[48] Thus did the barbiturates become ubiquitous.

As the uptake of the barbiturates soared, certain disadvantages started to emerge that had not been apparent to an earlier generation of physicians. Misuse haunted the barbiturates. Out of rage over his insomnia, for example, French novelist Marcel Proust once took an entire box of Veronal in addition to Dial (allobarbital) and opium—"and I didn't sleep but suffered horribly."[49] Proust was a heavy barbiturate user, and his moment of exasperation poses the question: Were these drugs addictive?

Then there is the issue of suicide. So much did the Veronal suicide become a literary trope that the Bayer company considered requesting

Vienna playwright Arthur Schnitzler not to have his heroes kill themselves with it.[50] But how often were barbiturates in fact used for suicide?

Before the Second World War, concern about the barbiturates' potential use as suicide drugs was tempered by the fact that they were not as wildly overprescribed as they were in the postwar years. To be sure, murmurings about the dangers of these new "hypnotic drugs" were uttered at a meeting of the psychiatry section of the Royal Society of Medicine in December 1933, yet Ronald G. Gillespie, physician for psychological medicine at Guy's Hospital in London, "strongly contested the views which had been put forward as to the danger of therapeutic doses of these drugs. . . . He did not believe that there was a case on record where either a single dose of the barbiturates or a repeated dose of therapeutic magnitude had caused death in the absence of complicating factors."[51] A review several years later of the side effects of barbiturates did not even mention the risk of overdose or suicide.[52]

According to coroners' data, in the United States between 1928 and 1937, there had been 4,493 suicide deaths from drugs and poisons, of which 363, or 8.1 percent, were owing to barbiturates. This is not a high figure for 10 years in a country that numbered 123 million in population in 1930. An increase in the absolute number of barbiturate deaths over that decade is meaningless because it does not control for increasing usage. Census Bureau data and statistics from the Metropolitan Life Insurance Company, both for the mid-1930s, also show a low proportion of drug suicides from barbiturates.[53]

Later statistics did establish that the barbiturates had a suicide rate that was far higher than that of any other drug class.[54] Yet two points: First, in terms of the absolute number of deaths, the total was rather low; and although of course any deaths are too many, the pluses and minuses for public health of removing an important drug class must be weighed. Cancer drugs, after all, carry a considerable mortality. Second, it was not those with insomnia but those with melancholia who committed suicide with the barbiturates. As Louis Lasagna, then at the Johns Hopkins University Department of Pharmacology, argued in 1957, ". . . It is hard to conceive of a compound which has definite hypnotic potency . . . which cannot cause death if taken in sufficient quantity."[55] The number of patients with insomnia taking barbiturates was far higher than the number of melancholic patients taking them who were inclined to suicide.

What about addiction? The evidence of the addictiveness of the barbiturates was certainly not overwhelming. In 1934 a family physician from Bournemouth, England, told the neuropsychiatry section of the British Medical Association, "In thirty-five years' experience he had never seen a case of habit from the use of barbiturates."[56]

Somewhat later, in 1964, Leonard Goldberg, an addiction specialist at the Karolinska Institute in Stockholm, figured out the relative addictiveness of the barbiturates compared to other drugs:

- "Dependence created on therapeutic dose"? No, in contrast to narcotics.
- Risk on use? 0.1 percent, in contrast to alcohol 2–3 percent, or morphine 50–70 percent.
- Severity of sudden discontinuation syndrome? Here the barbiturates ranged from "slight" to "marked," depending on the drug.
- Frequency of addiction per million users? 200–500, in contrast to 5,000–20,000 for alcohol.[57]

Then, in a Congressional hearing in 1966, Gane's Chemical Works in Carlstadt, New Jersey, which had been producing barbiturates since 1928, reported that for the past 37 years it had "no record of abuse within its own employment. To date, Gane's has no positive or substantive record of abuse among its customers."[58]

Clearly, the barbiturates had to be used cautiously. But hysteria of the sort that reached fever pitch in the 1960s about barbiturate abuse and addiction was not justified either. The whole addiction dialogue shifted in 1964, as what had previously been "addiction," with its driven drug seeking, now became "dependence," a much broader and looser framework onto which many additional drugs previously deemed innocuous could be tacked. The World Health Organization, which engineered this change, said, "The component in common appears to be dependence, whether psychic or physical or both. Hence, use of the term 'drug dependence' . . . has been given most careful consideration."[59]

In 1970 the Controlled Substances Act gave the Department of Justice the authority to classify drugs deemed capable of abuse on the basis of a schedule of dangerousness, with schedule I being the most dangerous (for drugs with no medical use, such as heroin) and schedule IV the less dangerous (such as most sleeping medications, or hypnotics); a brief schedule V allowed for even less menacing substances such as cough medicines with codeine. In 1972 the DOJ's Bureau of Narcotics and Dangerous Drugs announced it was moving the barbiturates from schedule III to the more stringent schedule II of the Controlled Substances Act, right alongside the narcotics and methamphetamine.[60] This was essentially the end of the barbiturates in the North American world for any purpose save prescribing phenobarbital for epilepsy.[61] They remain even today widely prescribed in the developing world, however.

On balance, the barbiturates were vastly superior to anything else available when they were introduced in the first half of the twentieth century. The short-acting barbiturates remain excellent hypnotics and short-term anesthetics. Like any successful drug class, they became vastly overprescribed. Psychiatrist Max Fink remembers his days in the mid-1940s as an intern in the psychiatric wards of Bellevue Hospital in New York:

> We gave barbiturates to anybody who screamed. Anybody who was mute or catatonic or not eating or screaming, you gave barbiturates, like you gave [the antipsychotic] Haldol years later. . . . There was nothing else except morphine, which you didn't want to use. We also had ECT for people who were screaming. This was horrendous but you have to ask yourself what Bellevue was like in 1944 or '45. Some of the patients on barbiturates died if your dose wasn't right. They stopped breathing. You said—"oh well" and filled out an accident report. Don't smile, it was a very different world.[62]

Did the disadvantages of barbiturates truly outweigh the benefits of careful therapeutic use? Was the ratio between risk and benefit sufficient to warrant dumping almost the whole drug class into the sea? This has never really been resolved. Given the herd behavior in psychiatry, the rush away from the barbiturates following their schedule II listing (a classification that all but shouted "addiction!") was almost as dramatic as their embrace. Yet the question is worth pausing over today, as we contemplate the contemporary dilemma of psychopharmacology and ask whether the past has anything of value to offer.

Amphetamines

History's first true antidepressants were the amphetamines. As stimulants, they appear to have an elective effect on low mood (but make anxiety worse). So they are not just general sedatives, like barbiturates, in the basin of nonmelancholic mood disorders, but act on nonmelancholic depression in particular. This is generally recognized among psychopharmacology insiders today. In 1996 Jules Angst, director of psychiatric research at University of Zurich, told psychiatrist David Healy, "I'm not convinced about this whole matter of selective clinical profiles for antidepressants. An exception may be amphetamine. I have treated many depressives with amphetamines, as have others like Nathan S. Kline, Donald F. Klein [both pioneering psychopharmacologists in New York] and others. In the early 1950s opium and amphetamine were the main drugs used to treat depression."[63] Yet today this is not widely discussed in public. Rare are the articles about amphetamines for medical purposes other than hyperactivity and narcolepsy (acute daytime sleepiness). And good luck if you want a grant for research on this subject from the U.S. federal government.

The amphetamine story began in 1887, when Lazar Edeleano, a Romanian doctoral student in chemistry in Berlin, synthesized a "PEA" molecule.[64] PEA means phenyl-ethyl-amine, or a drug having a phenyl (six-carbon ring) head, plus a two-carbon chain (ethyl) as a body, and finally at the tail end a nitrogen-hydrogen ("amino") group. PEA molecules are highly psychoactive because they conform closely to the structure of the neurotransmitter norepinephrine. Nobody thought very much of Edeleano's molecule, which he named phenisopropylamine, and it sat on the shelf. (The term *amphetamine* itself does not surface until 1938; previously the molecule was known under a wide variety of chemical names.)

In the same year, 1887, Nagayoshi Nagai, a professor of ophthalmic surgery at the University of Tokyo, isolated the pure form of the alkaloid ephedrine from the ephedra plant.[65] Ephedrine has a PEA structure, with a slightly longer carbon-chain body to which an oxygen is attached as well as an amino. Ephedra had been used for many years as a stimulant in Chinese herbal medicine. Unfortunately, Nagai's initial discovery was not really perceived in the West, and ephedrine required rediscovering in 1923 by Ku Kuei Chen, a freshly minted PhD in biochemistry from the University of Wisconsin who had returned to China to lecture at Peking Union Medical College; American pharmacologist Carl Schmidt, also visiting at Peking Union, helped Chen establish that ephedrine's effects were similar to those of the hormone epinephrine, cleaning up the sinuses and active in asthma (but, unlike epinephrine, it could be taken orally). Lilly got ephedrine onto the market in 1926 for nasal congestion and bronchial spasm.[66]

In 1901, a Japanese scientist working in New York, Jokichi Takamine, isolated epinephrine from the cortex of the adrenal gland, touching off a huge wave of interest in medical treatments with epinephrine (adrenaline).[67] (Only much later was norepinephrine discovered to be a neurotransmitter.) Using epinephrine pharmacologically was described in 1910 in the classic article of George Barger and Henry Dale at the Wellcome Physiological Research Laboratories in London on what they called the "sympathomimetic amines," the PEA chemicals that stimulated the sympathetic branch of the autonomic nervous system.[68]

This brings us to the amphetamines, the PEA derivatives with manifest psychic activity. In 1910, MDA, or methylenedioxyamphetamine, the parent drug of "ecstasy" and known as "the love drug," arose in the test tube.[69] It was the first of the amphetamines. Today, it's a controlled substance, a hallucinogen. We are now on a direct PEA train that, if it travels slowly, leads to important medications, but if too quickly, to consciousness-transforming substances and street abuse.[70]

MDMA came next. Methylenedioxy*meth*amphetamine, called ecstasy or "Eve" among other names today, was patented by Merck in 1914, who conceived it as an anorexigenic, or appetite suppressant.[71] (The "meth" is italicized here to show the difference from MDA.) Neither MDA nor MDMA was ever marketed, but their potency as hallucinogens disposed them to street use.[72] Both conserve the PEA backbone, although their six-ringed phenyl group has a couple of oxygens attached to it. With MDMA, the tail hydrocarbon chain is longer by one carbon atom, making it even more reactive. (MDMA has excited some scientific interest today as a drug that causes surges of serotonin—as do many of the PEAs—hence having possible use as an antidepressant.)[73]

In 1919 Japanese chemist Akira Ogata synthesized methamphetamine, a drug known today as "speed," "crystal," and "ice," but which is also one of the most effective antidepressants ever created. It has a simple PEA structure, and can be produced by "reducing" ephedrine (i.e., stripping ephedrine of its oxygen). It was marketed in the United States in 1943 by Abbott Laboratories in Chicago as Desoxyn (generic name: d-desoxyephedrine hydrochloride, thus, ephedrine minus the oxygen), and discontinued by the firm in 1969. Abbott claimed the drug's superiority "over other sympathomimetic amines in producing euphoria and stimulation of the central nervous system."[74]

In 1919, as well, mescaline, another PEA derivative, was synthesized;[75] Philadelphia neurologist Silas Weir Mitchell had noted in 1896 the clinical effects of the natural form.[76] British sexologist Havelock Ellis rapturously described 2 years later its psychological effects as an "artificial paradise": "Unlike the other chief substances to which it may be compared, mescal does not wholly carry us away from the actual world, or plunge us into oblivion; a large part of its charm lies in the halo of beauty which it casts around the simplest and commonest things. It is the most democratic of the plants which lead men to an artificial paradise."[77]

This brings us back to Edeleano's amphetamine, or phenisopropylamine as he first named it. The story of his long-ignored 1887 discovery resumed in 1923 as Gordon Alles, a master's student at the California Institute of Technology, became interested in making epinephrine derivatives, for which commercial demand was absolutely booming in the treatment of asthma and hay fever. After finishing his master's thesis in 1924, he started working in the practice of George Piness, a Los Angeles allergist, on proteins for desensitization treatments. After finishing his PhD in 1926, Alles turned in earnest to epinephrine substitutes and decided to work with the PEA derivative phenylethanolamine, which differed from Edeleano's amphetamine only in having an extra oxygen ("hydroxyl") group but no methyl (CH_3) tail. When phenylethanolamine didn't work out, Alles resynthesized what was in effect amphetamine, unaware that Edeleano had done so many years previously.

In 1928 Alles experimented with the new compound on dogs in the Department of Physiology at the University of California; he saw that it produced a blood-pressure rise (which epinephrine-derivatives of course do) and that it was orally active, meaning that it could be swallowed without becoming deactivated (unlike phenylethanolamine). He gave it to some of Dr. Piness's patients, who experienced "exhilaration" and "palpitation"; in 1929 Piness and Alles presented these findings at the annual meeting of the American Medical Association.[78] Meanwhile, Alles was experimenting on himself, taking amphetamine orally and noting a prolonged blood-pressure rise plus a long night of wakefulness. "This made him realize," as the U.S. District Court for the State of New Jersey later brought out, "that the drug had a waking effect that was many times that which he had observed with ephedrine in similar dosage."[79]

On August 29, 1930, Alles applied for a patent. The following year the claim was disallowed, partly on the basis of Edeleano's earlier work, and only in 1932 did he finally get through a partial patent claim. In the meantime, the drug house Smith, Kline & French was also on the trail of amphetamine. Their chemist Fred Nabenhauer, inspired possibly by reports of the Piness-Alles paper in 1929, had synthesized a volatile liquid ("base") form of amphetamine trade-named Benzedrine that could be used in an inhaler for asthma; in 1932 SKF marketed the new inhaler. Two years later Alles and Smith, Kline & French reached a deal in which Alles signed over all his patent rights to the company in exchange for 5 percent royalties on Benzedrine sales.[80] In December 1935 the company brought out a nonvolatile crystalline form of amphetamine as Benzedrine Sulfate that could be taken in tablets, thus launching Benzedrine's career in nonasthma medicine. (In 1938 the Council on Pharmacy and Chemistry of the American Medical Association gave Benzedrine Sulfate the generic name "amphetamine sulfate," historically the first use of the term "amphetamine.")[81]

Clinicians studied the effectiveness of Benzedrine first in narcolepsy. In what was probably the first controlled trial for a psychiatric indication, Myron Prinzmetal and Wilfred Bloomberg, in the department of Medicine at Boston City Hospital, studied nine in- and outpatients with narcolepsy who were blind as to whether they were receiving, on an alternating basis, Benzedrine or ephedrine. The trialists established that Benzedrine was much more effective. Four of the patients experienced "complete relief from symptoms."[82]

Yet over the years it was as an antidepressant that Benzedrine derived its reputation. From the outset came reports of Benzedrine's effectiveness in nonmelancholic depression. Eric Guttmann was one of a small cluster of émigré Jewish psychiatrists from Hitler's Germany who were providing a swift upgrade to English psychiatry at the Maudsley Hospital in London. Alles had sent the Maudsley a shipment of Benzedrine, and Guttmann, who was a Rockefeller Research Fellow, and a colleague gave it to 25 patients with mixed disorders (the Maudsley did not admit psychotic patients). In May 1936 they said, "Our results with the drug in the mental field were unexpected, considering that it so closely resembles adrenaline [epinephrine] which produces anxiety. . . . The first psychic symptom which struck us was the talkativeness of our subjects. Almost everybody showed an increased tendency to talk, but the effect was most striking in depressive patients; they overcame their retardation, and several of them talked spontaneously to other people for the first time since their admission." The trialists also noted, "The most interesting feature was a change of mood, experienced in nearly every case. In no instance was anxiety produced or a depression deepened. The change was generally in the direction of euphoria."[83] In 1937 Guttmann and another colleague, William Sargant, in a larger partly placebo-controlled series, made clear that Benzedrine was for nonmelancholic depression, not melancholia. "Mild depression accompanied by retardation is the most favourable of all psychological disorders for benzedrine therapy."[84]

Meanwhile, in the United States, Abraham Myerson, head of research at Boston State Hospital in Mattapan, was giving Benzedrine to "normal and neurotic persons." He reported in October 1936 that, although the psychotic cases derived no benefit, "Benzedrine sulfate seems to have definite though limited value in combating the neuroses. . . . When used judiciously it is of value in lessening the distress and the depression and increasing the feeling of energy."[85] During his training at the University of Minnesota, Morris Nathanson administered a supply of amphetamine that Alles had sent him to 40 patients "who complained of exhaustion and who tired easily," compared to a placebo-control group of 25 with similar complaints. The Benzedrine patients in the study did brilliantly, responding with "a marked lessening of fatigue, an increase in mental and physical activity, and a distinct feeling of exhilaration."[86]

How about the drug's effects on frank depression? In August 1937 trialists at the Mayo Clinic in Rochester, Minnesota, reported on Benzedrine in 100 patients with "chronic exhaustion, depression and psychoneurosis." About four-fifths of the depressed and exhausted received a benefit, as opposed to fewer than half of the neurotics. "In some instances the results were spectacular."[87] The spotlight now turned on Benzedrine in depression and the next years saw many reports, the gist of which was that Benzedrine was quite effective in non-melancholic depression, much less so in melancholia. In 1948 the great pharmacologist Torald Sollmann at Western Reserve University in Cleveland concluded that Benzedrine was "useful as a symptomatic treatment of mild depressive states and somewhat against severe psychopathic depressions."[88]

Benzedrine exists in two isomers, or structural forms, usually "left" and "right" (dextro-). Amphetamine has a pharmacologically active right isomer, called dextroamphetamine, which has a more powerful effect than amphetamine with both isomers mixed together ("racemic" amphetamine). In 1939, with the help of Alles, Fred Nabenhauer at Smith, Kline & French applied for a patent for dextroamphetamine;[89] the patent was granted in 1942, and in 1944 the firm brought it out as Dexedrine Sulfate for "mild depression," thus differentiating it from Benzedrine's indications for "abnormal reactive depressions of mood."[90] In fact, the firm flogged Benzedrine as an antidepressant for the first time in an advertisement in January 1941: "Particularly appropriate in depressive states."[91] The term "anti-depressant" itself is used for the first time in 1947, in the firm's advertisement for the Benzedrine-analgesic combo Edrisal; Dexedrine becomes "the anti-depressant of choice" in 1948.[92] The amphetamines, increasingly referred to as "stimulants," thus become the first drug class to be delineated from the soup of nervousness as "antidepressants."[93]

In the meantime, methamphetamine, the most effective of all the stimulant antidepressants, was launched by Abbott Laboratories as Desoxyn, as we have seen, in 1943. The company billed it as having quicker action, longer duration, and fewer side effects than other agents, but did not indicate it specifically for depression.[94] Numerous other methamphetamines came onto the market, such as Burroughs-Wellcome's "Methedrine" around 1950, which was offered as an antiobesity drug, not as an antidepressant.[95] Indeed, antiobesity and not mood was the indication of the future, and among the many competing brands of methamphetamine available in the early 1950s, depression sounded a minor note.

But among the psychiatrists, internists, and family doctors treating depression, there was a good deal of thinking that methamphetamine was an excellent antidepressant. Jean Delay, professor of psychiatry in Paris and France's foremost psychopharmacologist, differentiated in 1949 between (1) the sodium barbiturates such as Amytal, "'psycholeptic' since they produced a lowering of intra-psychic tensions and are depressants of psychological tonus," and (2) methamphetamine, "a 'psychogogue,' increasing intra-psychic tension and acting as a stimulant." Both were useful in the treatment of something like depressive stupor: Amytal decreased anxiety and let the patient express depressive ideas; methamphetamine "by increasing the anxiety, forces the production [of these ideas]."[96]

Of 219 depressed in- and outpatients in several Bristol hospitals whom Gerald Rudolf, an experienced consultant psychiatrist, treated with methamphetamine in 1955, 82 percent improved, almost half of them markedly so. He concluded that methamphetamine was "the preparation of choice" in depression.[97] An editorial in the British medical weekly *Lancet* that same year said, "For the treatment of depression the value of the amphetamine group of drugs is now established. . . ." Specially recommended were dextroamphetamine and methamphetamine.[98]

Yet depression was not the only indication for methamphetamine. It seemed of utility in the treatment of "post-traumatic anxieties," the ancestor of posttraumatic stress disorder (which was born with *DSM-III* in 1980). This therapeutic thread began at the Psychiatric Division of Bellevue Hospital in 1946, as psychotherapeutically oriented clinicians used methamphetamine to get their patients to disclose "previously unobtainable material."[99] In 1952 at Roffey Park Rehabilitation Centre in Horsham, England, occurred the frank abreacting of traumatic memories:

> A lorry-driver, aged 23, had been involved in a road accident
> 3 months before admission. There was a posttraumatic amnesia of
> 48 hours. Under methedrine [methamphetamine] he abreacted
> violently, the patient reliving the experience he underwent when
> his lorry blew up in flames. Not only was this incident recalled,
> but the drug uncovered a comparable bombing experience during
> a severe London airraid, the patient reliving the terrors of being
> buried in a burning house.

He recovered well on methamphetamine, as did several other such patients at this trauma hospital.[100]

After this promising beginning as a member of the therapeutic armamentarium, methamphetamine underwent, of course, a vast evolution, becoming a drug of calamity when consumed without an appropriate medical indication. There is little evidence that the patients for whom it was legitimately prescribed went on to abuse it. But evidence of the damage that street "meth" has inflicted on American society confronts us today at every turn. This terrible epidemic has many causes, but not one of them was its proper provision for suffering humanity. Nonetheless, the baby was thrown out with the bathwater. By the new millennium, methamphetamine, once prescribed benignly and confidently, was seen as so addictive that even a single dose would launch you toward a lifetime of ruin. "So addictive that one fix can get you hooked!" shrieked the *Financial Times* in 2005.[101] Thus do urban myths displace medical therapeutics.

There is one last moment to describe in the early story of amphetamines: their combination with barbiturates to make them more tolerable for patients, and possibly more effective. The 1950s were the golden years of combo therapies. The idea of tempering the pick-me-up (but hyperdriving) power of amphetamines with the calming of barbiturates was irresistible, and some of the most widely prescribed drugs in medical practice were these amphetamine-barbiturate combos.

The logic of this particular combo goes back to 1938 when Benjamin Cohen at the Grafton State Hospital in Massachusetts and Abraham

Myerson, at Boston State Hospital, proposed a combo of barbiturate and amphetamine in epilepsy. Phenobarbital alone greatly reduced the incidence of seizures, but the trialists added Benzedrine to forestall the "extreme drowsiness and ataxia" that phenobarbital caused. "These untoward results cleared up rapidly without unfavorable effect upon seizure incidence."[102]

In 1939, Edward Reifenstein and Eugene Davidoff at Syracuse University started getting good results in "schizophrenia" by giving, on alternate days, Amytal orally with Benzedrine intravenously. "To date sixteen cases have been treated and of these eight have been discharged to their homes."[103] (Remember that in those days any symptoms that even smelled of psychosis were called "schizophrenia.") Later in 1939, Myerson took up the use of the combo in depression: "We have shown that the narcotic effects of Amytal can be offset by amphetamine sulfate." Further: "No combination of drugs . . . has anything like the value of . . . Amytal in combination with amphetamine sulfate in the treatment of depression."[104]

Beginning in 1942, Jacques Gottlieb at the University of Iowa had been working systematically with various combinations of Amytal and Benzedrine in schizophrenia and depression, injecting them one right after the other. Best results in depression occurred when the two drugs were given "in mixture."[105] Essentially, the investigators had invented the combo themselves. In 1949 Gottlieb said that the results of giving the two drugs in combo were really terrific: "a synergistic effect occurred." But there was a caveat: "Not all patients will respond to the medication; about 10 percent fail."[106] Where is the antidepressant today that is effective in 90 percent of the patients?

Years later, in 1962, Hannah Steinberg, professor of pharmacology at the University of London (in fact, worldwide the first female professor of pharmacology), found that Gottlieb was right, that amphetamine together with the barbiturate cyclobarbital did in fact have a synergistic effect: "The results of the present experiments therefore suggest that an amphetamine/barbiturate drug mixture can produce a pattern of effects which is different from that produced by either constituent separately."[107] But the finding was little followed up, for by this time the world was reeling in horror at the "dependence" that use of the two drug classes supposedly fostered with ease.

In 1948 Smith, Kline & French brought out the first amphetamine-barbiturate combo for commercial use. Called Benzebar, it was a mixture of phenobarbital and Benzedrine, "combin[ing] the unique anti-depressant action of Benzedrine Sulfate and the mild sedation of phenobarbital."[108] Benzedrine, of course, was the company's own drug while phenobarbital had long gone off patent, so commercially the combo worked well.

Two years later, in 1950, Smith, Kline & French launched the combo that would be among psychiatry's greatest hits in combining barbiturates and amphetamines: Dexamyl, a mixture of Lilly's Amytal and Smith, Kline & French's Dexedrine. Why the firm decided to buy an Amytal license is unclear, possibly because Amytal was proving among the most popular of the barbiturates. The company claimed that Dexedrine "because of its 'smooth' and profound antidepressant action" plus Amytal "because of its calming action" relieved "nervous tension, anxiety and agitation."[109] Launched in the United Kingdom as Drinamyl, Dexamyl proved a mainstay of American family medicine in the 1950s, and Smith, Kline & French's ads showing smiling actresses on Dexamyl while vacuuming the home featured later in feminist indictments of how the "tranquilizers" had contributed to the oppression of women. (Neither part of the combo, of course, was a tranquilizer.) Dexamyl was initially regarded as so innocuous that in 1963 the Food and Drug Administration considered making it available over the counter.[110] Yet in the 1970s it fell victim to the FDA's cleanout of combos involving either amphetamine or barbiturate.

Looking back, the amphetamines (especially methamphetamine) and barbiturates could indeed be abused and were, alas, frequent sources of street addiction. But for patients for whom these drugs were legitimately prescribed, they worked in ways that later generations of drugs have not been able to replicate: Depressed and insomniac patients got well and stayed well for years on them without becoming dependent. They, too, are a reminder that effective drugs were available before the "era of psychopharmacology"—that concentrated wave of psychopharmaceutical research and development during the 1950s—was in full swing.

3

The First Drug Set

"If our descendants should ever look back at the present era in psychiatry, they would probably call it the age of psychopharmacology," said
Harry Pennes, research director of a psychiatric hospital in Philadelphia, at an after-dinner meeting at the New York Academy of Medicine
in 1956.[1] The remark was prescient. Between 1951 and 1959 a set of
drugs was introduced into American psychiatry that even today has
never been bested. This discovery so early of drugs that truly work is a
remarkable development. One would not normally expect the first attempts at drug discovery to remain superior to those that came along a
half century later. There is no counterpart anywhere else in medicine; it
is as though the airplanes of the Wright brothers have continued to
best today's Boeing jets. In cardiology, cancer medicine, or any other
medical field, we are accustomed to progress, to steady improvement,
and to building upon the blocks laid down by previous generations. In
psychopharmacology, such progress has not happened. If anything, we
have lost knowledge, as the drugs available today are in no sense an
improvement upon the pioneer generation of drugs whose efficacy *we
have forgotten*.

In 1951 meprobamate, the first big success of the "tranquilizers,"
was synthesized. In 1959 the new tricyclic antidepressant imipramine
reached the American market. Between these bookends came a series
of other important drugs for tension, anxiety, depression, and psychosis. These drugs together represent the first drug set,[2] a group of pioneering psychopharmaceuticals that true progress would sooner or
later have relegated to the sidelines.

Today, they are on the sidelines all right—not as a result of progress but in part as a result of patent expiration. Other factors play a significant role as well, about which later chapters will elucidate, but the sad truth is that drugs of even superior benefit are no longer promoted as soon as their patents expire, at which point the drugs are adopted by generic-drug companies that rush into the market but do not advertise. Otherwise pharmaceutical sales representatives move on to the next set of patent-protected offerings and the older drugs become largely forgotten, not perhaps by older practitioners who remember and trust them, but by the younger generation that fails to learn of their use while in training. It is of course possible that newer generations of drugs still under patent will be superior to those they are replacing. But it is also possible that they will be worse. Actually, it's sort of a flip of the coin, given that therapeutic safety and efficacy are beside the point in the patent system, where the objective is marketplace exclusivity. In psychopharmacology, the coins have mainly come up tails.

In the early 1950s, it was as though someone had opened a faucet. "Since 1954, 32 tranquilizing agents have been synthesized," said the *Pink Sheet*, a tip sheet for pharmaceutical industry insiders, in 1962.[3] At the Food and Drug Administration, there was discontent. "The work load in reviewing NDAs has been increasing appreciably both in volume and complexity," complained one bureaucrat to the FDA commissioner in 1958.[4] (The NDAs, or New Drug Applications, submitted by pharmaceutical manufacturers seeking FDA approval for the launch of a drug, often extend to hundreds of volumes of data.) Lamented FDA brass a bit later, there are only two psychiatrists at the agency doing drug reviews![5] A revolution in psychopharmacology was swamping the system.

What were all these new drugs good for? In psychopharm, nobody really knew. The conventional illness categories of U.S. psychiatry in the 1950s didn't seem to fit the new agents very well. What drugs were specific for "psychoneurosis," the commonest psychoanalytic diagnosis of the period? "We have so many drugs whose effects we do not properly understand," said Frank Fish, professor of psychiatry in Liverpool, in 1959. "And we have sometimes very little idea of precisely what the condition is that we are trying to treat." He compared the current situation to "what might have happened had somebody introduced simultaneously five powerful antibiotics in the middle of the eighteenth century."[6]

Let's look at the new drugs closely. What effect do they seem to have on the patients?

The Tranquilizers

The term *tranquilizer* did not originate in but is indissolubly linked with "the age of anxiety," the 1950s. Yet let's not overcredit. The anxiety focus came from psychoanalysis, a nineteenth-century doctrine that reached its fulsome blossom in the 1950s. The king of the tranquilizers, meprobamate, was launched only in 1955. But as early as 1949 anxiety was the big theme at the annual meeting of the American Psychopathological Association, the weather vane of what's in for American psychiatry; two heavy guns at the New York State Psychiatric Institute—Paul Hoch and Joseph Zubin—edited the volume that came out of that meeting.[7] So even though these drugs may have epitomized the age of anxiety, they didn't whelp it.

Nevertheless, it was the tranquilizers that initiated the first drug set. The classic tranquilizers were meprobamate, chlorpromazine, and reserpine. The tranquilizers thus included agents from drug classes that would later be considered quite distinct: meprobamate was later classed as an anxiolytic (antianxiety), reserpine and chlorpromazine as antipsychotics. Was the tranquilizer concept just the result of initial stumbling at the beginning of the psychopharmacologic revolution? Or was there something of value here that we have lost sight of?

Mephenesin

It is the Second World War. Frank Berger, a Jewish refugee from Nazi Germany who was born in Pilsen, Austro-Hungary, in 1913 and graduated in medicine in Prague in 1937, has made his way to England and taken a job with British Drug Houses. Having a strong background in chemistry, he directs in 1946 the pharmacological study of a drug called mephenesin, a glycerol ether synthesized in 1908.[8] "So before we gave it to a human, we gave it to mice and dogs and cats to see about the toxicity of the drug and what would happen," he said. "They all fell asleep, became unconscious, and came back. After big doses, they came back after twelve hours or more of unconsciousness. Dramatically. Anybody who sees that dog would not argue that mephenesin is like barbiturates," which in similarly large doses would kill the animal.[9]

In mephenesin, Berger had discovered modern history's first "tranquilizer," a drug that relaxed muscle, calmed the mind, and conferred the balm of sleep, without causing daytime sedation. He did not, however, realize at first the importance of his discovery. He then did some research adding mephenesin to anesthetics to observe its muscle-relaxant qualities. He also successfully used mephenesin to diminish the cramps and spasms in tetanus. At this point he didn't think that mephenesin acted on the brain.[10]

Then in 1947 he immigrated to the United States. Berger's first post was at the University of Rochester Medical School in the department of pediatrics. It was the only job he could get at the time. Many of the patients had diseases involving movement disorders, such as cerebral palsy. Berger said to himself, "Let's try mephenesin on some of these." He had great success. Later he said, "I had never seen anything like mephenesin. I wanted to pursue this. The only thing wrong with it is, it's not long acting. If you give it to a patient with cerebral palsy, it will diminish the shaking and tremors for half an hour completely. Then it will gradually come back over three or four hours."[11]

Berger didn't have a solid British patent for mephenesin. Squibb became interested in the drug, and learned that it allayed anxiety as well as relaxed muscle spasms;[12] the FDA approved it in September 1948 and Squibb brought it out in 1954 as Tolserol. Quoting from a clinical trial published in the *Journal of the American Medical Association* in 1949, the company claimed it as ". . . the only drug we have seen that allays anxiety without clouding consciousness."[13] It was also useful in the treatment of alcoholics: Wean them off alcohol and onto mephenesin, then withdraw them from the mephenesin. Squibb told Berger, "Look here, your British patent is no good. We won't pay you any royalties, and if you don't like it you can sue us."[14]

Decades after these events and after everyone had forgotten about mephenesin, Berger—by this time a distinguished figure in psychopharmacology—said somewhat ruefully, "Mephenesin was *the* product." He considered it superior to all the antineurotic drugs that came later. "It's the drug that totally works."[15] As far as Berger was concerned, the apex of the mood drugs had been reached with the very first attempt.

Reserpine

Although mephenesin was the first tranquilizer, it wasn't billed as one.[16] Philadelphia psychiatrist Benjamin Rush initially used the term *tranquilizer*, early in the nineteenth century, to refer to a chair into which mad patients were strapped.[17] The word then went out of fashion for the next century and a half, when the modern use of the term was initiated by Ciba pharmacologist Frederick F. Yonkman in 1953 in an internal company discussion.[18] "Tranquilizer" was first aired publicly later that year in an ad for Ciba's new antihypertensive product Serpasil, a brand name for the alkaloid reserpine from the *Rauwolfia serpentina* plant. "Now a safe tranquilizer–antihypertensive," the company trumpeted in 1953.[19] Thus the word *tranquilizer* was first used in connection with cardiology, not psychiatry.

Yet it was difficult for trialists to overlook that this antihypertensive drug also produced "a calming, tranquilizing effect, without the drowsiness so frequently associated with barbiturates," as Riker Labs claimed in 1953 of its product "Rauwiloid," an alkaloid fraction of the *Rauwolfia serpentina* plant.[20] Boston cardiologist Robert Wilkins, who undertook the first clinical study of reserpine, reported comments of hypertensive patients, such as, "I've never felt as well," "I haven't felt this good for years," "Nothing bothers me anymore," and "I just don't give a damn." Wilkins added, "Of course, this is gratifying to the physician, but more important, it may give an indication of how the drug may act not only in the neurotic hypertensive but in other neurotic patients as well. I have told many psychiatrists . . . that '*Rauwolfia* is good psychotherapy in pill form.'"[21]

In 1954 Riker Labs linked the concept of "tranquilizing" to frankly psychiatric indications in an ad for its new drug "Rauwidrine," a combo of Rauwiloid and amphetamine: "Mood elevation needed? Here is a better approach." The company praised "the "tranquilizing, mildly sedative action of Rauwiloid" combined with the stimulant effects of amphetamine. Nothing was said about hypertension.[22] This marked the beginning of the era of advertised tranquilization in psychiatry.

Tranquilization was not just a marketing concept but was believed at the time to have an underlying scientific validity. When in 1957 the FDA sued State Pharmacal, a Chicago firm, to stop advertising their over-the-counter sedative "Tranquil" as a "tranquilizer," it was on the logic that tranquilizers were something more than sedatives.[23] The FDA believed there were four groups of tranquilizers: phenothiazine derivatives such as chlorpromazine (Thorazine); rauwolfia and its alkaloids such as Serpasil (reserpine); antihistamines with a diphenylmethane structure, such as benactyzine, which Merck brought out in 1957 as the "antiphobic" Suavitil; and meprobamate-style agents.[24] It is thus interesting to see these highly diverse groups of drugs gathered together under the same umbrella on the grounds that they produced "tranquilization," a concept that has now vanished from psychopharmacology. But much else of value has vanished as well.

Methylphenidate

It is difficult for clinicians of the twenty-first century to accept that they might be offering their patients medications that are less effective than those available in the past. But the historical evidence is difficult to overlook.

In the early 1950s, a stream of new psychiatry drugs began to pour onto the market, although the psychoanalytically oriented psychiatrists of the day were really the last to prescribe them, and family doctors and internists the first. Today, the well seems to have run dry and new drugs in psychiatry are seldom. It seems astonishing that in the 1950s and early '60s medicinal chemistry could have devised so many agents that conferred a benefit and had few conspicuous side effects. Granted, these early drugs didn't have to run the gamut of animal safety tests and randomized placebo-controlled clinical trials that are required today, but they did undergo some investigation that, along with informed clinical opinion, served as valid sources of evidence that the effectiveness of these drugs was not in doubt, especially their impact upon depressed mood.

In 1951, Schering Labs brought out the first of the nonbarbiturate drugs for insomnia and anxiety. Dormison (methylparafynol), synthesized in Germany in 1913, had a modest uptake in the United States. A modified version, synthesized in 1955 by British Schering and launched that same year in France as N-Oblivon, enjoyed huge success.[25] The drug was quickly elbowed aside by the benzodiazepines after 1960 and forgotten. But it's a sign that what were now being called the tranquilizers were picking up.[26]

In 1954 Ciba launched a drug against depression of much greater historical heft, even though its antidepressant activity later became forgotten in the furor about hyperactivity in children: Ritalin (methylphenidate). It was marketed as a stimulant rather than a tranquilizer, although it fit the part. The story begins in 1944 when Leandro Panizzon, one of Ciba's medicinal chemists in Basel—born in 1907 and raised in Milan—was synthesizing nitrogen-containing compounds. Ciba's in-house pharmacology showed it to be a mild stimulant—indeed it had an amphetamine-like structure. Because it was almost a matter of honor in those days that chemists experimented on themselves, Panizzon and his wife Marguerite both took the new agent. It made no particular impact on him, but Marguerite felt excited and adventuresome under the drug's influence. "I used to take it before a tennis match," she later said. Ritalin was in fact named after her ("Rita").[27] Ciba marketed it in Switzerland as a "psychotonic" in 1954, and brought it out in 1956 in the United States from its headquarters in Summit, New Jersey, as a drug "to lift the depressed patient up to normal without fear of overstimulation"[28] (a disadvantage of the amphetamines). By 1957 Ciba was flogging it as a "mild smooth-acting antidepressant and stimulant."[29]

There was evidence for this claim. In animal studies, Ritalin reversed the side effects of reserpine in monkeys[30] (reserpine caused a depression-like syndrome, and reversing it was a standard pharmacological test of antidepressant efficacy). In the first clinical trial, in 60 patients on a general medical ward in the Berlin-Charlottenburg Municipal Hospital in 1954, the drug caused considerable increases in mental aptitude, as measured in math experiments, plus produced a "good to euphoric" mood in three-quarters of the patients.[31] The amount of Ritalin imported to the United States rose from 22 pounds in 1954 to 1,215 pounds in 1955,[32] and it was in the United States that the main work was done establishing Ritalin as an antidepressant.

In 1955, at the Traverse City State Hospital in Michigan, there were about 500 patients on the antipsychotic drug reserpine, many of whom fell into reserpine-induced depressions or were sedated to the point of seeming asleep all the time. Of the 25 given a reserpine–methylphenidate combo, 22 improved. "Some have even been sent home. . . . In our opinion," the study concluded, "phenidylate [methylphenidate] is well worth further clinical trial as an analeptic [stimulant], particularly in the chronic, regressed, negativistic psychotics." Many of these backward patients may have had psychotic depression. The Traverse City statistics were eye-openers.[33]

Evidence started to accumulate of Ritalin's effectiveness in fatigue and dysphoria, symptoms associated with the kind of nonmelancholic patient in the community who today would probably be diagnosed with the catchall label of "major depression." Of 39 "fatigued, tired, depressed" outpatients in the private practice of Milwaukee physician Adolph Natenshon, 27 had an "excellent" response to Ritalin and 7 a "good." "Their worries seemed to disappear," said Natenshon. "They were alert, fatigue disappeared, and they could go all day without tiring."[34] Although these 39 patients, "depressed due to pressures of modern day living," were not melancholic, they certainly corresponded to the popular conception of depression in our own day.

In drug studies, special efficacy is spied in the "dose-response" relationship: the higher the dose, the better the response. Of 77 patients with diagnoses mainly of fatigue and neurotic depression seen at Hahnemann Medical College Hospital in Philadelphia in 1960, 44 percent of those on the 20-mg daily dose of Ritalin had a good response, 70 percent of those on the 60-mg dose.[35]

In those days there were few controlled trials against placebo, so the kind of data one might expect today are simply not available for these historic periods. Moreover, the few controlled trials that were undertaken enrolled typically such small numbers of patients (being "underpowered") that they were unable to spot anything less than penicillin-size differences. Nonetheless, there were some useful trials. In 1970 veteran psychopharmacologist Karl Rickels at the University of Pennsylvania studied Ritalin against placebo in 42 "mildly depressed" outpatients versus 34 on placebo. He and co-trialists found Ritalin significantly more effective than the sham drug. He concluded that Ritalin "may be of value in the treatment of mildly to moderately depressed patients who are treated by general practitioners, whose main target symptoms are fatigue, apathy, or anorexia. . . ."[36]

In 1957 the Council on Drugs of the American Medical Association found Ritalin "useful as a mild cortical stimulant in the treatment of various types of depression. . . . Neurotic patients appear to respond better than those with frank psychoses."[37] This judgment is really the bottom line: Ritalin was quite effective in nonmelancholic depression, rather less so in hospital-type melancholia.[38]

"Methylphenidate in 1956 was the first new drug used for the treatment of depressive states," said pharmaceutical market-researcher Paul De Haen in 1973.[39] It replaced the amphetamines, but when it became overshadowed by the tricyclic antidepressants, it was switched to childhood hyperactivity, its function as an antidepressant forgotten. Yet Ritalin is a reminder that there is gold in them thar hills, that much of the first drug set was quite useful in mood disorders.

Meprobamate

As the Ritalin story was unfolding, Frank Berger was searching for a longer-acting mephenesin, the drug with such salutary effects on cerebral palsy at the University of Rochester Medical School. Henry Hoyt, president of Carter Products, a company that had come up on "Carter's Little Liver Pills" in the nineteenth century (they were thought supereffective because they turned your urine green), was hunting for some way of getting in on the exploding psychopharm boom. In 1949 Hoyt invited Berger to come from Rochester to Carter's prescription pharmaceutical subsidiary Wallace Labs in New Brunswick, New Jersey. Carter offered Berger double what he received from the University of Rochester and told him to get cracking in the lab on lengthening the duration of action of mephenesin, or to find a related product. By 1951 he and Wallace Labs' chemist Bernard Ludwig, who had joined the firm 4 years earlier, had synthesized the molecule that would become the first blockbuster drug in psychiatry[40]—meprobamate—which Carter marketed in 1955 as Miltown, selling the license to Wyeth, who brought it out as Equanil. (Wyeth sold far more because they had a 900-person sales team and a "long, long reputation among doctors"; Carter had no sales force but extensive coverage in the medical press.)[41] The name Miltown was chosen after a village in New Jersey that Berger could see from his office in New Brunswick. Berger did well enough financially from his drug, but he did not become vastly wealthy because he had agreed to a 1 percent royalty rate at sales under seven and a half million dollars, and nothing over. This then seemed a lot, but it was not a shadow of the hundreds of millions of dollars the drug ultimately brought in.[42]

Methylphenidate (Ritalin) and meprobamate (Miltown) were quite different drug classes. Methylphenidate is a stimulant whose structure, a "phenyl-ethyl-amine backbone," is close to that of amphetamine. Meprobamate is a dicarbamate, a compound based on carbamic acid, composed of a simple nitrogen–carbon molecule. Yet meprobamate, like methylphenidate, was an effective agent for nonmelancholic depression.

Wallace Labs billed Miltown explicitly as a tranquilizer, and said that it was specific for anxiety. Effective in "anxiety, tension and mental stress" claimed the first ads in 1956.[43] It was Wallace's benactyzine–meprobamate combo Deprol, launched in 1958, that they marketed for depression. (Benactyzine is synthetic atropine, an anticholinergic that American Cyanamid had patented in 1946 and, as mentioned, Merck brought out as Suavitil in 1957; it was thought, like all anticholinergics, to have some antidepressant properties, and atropine was commonly used in Europe as an antidepressant.) Deprol is rather difficult to defend as a superior product, given that the psychopharmacologists of the day widely scorned it and the American Medical Association's Council on Drugs called it in 1971 "an irrational mixture," declaring it "not recommended."[44] Yet many practitioners have fond memories of Deprol, and it must have had qualities that escaped the academic psychiatrists.[45]

The blockbuster meprobamate itself served quite well as a mood drug, which makes it sound like an antidepressant but in fact it was probably best for "nerves," in that large space between antipsychotics and aspirin. Frank Ayd, chief psychiatrist at the large private psychiatric hospital Taylor Manor in Ellicott City, Maryland, and active drug trialist, later said in an interview, ". . . There are people out there who are not psychotic but who are very miserable and who are quite willing to pay good money and go to a lot of inconvenience to get some relief. They knew they were never going to end up in institutions, although they often feared that, but they knew it was impacting on their married lives, social lives and their ability to work. . . . God knows, there was enough overwhelming evidence that the barbiturates were not drugs that you could give out in a cavalier way for a minor condition." This was the advantage, he said, of meprobamate. "So now when you had meprobamate with very small companies in New Jersey and then Wyeth of course had connections, international and what not, it became world wide very quickly."[46]

Meprobamate did well in trials. Lowell Selling, a psychiatrist in Orlando, gave it to 187 patients with problems of various descriptions who came into his office between January 1953 and April 1954. In the course of the study, he dispensed over 54,000 tablets of the drug (four tablets per day was the standard dose). Ninety-five percent of those with tension improved or recovered; anxiety, 90 percent; involutional (midlife) depression, 80 percent; and so on. He found no withdrawal problems in the patients.[47]

Leo Hollister at the Veterans Administration Hospital in Palo Alto, California, among the best known investigators in the young field of psychopharmacology, gave meprobamate or a placebo to 37 inpatients; he also tried the drug in an open (uncontrolled) study of a further 191 chronically hospitalized patients. Results in the controlled trial: In the placebo arm, 2 of 15 improved (13 percent); in the meprobamate arm, 13 of 22 improved (59 percent). In the open trial: Of patients with affective disorders, 74 percent got better, as did 74 percent of those with anxiety; 40 percent of those with "mild" schizophrenia also improved. Hollister concluded, "The results from treating patients with anxiety reactions or affective disorders were quite gratifying. In these patients meprobamate appears to be the drug of choice."[48]

Meprobamate found all kinds of uses. Here is Arthur J. McComiskey, an ear-nose-and-throat specialist in New Orleans, testifying at an FDA hearing in 1966: "I see quite a number of people who feel they just can't swallow, they say they have a lump in their throat, anything from a lump in their throat to a ball, or a cocklebur, some of them even say a pine cone." So he checks them out, does maybe a bit of throat dilatation, then reassures them and gives them something to let them relax. "Most of all I think the medication [meprobamate] I give them to relax, to relieve anxiety does more for them than my actual treatment. I have seen it work again and again." Other of Dr. McComiskey's patients fear they can't breathe. "They are usually terrified and feel they are going to smother that night. I not only have to assure them but give them something to let them relax and lay this thing aside. That is where I use meprobamate too. . . . They absorb it all and get a good result with it, and they can go to bed. . . ."[49]

An imputation that haunted meprobamate from the beginning was addictiveness. This would result in a vastly unfair FDA hearing in 1966, discussed in the next chapter. Yet from the get-go, the scientific evidence of meprobamate's addictiveness was meager. A typical study: In 1957, Joseph Borrus, a psychiatrist in New Brunswick, found meprobamate free of addiction problems. Nor did he find evidence of tolerance, that is, of patients needing increasing doses to get the same effect, or of withdrawal difficulties: ". . . In a few instances, approximately 1 percent, a strong dependence upon meprobamate will take place with a definite reluctance to give up the drug. This usually occurs in extremely dependent, emotionally immature persons who will grasp upon any means to maintain themselves free of their inner tension. . . . The vast majority of patients, perhaps 75 to 85 percent in my own experience and that of others, will discontinue using meprobamate as they begin to feel better." The remaining group "will discontinue gradually at the physician's suggestion."[50]

In a study in 1964, Leonard Goldberg, an alcoholism researcher at the Karolinska Institute in Stockholm, found that, unlike heroin or morphine, meprobamate did not create dependence at therapeutic doses, and that the risk of dependence was less than 0.1 percent, far less than the dependency potential of alcohol. When dependency occurred, the time to its onset was measured in months rather than weeks as for other drugs (alcohol, however, was measured in years, heroin in days); the frequency of dependency per million users was on the order of 1–10, as opposed to 5,000–20,000 for alcohol.[51] Frank Berger later said, with something of a snort, of the SSRI antidepressant paroxetine (Paxil), "Paxil is truly addictive. If you have somebody on Paxil, it's not so easy to get him off. . . . This is not the case with Librium, Valium and Miltown."[52]

The uptake of meprobamate was stunning. In the months after the drug's marketing in 1955, as Frank Ayd later remarked, "the demand for Miltown . . . far exceeded that for any drug previously marketed in the United States. For a time [television comedian] Milton Berle was renamed Miltown Berle, magicians pulled Miltown instead of rabbits from their magical hats . . . and drugstores displayed signs reading 'out of Miltown.'. . ."[53] By 1965, around the time of the first break in the Miltown sales curve under hammering from the benzodiazepines, Carter-Wallace (as the firm became known) had sold about 14 billion tablets of meprobamate, supplying drug for around 500 million meprobamate prescriptions written in the United States for some 100 million patients.[54]

More than anything else, it was the tremendous sales of meprobamate that crystallized a political reaction against "the tranquilizers." At the generally hostile hearings of the Senate Appropriations subcommittee in June 1957 on the budget of the National Institutes of Health, psychiatrist Nathan Kline was the only witness to defend meprobamate, particularly against media statements "about side effects and withdrawal symptoms."[55] At hearings that Estes Kefauver, Democratic senator from Tennessee, convened in 1960, a horrified Kefauver remarked that in the United States alone 500 tons of meprobamate had been produced in 1958, "enough to give every adult male in the United States 40 hours a week of medication of this drug."[56]

The three drugs that symbolized the tranquilizer era had all been launched in or close to 1955: meprobamate, the antipsychotic reserpine, and the antipsychotic chlorpromazine. Although other drugs were called tranquilizers as well, these were the core products. They were seen as anchoring a spectrum of tranquilization for nervous conditions ranging from psychosis to nonmelancholic depression and anxiety, with chlorpromazine at one end in the "serious drug" category, and meprobamate at the other for the griefs of "everyday practice."[57] Later, science would distinguish between antipsychotics on the one hand and anxiolytics and antidepressants on the other, three separate categories, never shall they meet. But throughout most of the 1950s they were all lumped into one: the tranquilizers. In 1966 Ayd stated at the FDA hearings on meprobamate that, of these big three, reserpine and chlorpromazine were "major tranquilizers"—not everybody's cup of tea. "You would not normally prescribe such drugs for the anxiety patients. All we had for them was the barbiturates. When meprobamate came along . . . this was a welcomed addition. This is one of the reasons why in a very short period of time the whole world . . . began to prescribe both the major and the minor tranquilizers." These drugs meant "the ability of psychiatric patients to be treated in general hospitals, or in the office without even the necessity of going into a hospital."[58] This was significant progress.

Dissolving the Tranquilizer Unity

In the late 1950s the tranquilizer spectrum started to be hammered apart with the reification of specific drug categories such as antipsychotics, antidepressants, and anxiolytics as separate classes for distinct diseases. But this dissolving of the tranquilizer unity actually began as early as 1955 when Paris psychiatry professor Jean Delay christened the phenothiazines as *neuroleptics*, a drug class that included chlorpromazine as well as reserpine.[59] It was a drug class capable of producing "neurologic manifestations," as Delay's assistant Pierre Deniker defined the term.[60] An intermediate step was differentiating "major" from "minor" tranquilizers, by the World Health Organization in 1958, a distinction that carried well into the 1960s, as Frank Ayd's statement just quoted indicates.[61] Canadian psychiatrist Heinz Lehmann suggested the term *antipsychotics* for the neuroleptics in 1961.[62]

Other terminology also vied for currency. The term *antidepressant*, as noted in Chapter 2, had existed since the commercial publicity for the amphetamines in the late 1940s, but it was not generally accepted in psychiatry at that point. The term acquired the keys to the city only with the American launch of imipramine (Tofranil), the first of the tricyclic antidepressant drugs, in 1959; initially called a "thymoleptic," it was relabeled "antidepressant" in 1960.[63] Four years later, *antianxiety* surfaced as a separate category with Hoffmann-La Roche's advertisements for Librium (chlordiazepoxide), a member of the benzodiazepine class that the company insisted were not tranquilizers.[64]

All these terms represented the splintering of the unity of "tranquilizer." Indeed, the very existence of a concept such as "tranquilizer" menaced the effort to cut psychiatric illness into neat nosological categories and to assign a pharmaceutical treatment for each.

Chlorpromazine and the Phenothiazines

Yet the concept of tranquilizer was validated in the usefulness of chlorpromazine and other phenothiazine antipsychotics as antidepressants. Antipsychotics as antidepressants: a fateful notion, for if the concept had survived, the subsequent division of illness into separate categories might not have occurred; and later developments do indeed appear as a colossal historic error, the separation of a bucket of water into neat compartments for purposes of commercial advantage. But in the first drug set, the new phenothiazine antipsychotics often worked beautifully as antidepressants. This is not to say that all antipsychotics serve as antidepressants and vice versa. Many agents in each class convey little benefit in the other. But there's enough overlap to suggest that in both highly heterogeneous groups—depressives and psychotics—there are subgroups that overlap and may be identical.

The first antipsychotic in psychiatry was not chlorpromazine but a predecessor called promethazine (marketed in the United States in 1951 as Phenergan). The French drug house Rhône-Poulenc synthesized it in 1944 as part of a whole series of phenothiazine antihistamines they hoped to clean up with.[65] Of course nobody called it an antipsychotic in those days because the term had not yet been coined. The French phrase for this new drug class was *neuroplegics*, literally drugs that struck the neurons of the brain. Promethazine, the first of the neuroplegics, was used in French mental hospitals in the early 1950s.[66] Yet promethazine, though useful as a sedative in psychotic patients, was not terribly effective; it was said to make the patients so sleepy they could hardly move, and they were worse when they woke up.[67] Promethazine was forgotten in psychiatry as soon as Rhône-Poulenc, once put on the psychiatry trail, synthesized a much more powerful member of the antihistamine series: chlorpromazine.

In a story too well known to merit much retelling, chlorpromazine was used for psychiatric indications for the first time in France in 1952.[68] It was approved in the United States by the FDA in March 1954 and launched as Thorazine for "intractable pain" and vomiting. Only in July 1955 did Smith, Kline & French begin indicating it for psychiatry. The first ad: "Thorazine reduces need for electroshock therapy."[69]

Chlorpromazine was marketed in Europe as Largactil, or a drug having a large action, which was literally true: Chlorpromazine is effective for a wide variety of illness conditions, not merely for hallucinations, delusions, and psychotic agitation. It does abolish hallucinations and delusional thinking, and sedate the assaultiveness, the pacing, and the general agitation of many patients with schizophrenia. Its antipsychotic action is certainly no myth. "Anyone who would have bothered to spend just two nights on call prior to CPZ [chlorpromazine] on an admission service of a psychiatric hospital would have to be blind and deaf not to see what the introduction of CPZ did," said one senior psychiatrist.[70]

Yet chlorpromazine, and many of the other antipsychotics in the phenothiazine class, was also effective against pain, and was used, for example, as an obstetrical analgesic.[71] It is a splendid antianxiety drug, and probably the treatment of choice in severe anxiety—if one is prepared to accept, in low doses, a less than one percent risk of extrapyramidal motor symptoms (e.g., tremors, rigidity) in the balance. It is also an effective antidepressant, and as we scan the first drug set for evidence of antidepressant action that was later forgotten or minimized in the craze for later patent-protected agents, we must glance at the antipsychotics as antidepressants.

A qualifier: Electroconvulsive ("shock") therapy, originated in 1938, remains the most effective treatment of serious, melancholic depression. So reprising the usefulness of antipsychotics in depression might unwittingly convey the impression that they represent a superior treatment. They do not. Jean Delay, in whose Paris clinic chlorpromazine was first tried systematically, pointed out in 1955 the drug's tremendous success in treating mania, sudden-onset psychosis, and schizophrenia. It was unsuccessful, however, in treating eleven depressed patients who then responded to ECT.[72]

But not everybody wishes to undergo ECT, owing to the great stigma that is attached to it.[73] Antipsychotic treatment of depression should be considered only in those patients in whom a good seizure through ECT cannot be obtained, as occurs in those with alcoholism, or when for cultural reasons ECT is rejected. For many with depression, chlorpromazine represents an effective treatment option. Jean Sigwald in Paris discovered this with his outpatients in 1953, a year after the drug's first trials. In eight cases of "melancholia with anxiety," Sigwald had very good or good results in five. A typical patient was

> a woman of 46, experiencing an anxious melancholia for eight
> months, suicidal ideation with a plan, mental and physical
> slowing. From May 1952 on, for 37 days, we gave her 125 mg
> of chlorpromazine a day, a dose that we had to reduce to
> 100 mg following somnolence and tachycardia [accelerated
> heart rate]. In a few days the melancholic state disappeared, her
> suicidal ideation vanished completely, and the resumption of her
> earlier daily routines occurred progressively, becoming complete.
> We saw the patient nine months after the beginning of the
> treatment, and are maintaining her with a daily dose of 25 to
> 50 mg.

Sigwald said of the trial as a whole, "In general, chlorpromazine treatment almost always improves the patient's mood, and one observes the disappearance of sadness and depression, in some cases giving way to a certain euphoria."[74] Later, he called chlorpromazine "the insulin of the nervous."[75]

Among the "neurotics" in the practice of English psychiatrist John Hutchinson, "The patients who benefit from [chlorpromazine] most are those who suffer from mixed states of anxiety and depression," he said in 1956. "The states of agitated depression seen frequently in middle-aged patients respond dramatically to Largactil therapy. Deep intramuscular injections of 50 mg. up to twice daily bring the condition swiftly under control." Admittedly, this is qualitative testimony, not a quantitative finding based on the random assignment of patients to a treatment and a control group. But clearly from Dr. Hutchinson's perspective, chlorpromazine was close to a miracle drug in his older depressed outpatients.[76]

These early investigators were often ecstatic about the results of chlorpromazine in schizophrenia, yet in the same breath they might mention their depressed patients. When Basel psychiatry professor John Staehelin convoked a symposium on chlorpromazine in November 1953, there was great enthusiasm about its effect in schizophrenia. Yet his staffer Paul Kielholz pointed out that it was really quite effective in endogenous, or melancholic, depression as well.[77]

Having read a Rhône-Poulenc brochure while in the bathtub, Heinz Lehmann decided to introduce chlorpromazine in 1953 to several patients at the Verdun psychiatric hospital in Montreal where he served as director:

> We included schizophrenics, depressed patients and we also had some organic dementias; we didn't know who to give it to. We gave it for agitation. . . . And two or three of the acute schizophrenics became symptom free. Now I had never seen that before. I thought it was a fluke—something that would never happen again but anyway there they were. At the end of four or five weeks, there were a lot of symptom-free patients. By this I mean that a lot of hallucinations, delusions and thought disorder had disappeared. In 1953 there just wasn't anything that ever produced something like this—a remission from schizophrenia in weeks.

But then Lehmann added "something which is not often mentioned nowadays [1996], but quite a few other investigators had found the same: there were quite a few depressed patients who got better too, quicker than they would ordinarily have done."[78]

Lehmann thought little of ECT. But many ECT practitioners started adding chlorpromazine to their treatment of depression. In 1955 Douglas Goldman, director of the Longview State Hospital in Cincinnati, described a 35-year-old woman with a history of manic-depressive illness who had been on small doses of chlorpromazine. She then tried to commit suicide by driving her car into a tractor-trailer truck, an outcome avoided only by the skill of the truck driver. Afterward, "Patient told her husband she had planned her demise at home, but apparently the opportunity afforded by the truck seemed immediately attractive." Goldman gave her a course of ECT, continuing the chlorpromazine at 300 mg a day, whereupon she recovered. Goldman said, "It was entirely clear to those taking care of the patient, that the combination of chlorpromazine with electric shock treatment accelerated significantly her recovery from the depressive state."[79]

However compelling these stories and data from open trials, they do not represent the gold standard of psychiatric evidence, the randomly controlled trial, or RCT. In 1962, Max Fink and Donald Klein at Hillside Hospital in the New York borough of Queens, where Fink was director of the Department of Experimental Psychiatry, provided definitive evidence of the efficacy of the phenothiazines as antidepressants. Between October 1958 and October 1959, in the largest placebo-controlled study ever done in one place up to that point, they randomly assigned two hundred patients referred for pharmacotherapy to a phenothiazine antipsychotic or to the new tricyclic antidepressant imipramine. They were stunned by the results from the phenothiazine group: "The greatest change occurred in the patients who had the greatest affective expression. . . . The depressive state was markedly alleviated, although a mild apathy persisted."[80] This report was an early warning flare that the distinction then being established between "depression" and "schizophrenia" might be an artificial one, and certainly that the phenothiazines were not specific for "schizophrenia."[81]

Nonetheless, the distinction between "antidepressants" and "antipsychotics" in the late 1950s shattered the concept of "tranquilizers," despite the fact that many new drugs, it turned out, could be launched as either (and thus were de facto tranquilizers). Among French researchers, the phenothiazines were seen as having strong antidepressant activity. As Jean Delay's associate Pierre Deniker told an English audience in 1959, "Some of the new neuroleptics . . . seem to have a definite effect on depressive states. Levopromazine [levomepromazine] has been commonly used."[82] The supposed neuroleptic levomepromazine, synthesized by Rhône-Poulenc in 1958 and launched in France as Nozinan, went on to acquire a reputation as an antimelancholic.[83]

Sometimes, the choice of whether to identify an agent as an antipsychotic or antidepressant was more a business decision than a scientific flip of the coin. When Pfizer[84] developed thiothixene in the mid-1960s, they had little idea of the drug's uses. Nathan Kline said, "We ran trials on thiothixene when it first came out and the manufacturers did not know what it was good for; [the trials] showed that it was quite effective as an antidepressant. They subsequently produced doxepin, marketing that as their antidepressant and switched thiothixene to use in the treatment of psychotics."[85] Indeed, when Pfizer floated thiothixene as Navane in the United States market in 1967, it was for "acute and chronic schizophrenia."[86] The story is actually even more colorful, for when Pfizer produced doxepin (Sinequan) in 1969, they are said to have envisioned it as an anxiolytic, then switched it to an antidepressant.[87] For Pfizer, the concepts of anxiolytic, antidepressant, and antischizophrenic really turned out to be marketing slogans.[88]

Drugs marketed as antipsychotics often beat recognized antidepressants and anxiolytics in depression trials. In 1966 a team led by John Overall at the University of Texas Medical Branch at Galveston—and including pioneer psychopharmacologists Leo Hollister in Palo Alto and Veronica Pennington in Jackson, Mississippi—concluded that anxious depression was really quite different from retarded depression. The logic: the antipsychotic drug thioridazine (Mellaril)—a latecomer phenothiazine (1959) to the first drug set—had soundly beaten the tricyclic antidepressant imipramine (Tofranil) in anxious depression; yet in retarded depression imipramine beat thioridazine.[89]

There was lots of evidence that the supposed antipsychotics of the first drug set made serviceable antidepressants.[90] When Saul Rosenthal and Charles Bowden at the University of Texas Medical School in San Antonio put thioridazine head to head with the antianxiety drug diazepam (Valium) in 1973, thioridazine "was significantly superior to diazepam in a group of symptoms representing depressive symptomatology, including suicide, psychomotor retardation, helplessness, worthlessness, and guilt feelings."[91] Valium, unsurprisingly, did well in this trial as an antianxiety drug, yet Valium also had a long history of effectiveness in nonmelancholic depression. It is interesting that in both these trials, thioridazine, an "antipsychotic," was able to treat depression effectively; in theory depression was a quite different disease from schizophrenia.

Thus, the tranquilizer concept of the first drug set turned out to be quite robust; drugs belonging to different therapeutic categories—such as antidepressant, antianxiety, and antipsychotic—were actually more or less interchangeable. How could this be, in disease categories that in theory, by the late 1950s, were increasingly considered mutually exclusive and homogeneous?

Energizers

In 1957 Hoffmann-La Roche secured from the FDA a depression indication for iproniazid, their drug brand-named Marsilid, that had been on the market for tuberculosis since 1951. Marsilid worked in psychiatry by inhibiting the action of a brain enzyme, and was the first of the antidepressants with efficacy in melancholia. It was not initially billed, however, as an antidepressant. Belonging to a class called "monoamine oxidase inhibitors" (MAOIs), it was called instead an "energizer." Energizers were not tranquilizers. They would later be considered antidepressants, as the energizer concept fell flat. But the marketing story at launch was that they supplied energy, like the amphetamines, rather than fight depression.

The MAOIs were the first drug class based explicitly on a theory: that the biological brain "amines" such as serotonin and norepinephrine were neurotransmitters, and that correcting imbalances in neurotransmitters could make psychiatric illness better. In an advertisement in 1957, Hoffmann-La Roche flogged Marsilid as "an amine oxidase inhibitor which affects the metabolism of serotonin, epinephrine, norepinephrine and other amines."[92] How it works: These neurotransmitters are discharged by the upstream neuron into the synapse, the space between upstream and downstream neurons, in order to make the downstream neuron fire. In the world of academic psychopharmacology, the theory was that psychiatric illnesses were caused by too little norepinephrine and serotonin, so here's a great idea! We'll prolong the presence of the amine neurotransmitters (the "monoamines") in the synapse by inhibiting the action of the enzyme that destroys them, namely, monoamine oxidase. Hence, the presence of these vital monoamines in the synapse would be prolonged to do good; fewer would be taken back up into the upstream neuron (via the reuptake mechanism), and mental illness would be checked. Thus the concept of the monoamine oxidase inhibitors as therapeutic agents was born, although the first reference to monoamine oxidase inhibition appeared almost 20 years earlier, in 1938, when John Gaddum, then at University College London, said that the drug ephedrine increased the amount of epinephrine by inhibiting amine oxidase.[93] Even today, it's not clear whether this concept of reuptake inhibition offers the open sesame to the neurochemistry of psychiatric affliction.[94] But it makes a good story, and billions of dollars worth of drugs—latterly the selective serotonin reuptake inhibitors (SSRIs)—have been sold in its name.

The real story of iproniazid and the MAOIs is as follows: Hoffmann-La Roche had procured large supplies of the chemical hydrazine used as rocket fuel in Germany during the war.[95] On the basis of this supply, the company synthesized two antituberculosis drugs from isonicotinic acid hydrazide, and launched them in 1951: isoniazid (Rimifon) and iproniazid (Marsilid). An early trial of iproniazid took place at the Sea View Hospital, a sanatorium in the New York borough of Staten Island.[96] The Sea View trials were a success; the drugs reversed the systematic toxicity of tuberculosis; the patients' fevers subsided, and they began gaining weight. But there was one problem: In addition to the expected side effects such as muscle twitching and hyperreflexia, many of the patients became "mildly euphoric."[97] TB is not a fun disease, yet later news accounts had patients dancing about the halls at Sea View.[98]

In the meantime, Swiss chemist E. Albert Zeller, at Northwestern University in Chicago, had discovered in 1952 that iproniazid, but not isoniazid, inhibited the action of the enzyme monoamine oxidase.[99] Interest in the monoamines was just starting to quicken in psychiatry in these years, and any drug that had an effect on a brain chemical was going to be scrutinized clinically. But in 1953 Gordon Kamman, at the Fergus Falls State Hospital in Minnesota, put iproniazid into a group of chronic schizophrenic patients and found it virtually useless.[100] Three years later, George Crane, at the Westchester Division of New York's Montefiore Hospital, supplied a dyspeptic account of the "psychiatric side-effects of iproniazid": "Concomitant with changes of outward behavior [hyperactivity, euphoria] were ambivalence and hostility, particularly evident in the female patients."[101] Normally, such negative reports would put an end to a proposed psychiatric indication. Yet interest in psychiatric uses of iproniazid continued to percolate.

The question of who in fact *did* discover the psychiatric uses of MAOIs is clouded in mystery. Nathan Kline's name is usually associated with the discovery, but here the trail becomes foggy. Did pharmacologist John C. Saunders, then a research associate at Ciba's offices in Summit, New Jersey, really claim at a conference in 1955 that his work on reserpine had led him to the monoamine theory of depression? He later said, in another conference in 1958, that it was he who earlier had proposed "the application of amine oxidase inhibitors to psychiatry on the theoretical basis of their action on amine metabolism in the brain, with the probability that they would alleviate depressions."[102] Kline himself, director of research at Rockland State Hospital in Orangeburg, New York, was at the 1958 conference, and presumably sat in the audience as Saunders, by now also working at Rockland,[103] said he had made this earlier claim—a big claim, essentially to have discovered the role of neurochemistry in psychiatry. Unfortunately, the transcript of the 1955 conference made no note of Saunders's participation.[104]

Meanwhile, a second powder trail: In 1955, Alfred Pletscher, a scientist at Hoffmann-La Roche's Basel headquarters, was a visiting scholar in Bernard Brodie's lab in the National Heart Institute at Bethesda, Maryland, a lab that was rather surprisingly doing research on psychopharmacology. Kline visited Pletscher, who told Kline about the new drug iproniazid and its promise in psychiatry.[105] Kline is said to have experimented first on himself. Then in 1956, together with Saunders and Harry P. Loomer, who was head of the clinical service at Rockland State, Kline administered the drug to 17 chronic female patients in the hospital who were "withdrawn, regressed, deteriorated, colorless, and of flattened affect." Kline also gave iproniazid to patients in his private practice in Manhattan. At the end of 5 weeks, 47 percent of these chronically depressed patients had improved; by 5 months "a minimum of 70 percent of the patients have shown measurable response." These results, reported in 1957, were pretty impressive, given that hitherto only ECT worked in such a population. The authors billed iproniazid as a "psychic energizer." Loomer was senior author of the paper, then Saunders, then Kline.[106] (George Simpson, at Rockland State at the time, recalls them as such sloppy researchers that, "It was remarkable that they ever discovered anything.")[107]

Just prior to the publication of their results, Frank Ayd reported early in 1957 that he had given Marsilid to 39 psychiatric patients at Franklin Square Hospital in Baltimore who had a mixed bag of diagnoses. He found that over half of them "did not benefit from this drug."[108] When Kline saw this negative one-pager in the *American Journal of Psychiatry*, he "blew his cork," as Ayd said later. Ayd told Kline,

"Nate, the truth of the matter is I didn't know you were working with iproniazid. This was an idea that came from the Chief of Medicine who works with TB patients and I just tried it."[109]

Kline henceforth announced himself to be the discoverer of the effectiveness of the MAOIs in psychiatry. For this achievement he received the coveted Albert Lasker Award for Clinical Medical Research in 1964 (he had received a first Lasker Prize in 1957 for discovering the effectiveness of reserpine in psychiatry). Loomer and Saunders, their noses very much out of joint, sued to share in the monetary award. Loomer dropped out of the action, but Saunders ultimately collected a third of the prize.[110]

Curiously, Kline was said to have had "quite a job" convincing Hoffmann-La Roche to go for the psychiatric indication. According to London psychopharmacologist Merton Sandler, who was more or less an eyewitness, Elmer Severinghaus, medical director of the American branch of Roche, "was unimpressed by the case Kline put forward and vetoed further clinical study of the problem." But Kline went over Severinghaus's head, had lunch with G. David Barney, the president of the American office of Hoffmann-La Roche, and persuaded him to move forward on a pilot study.[111]

Subsequently, the evidence of Marsilid's effectiveness in psychiatry was substantial. In 1959, C. M. B. Pare and Merton Sandler at the Bethlem Royal and Maudsley Hospitals in London conducted the first large controlled trial of Marsilid, finding that, in 50 depressed patients "who had been considered suitable for electroconvulsive therapy," 26 were improved, 12 of them due to the drug and in some cases quite dramatically so. "Perhaps of most interest," they said, "is the question whether iproniazid is a general euphoriant or whether it acts only on patients whose depression is due to a specific metabolic abnormality which has yet to be identified. The striking response to iproniazid noted in some patients compared with the apparent ineffectiveness of the drug in others suggests that the latter may be true."[112] It is a striking comment on the failure of clinical psychopharmacology to progress that 50 years after they penned those lines, the biochemistry of depression remains a riddle.

By 1958, much experience had been collected. People spoke of Marsilid as eliciting a "Mona Lisa smile."[113] Carl Breitner, at Arizona State Hospital in Phoenix, concluded that "catatonic schizophrenia" and severe depression were really the same illness because both responded well to Marsilid and ECT[114]—this at a time when the only consistently effective treatment for catatonia and melancholia had been ECT. At

Mercywood Neuropsychiatric Hospital in Ann Arbor, over 70 percent of the patients with psychotic depression did well on Marsilid. (Today, there is no drug with remotely comparable effectiveness in this condition.)[115] Said Zale Yanof, a Toledo, Ohio, internist at a symposium in 1958, ". . . I soon found that the Marsilid effect was one that I had never seen clinically before. It is a potent psychic energizer and remarkable mood normalizer. . . ."[116]

In a trial beginning May 1957 of 142 psychiatry outpatients, Boston psychiatrist Samuel Joel discovered Marsilid to be the first drug effective in obsessive-compulsive disorder. Kline had already mentioned this anecdotally,[117] but Joel presented the numbers more systematically. "A group of six severe obsessive-compulsive cases have shown marked improvement with iproniazid treatment, where other therapies were ineffective."[118]

Kline himself gave Marsilid in high doses together with amphetamine for acute depression. One of his patients, "a professor of medicine in a well known university, despite annoying side effects, cannot be persuaded to reduce the dose of iproniazid below 75 mg, since he would 'rather suffer the side effects' and be free of the depression that has plagued him for twelve years than 'take any chances.'"[119] Kline's private patients on the Marsilid–amphetamine combo occasionally responded "in twenty-four to forty-eight hours."[120] (A horse named "Marsilid" won in the ninth at Belmont racetrack outside of New York on September 4, 1959.[121] It is tempting to think that its owner might have been among Dr. Kline's grateful patients.)

Marsilid seemed to have an elective effect not just in Nate Kline's "acute depression" but in melancholia as well, reducing the need for ECT by up to 70 percent, as Theodore Robie with a private psychiatric practice in East Orange, New Jersey, found in 1958.[122] Moreover, at St. Thomas's Hospital in London, medical staff preferred iproniazid in patients "showing somewhat atypical depressive states, sometimes resembling anxiety hysteria with secondary depression, who seem to be specifically and almost completely relieved of their disabling symptoms by iproniazid after the failure of all other forms of treatment."[123] This 1959 report, by two of the students of William Sargant, head of psychological medicine at St. Thomas's Hospital and one of the founders of biological psychiatry, was the beginning of the tradition of treating "atypical depression" with MAOIs.

So, Marsilid was a big therapeutic success, probably superior to any agent on the market today for serious depression or obsessive-compulsive disorder. It became almost a kind of cult drug, able to deliver therapeutic benefit in very sick patients who responded to nothing else. Unhappily, it was dogged by liver toxicity. In 1958 Hoffmann-La Roche sought to corral the problem by changing the recommended dose on the label. Practitioners could smell withdrawal coming; physicians at the Veterans Administration as well as the National Institutes of Health argued "that the product was so important in the treatment of certain mental health cases that it should remain on the market. . . ."[124] There existed, said the FDA in a private communication to a physician at the Philadelphia College of Pharmacy and Science, a core of "specialists familiar with its use . . . adamant in their opinion that Marsilid is a particularly useful drug and should be kept available for use where indicated." The risk of liver toxicity was, the agency said, about one per three or four thousand patients, with about a 20 percent fatality rate.[125] This jaundice side effect didn't appear "when the drug was used at high doses in over 300,000 TB cases," the *Pink Sheet* noted.[126]

Nevertheless, in January 1961 the FDA ordered Marsilid withdrawn.[127] It continued to be available for investigational purposes under a so-called IND, but was no longer in the pharmacies. An IND is FDA-speak for Notice of Claimed Investigational Exemption for a New Drug; they are filed by individual physicians seeking special permission to treat a patient with a drug not under an effective NDA, or New Drug Application.

Yet Marsilid's reputation as something of a wonder drug lingered on. In 1965 a psychiatrist in Batavia, New York, sought an IND for permission to treat Irene X, who had been a patient in Rochester State Hospital in 1958 because of "recurring psychotic depressions of an endogenous nature." Guy Walters, the director of Rochester State, told Mrs. X's treating psychiatrist in Batavia that, "Mrs. X failed to benefit from the usual anti-depressants and shock treatment, and she underwent a protracted hospitalization. Finally, in March 1959, she was started on Marsilid, 50 mgms. t.i.d. [three times a day] with remarkable improvement, and within a month, was released." Mrs. X stayed well on Marsilid for several years, but relapsed in 1962 after it ceased to be available; she was readmitted to Rochester State. "Since her readmission, Mrs. X has again received the gamut of accepted treatment for depression including Parnate [tranylcypromine], Tofranil [imipramine], Ritalin [methylphenidate], Elavil [amitriptyline], various tranquilizers and shock treatment, all without any lasting success." Now it was time, again, for Marsilid.[128]

By the late 1950s, a slew of other MAOIs had appeared, several with exceptional clinical promise. When the American Medical Association met in June 1959 in Atlantic City, Warner-Chilcott's Nardil (phenelzine) had just cleared FDA approval, Pfizer's Niamid (nialamide) was just around the corner, and Lakeside's Catron (pheniprazine) was in the wings.[129] "The entire group," said the *Pink Sheet*, "are regarded as potent agents, and are being watched closely."[130]

The rest of this story takes us beyond the 1950s and the first drug set. Yet it was in the 1950s that this drug class established its reputation, despite often horrendous side effects, as something of a miracle cure for mood disorders. There was a certain population out there, deuced hard to define, that responded beautifully to Marsilid. Mrs. X's story is clearly one example of this.

Moreover, intriguing little niche diagnoses bobbed to the surface, forgotten today but not necessarily inexistent, for which Marsilid proved effective. Leo Alexander, a noted Boston psychopharmacologist (and adviser to the U.S. government during the Nuremberg Trials), thought that "depression" was probably a cluster of different disorders. One of them was *anhedonia*, a "joyless inhibited state" that meant the inability to experience pleasure. He thought Marsilid a specific for that. Anhedonic patients were fatigued, listless, and filled with self-pity, unlike the self-reproach typical of melancholia. Alexander called this the "inert psychasthenic anhedonic reaction," echoing the "psychasthenia" of turn-of-the-century Paris psychiatrist Pierre Janet. In one group of 54 depressed patients, Alexander had 16 with psychasthenic anhedonia. Of these 16 patients, 88 percent responded well to iproniazid (versus 26 percent of the nonanhedonic depressed).[131]

Here's another niche diagnosis, today completely off the radar, whose responsiveness to Marsilid commands a second look: In 1959 Martin Roth, professor of psychiatry in Newcastle upon Tyne, described a syndrome he called "the phobic anxiety-depersonalization syndrome," involving patients who are "dependent and immature but also scrupulous, fastidious and inflexible."[132] The syndrome did not get taken into the official American diagnostic manual, *DSM-III*, in 1980. Yet it has wide international credence. In any event, the syndrome responds impressively to MAOIs. Thomas Ban said, "I've never seen a case of phobic anxiety-depersonalization for which MAOIs didn't work. What Martin Roth discovered *is* a distinct disorder."[133] Thus Marsilid served as a kind of psychopharmacologic torch for carving out diseases.

The MAOIs "opened new vistas for psychiatry," as Alfred Pletscher put it. "At a time when biological psychiatry was still in its infancy, the idea of treating mental disturbances, such as psychic depression, by interfering with biochemical processes in the brain, was quite sensational."[134] But by the summer of 1959, as the American Medical Association met in Atlantic City, there was one more development. "Very much in the limelight at last week's meeting," said the *Pink Sheet*, was "Geigy's Tofranil, an anti-depressive though not a monoamine oxidase inhibitor, cleared by the govt. a few weeks ago."[135] The MAOIs would shortly shuffle offstage because of rare "hypertensive crises," elevations of blood pressure that occur when monoamine oxidase is prevented from breaking down primary amines such as tyramine in the gut; these exaggerated fears represent the sort of herdlike behavior among psychiatrists that often unfairly sinks psychiatric drugs.

There now danced into the limelight a different kind of antidepressant entirely: the "tricyclics."

Tricyclic Antidepressants

The success of chlorpromazine wonderfully concentrated minds in the pharmaceutical industry. The discovery did seem capable of being reproduced. Chlorpromazine's phenothiazine nucleus—two phenyl rings held together with a nitrogen and a sulfur atom (giving the impression of three rings)—had been synthesized in 1883 by August Bernthsen in his laboratory in Heidelberg.[136] It was the basis of numerous dyes, and medicinal chemists were entirely familiar with it. To make chlorpromazine, Rhône-Poulenc's chemists had added a chlorine atom and a nitrogen-containing side chain. But there were plenty of other combinations, or "substituents," one could add to the basic model.

In the late 1940s the Geigy Company in Basel was following the same antihistamine trail that produced chlorpromazine. But not wanting just to duplicate the phenothiazine nucleus, in 1949 they took an "imminodibenzyl nucleus" (first synthesized in 1898, with an ethylene in place of the sulfur atom), then played around with the side chains, and put some of the resulting compounds into trials as hypnotics.[137] Among other trialists, Geigy was in contact with Roland Kuhn, a psychiatrist at the Münsterlingen Cantonal Asylum (Thurgau Canton) in Switzerland.[138] Kuhn, in his early 40s, had a strong interest in psychotherapy and philosophy and was anything but a psychopharmacologist. He had been losing confidence in psychoanalysis, and began to realize that many "neurotic" or "psychosomatic" patients were really depressed. But how to help them? Admitting them to hospital and doing ECT seemed a bit much to him. "How often I thought," he later said, "we should improve the opium treatment. But how?"[139]

Mindful of the success of chlorpromazine, in 1953 Kuhn contacted Robert Domenjoz, head of pharmacology at Geigy, and asked him if one of the earlier imminodibenzyl compounds they had looked at (G 22150) might be worth a second look. Yet 2 years later, in March 1955, Kuhn told Domenjoz that G 22150 had been ineffective in schizophrenia and manic-depressive illness.[140]

Sometime later that year, Domenjoz met Kuhn in a hotel in Zurich and showed him "a large sheet of paper on which were drawn about 40 chemical formulas of the substances which were available for clinical evaluation."[141] Kuhn said he wanted the molecule with the same side chain as chlorpromazine, and selected it from the chart. It was G 22355. Over the next year and a half Kuhn subjected G 22355 to trials for a number of different indications. It had some success in psychosis, but it showed an even more important feature: After putting G 22355 into around 150 patients, Kuhn wrote Domenjoz in August 1956 that it "has an obvious effect on depression. The vital depression visibly improves." Vital depression, a concept introduced by German psychiatrist Kurt Schneider in 1920, was a form of melancholia with severe physical sensations of pain and fatigue. Kuhn went on to tell Domenjoz, "The patients feel less tired, the sensation of weight decreases, the inhibitions become less pronounced and the mood improves."[142] Kuhn had, essentially, discovered the effectiveness of an important new agent in melancholia.

Yet Geigy was not really interested in Kuhn's discovery. Domenjoz remained fixated upon schizophrenia, and sent G 22355 out to a number of other trialists for further exploration as an antischizophrenic, saying nothing about Kuhn's discovery in depression.

In the meantime, the Second World Congress of Psychiatry loomed, to be held in Zurich in September 1957 (the first had been in Paris in 1950). Kuhn was invited to contribute a paper and wrote up his findings about G 22355, which Geigy had brand-named Tofranil, generically imipramine. When Kuhn gave his lecture at the congress, there were perhaps a dozen people in the audience and no questions were asked afterward. Among those present was Frank Ayd, who later said,

> Well, it was dramatic. Kuhn is a rather tall man, slender, very soft
> spoken, very cultured, very dignified and very erudite. . . . He didn't

say "this is a good antidepressant." He said "this is a good drug for depressed patients who have these symptoms. . . ." I'm not sure how many people in that room appreciated that we were hearing the first announcement of a drug that was going to revolutionize the treatment of affective disorders—and do more than that. If one thinks of what imipramine can do, it's not just an antidepressant, it's an anxiolytic, it's an anti-panic. We would have never had all these things if Kuhn hadn't given a very lucid and convincing paper. I'll tell you . . . you want to read the English translation of his paper—it's as good as the Gettysburg address.[143]

Published in the first week of September 1957 in the *Swiss Medical Weekly*, the paper reported a striking effect on depressive symptoms: "The patients become generally livelier, their depressive whisper voices become louder, the patients appear more social, the yammering and crying come to an end."[144]

When Tofranil was launched in Switzerland late in 1957—in the United States in 1959—it was described as a "thymoleptic," literally drugs that "take hold of the mood," a term long in use in Spanish psychiatry that Geigy had also been employing internally.[145] Geigy still did not really get behind the drug, however, and the next year, 1958, when Kuhn attended a psychopharmacology conference in Rome, the company representatives basically cold-shouldered him. The turning point came only when at the conference Robert Boehringer, one of the prominent Geigy shareholders (and an *éminence grise* in the firm), asked Kuhn if there was anything that might serve for his wife at home ill with depression. Kuhn recommended Tofranil; she readily recovered, and thereafter Geigy warmed to the drug.[146]

That Rome conference, the first International Congress of Neuro-Pharmacology in September 1958, was interesting for another reason. There, a group from the Parisian Val-de-Grâce military hospital presented a paper in which they reported finding in their depressed patients who had been given imipramine "a resumption of contact with the outside world, a suppression of internal inhibition, liberation from anguish [by which the French usually meant somatic anxiety]."[147] A year earlier, Geigy had given Jean Delay and his disciples at the Ste Anne Mental Hospital in Paris a supply of imipramine to try, but having never heard of Geigy, Delay evidently dismissed the drug from his mind.[148] Upon seeing at the Rome conference that they had been neatly scooped by the Val-de-Grâce group, Delay is said to have chewed his assistant Pierre Deniker out roundly in public for having had the drug for a year and not conducting trials.[149]

Internationally, the first big imipramine trial was Heinz Lehmann's in Montreal, published in October 1958. Lehmann had little use for statistics, preferring, like Kuhn, the close daily observation of his patients (rather than the use of rating scales in large trials). Lehmann concluded of his results: "In the setting of a closed hospital we were able to give effective relief to most of our depressed patients with the drug alone [as opposed to drug plus ECT], even if they were greatly disturbed."[150]

In England, it was psychoanalyst Hilda Abraham, the granddaughter of Freud-intimate Karl Abraham, who conducted one of the first imipramine trials. She told Alan Broadhurst, who worked for Geigy's English branch, "I haven't ever really thought about using medication in the treatment of depression, can we talk about it?"[151]

In the United States, Joe Schildkraut remembers trying imipramine at the psychoanalytically oriented Massachusetts Mental Health Hospital in those years. "These drugs seemed like magic to me," he said. "I became aware that there was a new world out there, a world of psychiatry informed by pharmacology."[152] Said Don Klein of an early trial at Hillside Hospital in Queens, "We assumed [imipramine] would be some sort of supercocaine, blasting the patients out of their rut. Remarkably, these anhedonic, anorexic, insomniac patients began to sleep better, eat better, after several weeks . . . saying 'the veil has been lifted.'"[153]

Later in 1958, Jean Delay and Pierre Deniker did get around to conducting a controlled trial comparing imipramine to the MAOI iproniazid (Marsilid). In therapeutic terms, they showed about equivalent results: About two-thirds of "depressed" patients improved on each drug, although the responders to the oxidase inhibitors might have been a different group from the responders to the tricyclic antidepressants such as imipramine (which acted, it was later discovered, by inhibiting the reuptake of neurotransmitters). The investigators found among their 137 depressed outpatients that 74 percent of those with "melancholic depression" got better on imipramine. What to call this new drug? Delay and Deniker scorned Geigy's label *thymoleptic* and preferred instead "psycho-analeptics," or mood stimulants. At a March 1959 conference at McGill University in Montreal, they said, "It seems appropriate to class these drugs together as anti-depressive agents falling within the category of psycho-analeptics." *Psychoanaleptic* did not catch on any better than *thymoleptic*, but *antidepressants* did.[154]

There were numerous other small trials, most of which were un-controlled, a matter of secondary importance because even the few controlled trials enrolled so few patients as to make the comparison with placebo meaningless. The whole concept of statistical "power" had not yet caught on in psychiatry (as opposed to "statistical significance"—all these little trials were "significant"). Yet for what it's worth, in 1965 Jonathan Cole, director of the National Institute of Mental Health's Psychopharmacology Service Center, which undertook large controlled trials of new drugs, and Gerald Klerman, previously a colleague of Cole's at the PSC and now a faculty member at Harvard, undertook an overview of the 23 controlled studies that by then had been published on imipramine compared to another active drug or to placebo. They found the effectiveness of imipramine clear though not overwhelming: ". . . Sixty-five percent of the 550 patients treated with imipramine improved while thirty-one percent of the 459 control patients improved. On this basis, imipramine seems superior to placebo."[155]

What established imipramine as the mainstay of antidepressant therapy for decades was not really this margin over placebo. As Tom Ban points out, "What made imipramine acceptable for clinical use was that in some patients, however few, it really worked. If one took the patient off prematurely the patient relapsed, and if the patient who responded to imipramine for the first time had a recurrence episode, he/she responded again to the drug. The nagging question was and has remained how to identify the responding patient without exposing non-responding patients to the iatrogenic effects of antidepressants, and the expense involved in purchasing them."[156]

Which patients? It was exactly the same problem as with Marsilid: How does one define the group that will do well on them? It would certainly not be all patients with "depression." The view was gelling that imipramine—and the host of other drugs introduced over the next decade as tricyclic antidepressants (TCAs) in reference to their chemical structure of three fused rings—had some specificity for melancholia. As Fritz Freyhan, another member of the pioneering generation of psychopharmacologists who, like Heinz Lehmann and Frank Berger, were German-Jewish émigrés, told the same conference in 1959 at McGill University, where Delay and Deniker gave their above-mentioned findings: "Tofranil, by way of a crude analogy, may be compared with an antibiotic, the action of which only becomes apparent if it hits a suitable bacterial target. Thus, Tofranil can be thought of as a key which fits only certain keyholes. If it fits, it opens a door through which the depressive psychopathology departs and disappears." In Freyhan's own trial at Delaware State Hospital in Farnhurst, patients with classic "manic-depressive illness" did best on Tofranil.[157] At this conference there was a general agreement that, as Frank Ayd put it, "Tofranil is not a tranquilizer [like chlorpromazine] but instead a specific antidepressant."[158]

One more qualification: "The TCAs worked beautifully in melancholics," said Max Fink, in a conversation in 2006 looking back, "so long as they weren't psychotic melancholics."[159] Melancholic patients who are psychotic do not respond well to tricyclic antidepressants alone and require urgently electroconvulsive therapy or, if that is not available, other chemical agents such as an antipsychotic or lithium. (Whether a combination of antipsychotic and tricyclic is the right treatment remains unsettled at this writing.)[160]

But among drug treatments for nonpsychotic melancholia, the tricyclics were the treatment of choice. I have not made a great deal about their serious side effects, of which there were some, simply because later advocates of the SSRIs have overstressed the side effects of the tricyclics. Older readers who are clinicians may recall wrestling with cardiac arrhythmias induced by the tricyclics. But such serious adverse events were uncommon, and the most frequent side effects were "anticholinergic" in nature, such as dry mouth, blurred vision, and the like.[161] As with any drug class, one has to weigh therapeutic benefits against risks, and the benefits were great.

Alfred Pletscher attempted to account for Tofranil's "victory march" in the 1960s and after, when the MAOIs were vanishing from the radar. Kuhn's original observations, Pletscher said, had been confirmed by others: The MAOIs had already shown "that mental depression was a condition accessible to chemotherapy." Yet imipramine did not have the side effects of the MAOIs; and researchers in basic neurosciences were coming up with evidence that these tricyclic antidepressants affected brain neurotransmitters differently, which gave them a convincing story.[162]

Pletscher was right: The door that Tofranil had opened in the brain saw much of the kind of psychopathology rush out that the amphetamines, history's first mild antidepressants, couldn't touch.

Looking back, Alexander Glassman at the New York State Psychiatric Institute said, "Actually, in the old days, the drugs were very effective. The old tricyclics were very effective drugs. They certainly had side effects that killed people in overdose, but they were very effective compounds. And if you got a good blood level, we really were getting 75–80 percent of the patients that were hospitalized in those days for depression better."[163] This is not bad.

Lithium

By rights, lithium should come first in a discussion of the first drug set, because its effectiveness was discovered—or more properly rediscovered—in 1949, just around the same time as mephenesin. The use of lithium in psychiatry—as a hypnotic—was first described in 1870 by Silas Weir Mitchell, a socially prominent Philadelphia neurologist with a large private practice.[164] Lithium is an important treatment, remaining today the agent of choice for mania, and probably the preferred drug to prevent relapse in depression as well. Only in the 1960s did it start to be accepted in Europe, and only in 1970 was it licensed by the FDA for use in the United States. But, as a treatment for mood disorders the effectiveness of which has never been surpassed, it has a role in the first drug set.

How John Cade, superintendent of the Bundoora Repatriation Hospital in a suburb of Melbourne, made his discovery of the almost wondrous effectiveness of lithium in mania is familiar and won't be repeated here.[165] Full-blast mania is a terrible illness that in former times was often fatal, as the patients would simply agitate themselves to death. A treatment had arrived for it! Yet Cade's article in the *Medical Journal of Australia* in 1949 had almost no international impact.[166] At the time, lithium had recently come into bad odor as a cardiac drug, and most psychiatrists had little interest in prescribing it.

Other isolated and little-noticed reports followed Cade's article.[167] It was actually to the young Danish psychiatrist Mogens Schou (pronounced "Sk-oh" as in "hoe") that credit is owing for putting lithium on the international radar. In 1952 Erik Strömgren, head of the Aarhus university psychiatric clinic in Risskov, suggested to Schou that he look into Cade's findings. There had been a tradition in Danish psychiatry of using lithium that went back to physician Carl Georg Lange's work in 1886.[168] Schou had a particular interest in the subject, as his father, psychiatrist Hans Jacob Schou, had been interested in manic-depressive illness, and a history of the illness ran in Schou's family.[169] With the help of colleagues, Schou organized a double-blind trial, randomizing the patients to lithium or placebo with the flip of a coin; the results were published in a British journal in 1954. It was one of the early ran-domized trials in psychiatry. Previously, Schou said, the only effective treatment of mania had been ECT. "The lithium therapy appears to of-fer a useful alternative since many patients can be kept in a normal state by administration of a maintenance dose."[170]

Yet this important finding was almost drowned in a sea of British doubt. The most influential training center in the United Kingdom since the 1930s has been the Maudsley Hospital in London, where after the Second World War Aubrey Lewis was professor of psychiatry and Michael Shepherd an influential senior figure. The Maudsley had a his-toric tradition of skepticism about pharmacotherapy, and emphasized social and community, not biological, psychiatry. Lewis and Shepherd both were said to have scorned lithium treatment as "dangerous non-sense."[171] Lithium was in fact tricky to use without experience, which is probably the reason the revolution in psychopharmacology began with chlorpromazine and not lithium.[172] But these English clinicians exag-gerated its dangerousness. Shepherd sneered that Schou had so much faith in lithium that he put his whole family on it.[173] As for Schou's con-cept of "the prophylaxis of depression," Shepherd considered it risible.[174] Alec Coppen, at a different hospital across London, sought to explain these attitudes: "A lot of people who are in psychiatry are not really interested in the medical model. They went into psychiatry to get away from it. . . . Psychiatric illnesses are seen as a sort of . . . social illness that should be treated by social methods." Coppen called this "out-of-date science dating back to the 1950s."[175] But it was alive and well at the Maudsley, and threw a blanket of doubt over early lithium research.

Lithium arrived on the Continent earlier than in the United States. Of the main players, France was first to license lithium, as lithium gluco-nate, in 1961. For years previously, the French had swallowed "Docteur Gustin's Lithium," which, one observer speculated, was why you don't have a lot of manic-depressed patients in Marseille.[176]

Lithium's arrival in the United States occurred in the late 1950s, when Sydney-educated Samuel Gershon imported the lithium concept from Australia while working in Ralph Gerard's big program at Ypsi-lanti State Hospital in Michigan on the biology of schizophrenia, spon-sored by the National Institute of Mental Health and the University of Michigan. Gershon and Edward Kingstone, a young Canadian psychia-trist at the Allan Memorial Institute in Montreal, published almost simultaneously in 1960 on lithium in mania.[177]

Even before the appearance of these articles, in 1959 Ronald Fieve, a resident at the New York State Psychiatric Institute, became fascinated with Cade's and Schou's work. Aided by a Coleman flame photometer (introduced in 1958 to measure blood levels of this potentially quite toxic substance), Fieve and another resident began an open-label trial with lithium, which they procured from a chemical corporation in Connecticut. Fieve later wrote, "In 1964, when lithium was still commercially unavailable in the U.S., a psychiatric group at the University of Texas had heard of my work, and sent a manic professor to see me. He was psychotic, working on 40 papers and 2 books, euphoric, overtalkative and charming. After I treated him for several weeks with lithium, he returned to Texas completely normal in mood and behavior."[178] In 1966 Fieve reported on 19 manic patients they had treated with lithium: 44 percent "had good responses."[179] Two years later Fieve and coworkers said lithium had "a mild antidepressant effect" as well.[180]

To put lithium into patients, of course, it was necessary to get an IND from the FDA. Jonathan Cole was one of two clinicians in the Boston area with an IND for lithium, and was among the several psychiatrists who got Merle Gibson, head of psychopharmacology at the FDA, interested in approving the drug for broader use through the New Drug Application (NDA) process. Cole said, "The Rowell company, a pharmaceutical company in northern Minnesota [Baudette], was the first drug company to be interested in making up lithium carbonate in capsules for double blind placebo and whatnot. They were a small company that sat on a lake [Lake of the Woods] in northern Minnesota because some fish in the lake produced something like cod liver oil, and so they were way ahead of any other company. . . . Then finally the FDA talked Smith Kline French and Pfizer into marketing the drug." The FDA held up approval of Rowell's NDA until the two big companies were ready, and all three manufacturers' lithium carbonate entered the market in 1970.[181]

What Cole didn't say, but is also true, is that in 1969 the FDA greatly agonized about the approval of lithium, especially whether it should be used for long-term prophylaxis after an acute episode, or only for acute mania. As one insider put it, "there was a good deal of caution and a good deal of worry" about its long-term effects.[182] It was thus a systematic lobbying campaign by Frank Ayd and Oregon psychiatrist Paul Blachly, who threatened to prescribe it approved or not, that put lithium over the top at the FDA.

Over the years, no drug has made as much of a difference in the lives of patients with manic-depressive illness, now known as bipolar disorder, as lithium; it not only effectively treats the acute manic phase of the illness, but it also prevents relapse from both mania and depression. In 1971 an English group led by Alec Coppen established the extraordinary effectiveness of lithium in the prophylaxis of unipolar as well as bipolar depression.[183] It's not clear that these really are two different types of depression, and readers should take this distinction with a grain of salt. Melancholia is melancholia, whatever its polarity.[184]

Nonetheless, the distinction was thought important at the time. In 2000, Sam Gershon, looking back on the launch of lithium 30 years previously, said, "Lithium is in general the most effective medication for acute mania, producing improvement in about 70 to 80 percent of cases." Its effectiveness in the prophylaxis of bipolar disorder was also beyond doubt, he said. In short, "lithium is the most effective agent in the treatment of bipolar disorder."[185] Gershon made this comment at a time when the shelves of the pharmacies were becoming crowded with other mood stabilizers for the exploding number of people, including children, being diagnosed with bipolar disorder.[186]

In retrospect, "The miracle of lithium was not its treatment of acute mania," as Dennis Charney, a veteran psychopharmacologist then at Yale University, put it in 1995 at a meeting of the Psychopharmacologic Drugs Advisory Committee of the FDA. "Neuroleptics, and even high-dose benzodiazepines, are quite effective for the treatment of acute mania. . . . The issue is prevention of relapse." The committee was meeting to consider Abbott's application for the approval of its mood-stabilizer drug Depakote (divalproex sodium) for bipolar disorder. Charney thought it appropriate that this fact about lithium should be mentioned in the Depakote label.[187]

It wasn't.

Eureka!

Out of the first drug set came a story. The story's plot told of the relationship among neurochemicals, disease, and drugs: Imbalances in brain chemicals caused illnesses that could be cured by "reuptake inhibitors." It was a story that, rightly or wrongly, profoundly influenced the subsequent unfolding of events.

The MAOIs, as mentioned, were the first drug class to give the story overt marketing traction, starting with iproniazid (Marsilid) in 1957, but it actually began a few years earlier at the National Institutes of Health (NIH) with the development in 1955 of a machine, the spectrophotofluorimeter, that permitted the measurement of the fluorescence of a wide range of organic compounds. With this device, you could tell, for example, how much of a given monoamine neurotransmitter was present in tissue.[188]

Two members of the first drug set, the "tranquilizer" antipsychotic reserpine and the "energizer" MAOI iproniazid, were quickly shown to affect neurotransmitters. Indeed, much that happened later in the psychopharm story occurred in the name of neurotransmitters. The acme of the story in the 1990s featured serotonin, with drugs that selectively inhibited the reuptake of serotonin, or SSRIs, as the key to unlocking "depression." By then the neurotransmitter narrative, and serotonin in particular, had become badly bent out of shape as a marketing device. But the story was initially rooted in high-level science.

In 1954 Marthe Vogt, an émigré German-Jewish neuroscientist researching in Edinburgh, identified norepinephrine in the brain.[189] This was the first neurotransmitter to be discovered in central nervous tissue. That same year John Henry Gaddum and associates in the Department of Pharmacology of the University of Edinburgh identified the role of serotonin in the central nervous system. He had been led to this discovery because LSD blocks serotonin; Gaddum had taken LSD and had "been out of his mind for forty-eight hours"; thus, he thought serotonin might play a role in keeping us sane.[190] In 1954, as well, D. Wayne Woolley at the Rockefeller Institute for Medical Research in New York pointed a speculative spotlight at serotonin as playing a possible role in mental illness. Woolley reasoned like Gaddum: LSD caused a mental condition that looked like schizophrenia. LSD also blocked serotonin. Maybe mental illness was caused by a serotonin deficiency. He said, "If the hypothesis about serotonin deficiency is accepted, then the obvious thing to do is to treat patients having appropriate mental disorders with serotonin."[191]

Meanwhile, pharmacologist Bernard Brodie was accumulating a gifted group of younger researchers in the Laboratory of Chemical Pharmacology of the NIH's National Heart Institute in Bethesda, Maryland.[192] In 1955, Arvid Carlsson had come over from the Department of Pharmacology at the University of Lund in Sweden; Alfred Pletscher was on leave from Hoffmann-La Roche headquarters in Basel; Parkhurst Shore was also present, a freshly minted biochemist from Georgetown University, who had joined the Brodie lab in 1950. Brodie saw problems relating to neurochemistry as more interesting than those relating to the heart; he would give his junior colleagues freedom to study whatever they wished, then make interesting findings into group accomplishments (which had good and bad sides as at the end of the day some, such as Julius Axelrod, at the time a junior researcher in Brodie's lab and later Nobel Prize winner, felt rather ripped off). Among those findings was Pletscher's 1955 discovery that reserpine caused the neurons to dump their stores of serotonin.[193] This Pletscher finding, in the view of Vanderbilt psychopharmacologist Fridolin Sulser, "catalyzed the birth of the neurotransmitter era in neuropsychopharmacology and biological psychiatry."[194]

Why? What was the evidence that serotonin affected behavior? And thus could a drug like reserpine change behavior by changing neurotransmitter levels? It took another 2 years to generate a clear answer. In 1957 Brodie and Shore gave reserpine to rabbits, which depleted their serotonin, which in turn caused a "depression" of rabbit behavior. Reserpine's depressive effects had already been known for some time, but this research was geared toward understanding the biochemical mechanism behind those effects. Brodie and Shore hypothesized that if reserpine's dumping of serotonin is what brings about the drug's depressive effects, then would increasing the neurotransmitter cure the depression? They pretreated the lab animals with iproniazid and found that, sure enough, it protected them from depression when given reserpine. So iproniazid was an antidepressant. A photograph showed, on the left, two depressed rabbits that had been given reserpine without pretreatment with iproniazid; their eyes were closed. On the right were two rabbits that had been protected from depression by pretreatment with iproniazid; their eyes were open.[195] It is difficult to exaggerate the impact these discoveries had on the world of psychopharmacology and on drug discovery concepts in the pharmaceutical industry.

Thus, the edifice was now almost in place. In March 1960, at a meeting at the Ciba Foundation in London, Julius Axelrod, now in the Laboratory of Clinical Science at the National Institute of Mental Health, a lab that rivaled Brodie's, showed that reserpine, among other drugs, caused the central nervous system to dump norepinephrine. He said, "It is possible that these psychotropic drugs produce their therapeutic actions by increasing the rate of destruction of liberated adrenaline and noradrenaline [norepinephrine]."[196] In 1961 Axelrod and coworkers demonstrated that the TCA imipramine acted by blocking the reuptake of norepinephrine in peripheral tissues and brain slices.[197] This gave norepinephrine a central role in nervous disease.

Two years later, Arvid Carlsson, now in the Department of Pharmacology at Gothenburg, provided evidence that antipsychotic drugs, like chlorpromazine, worked by blocking the receptors for dopamine, and to some extent, for norepinephrine.[198]

One more piece: In 1964 Axelrod and his colleague Jacques Glowinski confirmed that imipramine had the effect of blocking norepinephrine reuptake in the living brain. But chlorpromazine, they found, didn't block the reuptake of norepinephrine.[199] (So imipramine was confirmed as an "antidepressant drug," whereas chlorpromazine was confirmed as belonging to another drug class, acting, as Carlsson found, on dopamine; this research further disintegrated the notion of the "tranquilizers.") What was needed, therefore, was more "reuptake inhibitors." The hand now fit perfectly into the glove: Depression, caused evidently by a lack of norepinephrine, could be treated by giving imipramine to prolong the presence of norepinephrine in the synapse.

The drugs that worked had produced a theory that seemed to work.

Several developments had now occurred. First, as psychopharmacologist Brian Leonard put it much later, the drug reserpine was better understood as "depressogenic," meaning that by virtue of dumping serotonin and norepinephrine from the neurons, it was thought to cause depression. Second, a therapeutic drug, imipramine, was understood to inhibit the reuptake of norepinephrine, thereby making depressed patients better. So the logic seemed clear: You lose norepinephrine, you become depressed; you get more norepinephrine on board (by virtue of delaying its reuptake), you recover from depression. "For the first time," continued Leonard, "it was possible to provide a reasonable explanation not only for the mode of action of monoamine oxidase inhibitors and tricyclic antidepressants but also for the psychopathology of depression." Depression was caused by too little of a given neurotransmitter! This was the "amine theory of depression."[200]

Third, said Leonard, it was discovered (as we have seen) that chlorpromazine blocked the dopamine receptor, "opening up a new era of schizophrenia research." And fourth, the discovery that meprobamate "was an effective anxiolytic at doses that did not cause marked sedation soon revolutionized the treatment of anxiety."

"Thus," concluded Leonard, "by the mid-1960s major advances had been made in the effective treatment of the three major types of psychiatric disorder. For the first time in the history of psychiatry, it was possible not only to control the symptoms of these disorders with drugs but also to begin to establish the biochemical basis of the disorder."[201]

In fact, these drug discoveries were of sensational importance for understanding psychiatric illness and the basic nature of the human condition: Our personalities, our intellects, our very culture could presumably be boiled down to a sack of enzymes. As University of Chicago neuroscientist Ralph Gerard famously put it, "For every twisted thought there is a twisted molecule."[202]

But because of the great significance of these discoveries, it's important not to be swept away by the kind of reductionism that ultimately discredited psychoanalysis. Psychiatric illness at the end of the day does not reduce to disturbances in neurotransmission—powerful as the neurotransmitter concept is, it has the ability to fly out of control like a roaring fire hose if we lose sight of its place in the larger riddle of mental illness. At one conference in the early 1960s, a participant asked, "In the case of a schizophrenic who cannot read German but who buys a great number of books printed in German, would Marrazzi [the speaker] say that this might be an impairment of synaptic function?"

Amedeo Marrazzi, a University of Pittsburgh pharmacologist, replied, "It is obviously an impairment of synaptic function no matter how you look at it, because he operates only through his synapses."[203]

No, please, gentlemen. Let's not get carried away. Why this poor chap buys books he can't read goes beyond his dopamine levels.

But other, less triumphalist questions arise from the neurotransmitter revolution of the 1950s: (1) Why did these epochal scientific findings never become successfully translated into the discovery of superior drugs? and (2) Why did psychiatry and psychopharmacology permit their undoubted science to become debased in the service of commerce?

4
Power Play

What happened to these successful members of the first drug set? They had various fates, through all of which runs the common thread of indifference to science, the playing up of anecdotal risks rather than balancing the risk-benefit ratio for public health, and the willingness to use the regulator's awesome power for political purposes.

The Food and Drug Administration had been more or less a one-horse operation when in the 1950s and especially in the 1960s it vastly expanded to become eventually the major regulatory agency we know today. It solidified its authority largely by taking on the most popular drugs and beating their manufacturers as a way of expanding agency power. Not that there were any real problems with most of the drugs themselves, which tended to be safe, effective, and widely prescribed. It was rather that the agency aspired to emerge as the tough "new" kid on the regulatory block by knocking down some of the industry heavyweights. This is the story of how a federal agency won the power to dictate medical indications—meaning diagnoses—to the pharmaceutical industry.

A bit of background: the Food and Drugs Act of 1906 gave the Bureau of Chemistry of the Department of Agriculture regulatory functions, including the ability to prohibit interstate commerce in misbranded and adulterated foods, drinks, and drugs (a power, at least regarding drugs, that was almost never exercised except for narcotics). In 1927 the Bureau of Chemistry's name was changed to the Food, Drug, and Insecticide Administration, a clunker of a title shortened to the Food and Drug Administration in 1930. In 1938 the Federal Food,

Drug, and Cosmetic Act changed the scene considerably, giving the FDA the power to verify that drugs coming onto the market were safe. The mechanism for this verification was a New Drug Application (NDA), which a company would have to submit to the FDA, including proposed labeling for licensing. The "label" is bureaucratic shorthand for the instructions for use of a drug. The instructions are not actually printed on the bottle label but rather in the *Physicians' Desk Reference to Pharmaceutical Specialties* (PDR) and in handouts given to pharmacists.

In 1940 the FDA moved from the Department of Agriculture to the new Federal Security Agency, which in 1953 became the Department of Health, Education, and Welfare (HEW). In these years, as veterans recall, the FDA was "a real small scale operation," having a budget of only $5 million even in 1955. But that year, the first report of the Citizens' Advisory Committee of the FDA led to a big growth of the agency, and the workload began to shift from the inspection of poisoned seafood to the more rigorous inspection of NDAs—and to cracking down on companies whose products did not have an NDA (there were many such companies). Against this background of quickening interest in bureaucratic heavy lifting, in 1962 the Congress in the Kefauver-Harris Drug Amendments granted the agency sweeping new power to evaluate drugs for efficacy as well as safety.[1]

This new power turned out to have fateful consequences for the history of psychopharmacology: Government bureaucrats became able to destroy good drugs and to determine what doctors should prescribe for their patients. It was in such a power play that Carter Products' meprobamate, marketed as Miltown, and by Wyeth as Equanil, one of the most effective agents in the history of psychiatry, became denigrated as a dangerous, ineffective drug of addiction.

A Drug Becomes a Cause

This story begins, as so many do, with the uniquely American hysteria about "addiction."

A discussion about addictiveness had earlier surfaced within the federal government in 1942, when the FDA created a list of "habit-forming" drugs that must have a warning on the label. The mid-1950s saw the rebirth of this discussion when early in 1956 the FDA asked the National Research Council's Committee on Drug Addiction to determine what a "habituating" drug was and how it might differ from an "addicting" drug. This was becoming a hot subject, for it potentially involved putting addiction labels on the amphetamines and barbiturates.[2] A slew of new "tranquilizers"—it was the politicians who put the quotation marks on the drug class—were also coming onto the market, and it was inevitable that the addiction discussion slop over to them too.

One of them was meprobamate, and rumors of its addictiveness had been circulating in the federal government practically since the drug's launch in 1955.[3] The federal narcotic hospital of the Public Health Service (PHS), and the attached Addiction Research Center of the National Institute of Mental Health (NIMH), in Lexington, Kentucky, had been one prime source of the addiction talk. Staffer Harris Isbell had been a leading spear-carrier for the theory, thundering in 1956 against these "addicting" tranquilizers, a term that then embraced the budding phenothiazine drug class, including chlorpromazine, plus reserpine and meprobamate.[4] A whole gang of researchers at the PHS hospital and the NIMH Center in Lexington were keen to link the new drugs to addiction as well. Nathan Eddy, secretary of NRC's drug addiction committee, was said to be the guiding force behind a report on the tranquilizers in May 1957 that cautioned addictiveness.[5] Shortly after, his colleague Carl Essig, a neurologist at the Lexington facility, fingered meprobamate in particular, reporting withdrawal symptoms in patients at Lexington being treated for addiction.[6] His brief report became widely cited, which in turn touched off a small kerfuffle. Wyeth, which marketed meprobamate under the brand Equanil, pointed out that no nonaddict patient had ever been reported to be habituated to meprobamate.[7]

Others also tried to stem the rising tide of concern about the addictiveness of meprobamate and other drugs. In February 1957, Harry Anslinger, federal narcotics commissioner, told a House appropriations subcommittee that the tranquilizers were nonaddictive: "We have seen nothing in this orbit, and I am thankful, because I think these drugs, in relation to the mental health problem in this country, are of terrific value."[8] That should have ended the discussion.

As for the phenothiazines, it eventually became clear that they were absolutely not addictive because they were so unpleasant to take. Heinz Lehmann told a Senate subcommittee in 1960, "One should pay the patients for taking them rather than the other way around. . . . Sometimes they pretend to take them, and throw them away, and they swear they did take them, but nobody believes them."[9]

Yet addictiveness proved irresistible for Congress, and the federal civil service displayed its watchfulness on many occasions. In June

1957, at hearings on the National Institutes of Health budget, the Senate appropriations subcommittee "showed more interest in tranquilizers than in any other subject discussed." Was meprobamate addictive or not? Robert Felix, director of the NIMH, in furrowed-brow testimony told the subcommittee that "I cannot at this time say with certainty that it is not."[10] (At the hearings Nate Kline came out enthusiastically in favor of the drug.)[11]

Again, in 1958 Felix explained to a House subcommittee investigating tranquilizers that if meprobamate were addictive, it was in the manner not of narcotics but of alcohol and barbiturates. Felix's evidence: reactions on sudden withdrawal from high doses, which, he conceded, were "encountered only rarely in general clinical practice."[12] (Just as an aside, we encounter here one of the first references to the concept of "withdrawal symptoms," aggravating the illness by suddenly discontinuing the agent. But sudden discontinuation of virtually any drug affecting the brain will produce withdrawal symptoms, so that people who drink large amounts of Coca-Cola for the caffeine will get a withdrawal headache if they discontinue the beverage. We do not, however, place Coca-Cola on the list of schedule II controlled substances.)

Next step: In 1960–61 Senator Estes Kefauver held hearings on "administered prices" in the pharmaceutical industry, from which emerged the Kefauver-Harris Act of 1962 giving the FDA authority to monitor efficacy in new drug applications. We've already encountered Kefauver's expression of horror during these hearings at the volume of meprobamate sales: The 500 tons produced in 1958 alone, he expostulated, were "enough to give every adult male in the United States 40 hours a week of medication of this drug."[13] Never one to shy back from political meddling in medical practice, he also dueled notably with Carter Products' medical director Frank Berger, who had developed meprobamate. Kefauver was determined to extract from Berger an admission of addictiveness. A feisty Berger responded that there was little evidence of this in the literature and that 72 percent of physicians in the United States prescribed meprobamate: They couldn't all be irresponsible.[14]

Two years later, in a Senate subcommittee meeting in 1963, Senator Hubert Humphrey from Minnesota, who had once been a pharmacist in South Dakota and fancied himself an expert on drugs, had another whack at meprobamate, among other drugs. He scorned its popularity, "prescribed almost as freely as aspirin. . . . It seems almost unbelievable now, but there was talk of even selling it over-the-counter. It was advertised as '*non*-habit forming.'" Scandalous, said Humphrey, that "the early warnings were 'drowned out,' physicians have told the subcommittee, in the bombardment of advertising and public relations, urging use of the drug for every conceivable mental condition."[15] Clearly, there was need for Congress to intervene, thought Humphrey.

Where was the FDA at this point in the story? Before 1963, FDA leadership was not much interested in the addictiveness of pharmaceuticals. Under medical director Albert Holland, the agency had a reputation of not wanting to make waves with industry.[16] Holland's early warnings about the possible "addictiveness" of the tranquilizers were timid to a fault. He raised the red flag in a talk to the Chemists Club of New York City in November 1956, but said nothing would be known for "two or three years." Why might the tranquilizers be dangerous? Holland said that "without adequate psychotherapy, [they] may mask growing psychoneurotic symptoms."[17] Psychoanalytically oriented psychiatrists of the era found this much more convincing: The real problem with the new drugs was that they reduced the need for psychotherapy.

In 1960 the agency opposed putting a "habituation" warning on the label of amphetamines, on the grounds that there was nothing to fear in normal doses and that physicians already knew about "the possibility of the danger of habituation from injudicious use of the drug."[18] As late as 1964, the agency told a Houston law firm that they found methamphetamine to be "a useful drug."[19]

Yet a ginger group of more junior officers did turn their guns on specific drugs. The reality is that the top management of the FDA does not necessarily have much control of the agency, and the second tier of officers is able to behave more or less autonomously.[20] The second tier was mushrooming in these years, the staff of the FDA's Bureau of Medicine, which had responsibility for drug approval, soaring from 39 in 1956 to 108 in 1961.[21] In 1957 this junior tier stepped up its ongoing pressure to make the bromides prescription-only.[22] In 1960 another junior staffer, Barbara Moulton, resigned in fury after the chief of the bureau's New Drug Branch overruled her suspension of the New Drug Application of Wyeth's antipsychotic Sparine (promazine).[23]

Indeed, this second tier of officers was suspicious of the pharmaceutical industry as a whole and often sought to unravel the sinister combines of the drug magnates. When George Leong joined the FDA's Office of Scientific Evaluation in the 1960s, he said, "I continually heard—and still hear—people within the agency saying that we are in an adversary arena and have to maintain an adversary role with the industry.

As a scientist, this was quite new to me."[24] Louis Lasagna, a senior figure in American pharmacology, later looked back on "the adversary, confrontation posture of the past, where all too often the FDA monitors looked on industry folk as evil geniuses trying to subvert and delude them. And for their part, the industry people looked on the FDA people as obstructionists."[25]

It was into this buzz saw that meprobamate now tumbled. The second tier of officers, intrigued by dog research at the PHS facility in Lexington (discussed later in this chapter), became suspicious of meprobamate on grounds of addictiveness.[26] A background patter of reports from the district offices identified patients who were bona fide addicted to meprobamate. There were not many, but they did exist, and usually seemed to involve large doses taken over long periods. Jack S. in Seattle, for example, was divorcing his wife in 1961 because she "has become addicted to Miltown." Justifying his action, he noted that she had spent time in the Washington State Mental Hospital in Sedro Woolley in 1953 (2 years before meprobamate was launched) and in a private clinic in 1957. A local physician had been giving her prescriptions, and she had been receiving additional supplies from her psychiatrist's former receptionist and from her obstetrician's former receptionist. Any information the FDA might be able to provide would be useful during the divorce trial, said Jack S.[27]

How to evaluate these few reports? In a drug taken by over 100 million patients worldwide, how many cases of imputed addiction is a lot?

There was another factor. The FDA harbored suspicions of meprobamate not just because it might, or might not, be addictive, but because of its use in dodging a breathalyzer test. People had been known to take meprobamate after drinking in an effort to lower their blood alcohol. The science behind this is obscure, but the effect is apparently real: Meprobamate is said to prevent people from blowing drunk in a breathalyzer test. An officer of the traffic division of the Oakland Police Department told an FDA inspector in September 1960, "In the past nine months, the Division had come across thirteen cases of individuals driving under the combined influence of alcohol and the tranquilizers. . . . In these cases the alcohol level of the blood was very low and would not support a drunk driving charge. Miltown was the brand involved in most cases."[28]

After such early reports, the FDA's interest in meprobamate quickened, in fact, became obsessional. Every New Drug Application requesting approval to use the agent for new medical indications had to be minutely scrutinized. Of 16 NDAs approved in July 1963, 13 were for meprobamate while other applications lay stalled in the queue. (Every new indication, combination, or dose of an already accepted drug requires an NDA, or something like it, such as an Abbreviated New Drug Application, or ANDA.) Edward Grundlach, a pharmaceutical consultant in Miami, wrote later that year to FDA assistant commissioner Winton Rankin about meprobamate, "This drug, which your department has been continually approving over the last six months, has been prescribed so many millions of times by American physicians, the name has become an accepted part of the English language, it has become almost as well known to the laity as aspirin, it has made countless millions of dollars in profits for its originators—and it is only a mild tranquilizer." How can this totally useless expenditure of taxpayer dollars be justified, asked Grundlach. Important new drugs still awaited approval, "while your department plays jokes with Miltown."[29]

It got curiouser. In 1963 Arthur Ruskin, director of the FDA's Division of New Drugs ("Division" having now replaced "Branch"), told Commissioner George P. Larrick that it was high time for a revision of the meprobamate label. Ruskin forwarded a list of 22 purported meprobamate side effects, among which were "fatal suicide attempts," "withdrawal reactions," and "addiction, habituation," as well as "proctitis," "bronchial spasm," and "hyperthermia."[30] It is interesting that Ruskin wanted to discuss this with the commissioner himself, given that sorting out side effects for possible changes in a medication's label is normally not done at this high a level.

In the meantime, the climate in Washington on the issue of drugs and drug abuse was heating up. A few months before, in September 1962, the White House Conference on Narcotic and Drug Abuse had been convened by President John F. Kennedy. One does not usually associate the Kennedy administration with conservative social policy measures. Yet in 1962, Pat Brown, the Democratic governor of California, was facing Republican Richard Nixon in a reelection campaign. Given rising concern about drug use on the West Coast, Brown needed a tough-sounding bone to throw to the electorate. According to author Rufus King, Kennedy's desire to come to Brown's aid led the president to set up the White House Conference, where Brown shared front bill on the program.[31] What emerged from it was the President's Advisory Commission on Narcotic and Drug Abuse, a panel of appointed "experts" charged with assessing the extent and nature of drug abuse nationwide.

The composition of the commission was loaded toward the conservative regulatory side and away from the liberal, legitimate-use side, including among its seven members a retired judge as chair, two figures with backgrounds in criminal justice (FBI and Bureau of Prisons), an urban welfare commissioner, two physicians with backgrounds in social welfare, and one physician who directed a drug-abuse clinic in a New York hospital. These appointees were by no means stellar figures in addiction medicine or psychopharmacology: One expert had never heard of virtually any of the members.[32] Their bent was overwhelmingly toward criminalization, federalization, and suppression. (Among their numerous recommendations was that the Department of Justice take over the regulation of "psychotoxic drugs.")

In their final report, issued the month that the president who commissioned it was assassinated in Dallas, the commissioners divided into two groups what were, in their terms, dependence-producing drugs: "addicting and nonaddicting drugs." The addictive variety, they said, produced physical dependence; the nonaddictive, psychological dependence.

Among the addicting variety were the opiates and the "barbiturate-alcohol type." It was here that the growing social-conservative impatience with the new psychoactive drugs found ample expression, for among the sinister barbiturate-alcohol type ("convulsions and delirium on withdrawal") were meprobamate and the new benzodiazepine Librium (chlordiazepoxide).

Interestingly, among the presumably less dangerous "nonaddictive drugs," producing mere psychological dependence, were marijuana, cocaine, and methamphetamine.[33] Thus, the prestigious President's Advisory Commission on Narcotic and Drug Abuse had deemed meprobamate even more dangerous than cocaine and methamphetamine.

Taking Down Meprobamate

Following the President's Advisory Commission, in late winter 1965 Oren Harris, chair of the House Committee on Interstate and Foreign Commerce, held hearings on the "depressant and stimulant drugs," terms that were drawn from a skewed understanding of the scientific literature on the effects of drugs upon cells in the central nervous system. Amedeo Marrazzi, at the neuropsychiatry research labs of the Veterans Administration Hospital in Pittsburgh, had pointed out in 1961, "the only thing that can happen is that they [cells] can either be stimulated or depressed." Yet drugs that inhibited cells did not always produce sedative results in humans. Marrazzi: "It is not correct to believe that inhibition of the nervous system always results in decreased activity. . . . Likewise, excitation of the nervous system does not always result in increased behavioral activity."[34] Ignoring such distinctions, the politicians found it more convenient to believe that CNS "depressants" and "stimulants" caused either addiction-level sedation or "kicks," to use the early 1960s code word for what was later called a "high," and a bill incorporating these beliefs was written.

Everybody on the House committee agreed that the barbiturates and amphetamines, the main drugs among the depressants and stimulants, should be controlled. The committee invited witnesses, calling first FDA Commissioner George Larrick who, reading from a text prepared for him, switched the discussion deftly from the amphetamines and barbiturates to "the tranquilizers." "Authorities in the field," he said, "have taken the position that many of the tranquilizers are very close to the barbiturates in their effects. . . . Tranquilizers, like barbiturates, can cause tolerance and psychic and physical dependence. The addicting properties of meprobamate have been rather extensively reported in the literature." Larrick concluded that "the so-called tranquilizers are subject to abuse," and even though the bill didn't mention them, they must be controlled.[35] It is interesting how the dice were loaded here against science and in favor of a prefixed FDA agenda not intended by Congress, which wanted to control barbiturates and amphetamines.

The bill that Larrick was referring to was later enacted as the Drug Abuse Control Amendments (DACA) of 1965, stipulating that the barbiturates and amphetamines were to be listed as drugs subject to special controls. The amendments also provided that other, unnamed psychopharmaceuticals might similarly be controlled, their possession subject to felony charges, their prescribing by physicians and dispensing by pharmacists regulated in a variety of ways. Congress did not specifically embrace the list of the President's Advisory Commission or adopt Larrick's and other witnesses' proposals about controlling the tranquilizers. Although urged to name individually some nonbarbiturate drugs such as meprobamate and Librium, the bill, HR 2, neglected to do so. Harris disliked the notion of "abuse potential." He said during the hearings, ". . . What causes me some difficulty about legislating on the basis of a potential hazard is how far you are going to go, where are you going to stop?" Coffee? Alcohol? he asked. "I suppose there have been abuses in the use of aspirin. I suppose there can be abuse in most anything."[36]

Congressman Walter Rogers of Texas also smelled trouble with Larrick's recommendation: "Well, Mr. Larrick, of course, the thing that disturbs me is there have been some very terrible mistakes made in delegation of power. Now, we have a Constitution, and this is supposed to be the lawmaking power. . . . Yet there is a continuous and a consistent demand by departments downtown for Congress to delegate its powers to those departments downtown. Now, those departments downtown are not primarily responsible to the electorate."[37]

But FDA bureaucrats rushed to assure Congress that "potential for abuse" would not become a general hunting license. It was a classic case of bait-and-switch. During the hearings, William Goodrich, FDA assistant general counsel and a driving force behind expanding agency authority, explained that "potentiality for abuse" meant only the most flagrant public menaces, such as LSD and methamphetamine inhalers against which, he insisted, the agency had been previously powerless.[38] Larrick went even further, assuring the House committee that only those drugs producing "escapes from reality" would be considered to have "potential for abuse."[39]

That was the bait. Next came the switch. On January 18, 1966, Larrick's successor James L. Goddard, the aggressive new FDA chief who had begun his tenure that month, determined that a number of other pharmaceuticals termed "depressant and stimulant drugs" be subject to Drug Amendment controls, one of which was meprobamate; among other drugs, Librium and Valium, the first of the benzodiazepines, were also to be listed.[40] None of these drugs could be construed as the flagrant public menaces identified the previous year—none produced "hallucinations" or could be compared to methamphetamine. In response, meprobamate's manufacturer Carter-Wallace, as Carter Products was now known, and the Librium and Valium producer, Hoffmann-La Roche, both appealed this decision to list these enormously popular and profitable drugs, and the FDA scheduled hearings on meprobamate to begin in June 1966.[41] The Librium-Valium hearings would begin in August.

The promise of such hearings had been one piece of the bait that the FDA had dangled before Congress in 1962 to get the Kefauver-Harris bill passed, legislation that greatly toughened the agency's authority. Critics said the bill would make drug approval dependent on the whims of a single individual. Not true, the FDA responded in September 1962: Firms could force hearings. "If [the manufacturer] is not then satisfied with the ruling, he can carry the case to the Federal courts."[42]

As hearings loomed in 1966, the FDA activated the Advisory Committee on Abuse of Depressant and Stimulant Drugs, struck a year previously, to help determine which additional drugs should be singled out.[43] It was headed by University of Michigan pharmacologist Frederick Shideman.[44] The committee decided at its first substantive meeting in April 1966 *not* to recommend that the "minor tranquilizers," among which would have been meprobamate, be placed "under the controls of the Drug Abuse Amendments."[45]

Yet the FDA had already taken the decision to go after meprobamate in January, and the committee's deliberations were really window dressing, mainly of interest as an insight into FDA thinking. The acting chief of the FDA's Bureau of Medicine, Paul Palmisano, appeared at the committee's meeting of June 13. What was drug abuse? Palmisano asked rhetorically. He said it was the use "of any drug affecting the central nervous system that deviates from the approved medical or social pattern within the country."[46] Thus, regardless of the endless later agonizing about animal models in abuse and addiction-maddened rats pushing foot pedals, the basic definition of abuse with which the FDA operated was exquisitely cultural and political: It would not include any of the accepted drugs such as alcohol, caffeine, or nicotine, but would include anything that Main Street didn't feel comfortable with. The switch was complete.

In the meantime, both sides had begun preparations for the hearings. Carter-Wallace was represented by Breed, Abbott & Morgan, a law firm at 1 Chase Manhattan Plaza. The firm's lead lawyer on the matter, William Hanaway, had already told the FDA back in January that the proposed agency implementation of the 1965 drug amendments went way beyond what Congress had intended. Hanaway said that in the report of the Committee on Interstate Commerce on "H. R. 2," the bill that became the DACA, Congress "was most explicit in stating that the Amendments were not aimed at drugs which were only occasionally, infrequently or sporadically abused." Carter-Wallace believed that meprobamate fell into that category, and their preparations for the June hearings were driven by an effort to gather expert testimony in support of that point of view.[47]

Yet from the very beginning, the FDA intended to bring down meprobamate. There was no question of organizing impartial hearings in a quasi-judicial process intended to get at the truth. As far as the FDA was concerned, at the end of the day meprobamate would receive the same status as the barbiturates and amphetamines, a drug identified as a danger to the public health and brought under the kind of control reserved for agents deemed addictive, habituating, and intended for use only under very tight restrictions.

The assault on meprobamate was to be part of a larger agency effort to assert itself against the pharmaceutical industry. To let Wyeth "know we mean business," we should seize oxazepam, an FDA official argued about another drug (Wyeth's Serax) around the time the meprobamate hearings were cranking up.[48] Pumped up by its new DACA authority, the agency was going on the offensive against oxazepam, a drug it had previously considered innocuous.[49]

Attacking hard was similarly to be the strategy against meprobamate. "We are acutely aware of the necessity for prevailing in the meprobamate hearing," Kenneth Lennington, at the FDA's Bureau of Regulatory Compliance, told the district offices. The districts were to find "instances in which meprobamate has been involved in complaints, buys not charged. . . . In short, we must have a record of instances in which meprobamate was tagged as having been connected with misuse or abuse."[50] The evidence against meprobamate, in other words, lay anything but ready at hand.

Similarly, the bushes had to be beaten to find suitable witnesses. In those days there were virtually no controlled trials that one could appeal to for guidance. So it boiled down to "clinical experience," distinguished figures of long experience telling about their personal impressions of drug safety and efficacy. Indeed, clinical experience, though not a replacement for doubly blinded controlled trials, is worth something. It was clinical experience that launched penicillin.

Therefore, in the month before the hearings began, the FDA began a frantic search for experts to serve as witnesses for the prosecution. It was the job of FDA officers such as Bennie Moxness at the Case Review Branch to locate experts who would declare meprobamate subject to abuse and a peril to the public health. Moxness phoned Robert Sharoff in the narcotic addiction service of Metropolitan Hospital in New York and asked for his views. Unfortunately, "Dr. Sharoff recollects only one case of Meprobamate habituation. . . . He does not feel that Meprobamate is a problem insofar as his Service in the Metropolitan Hospital is concerned. He has, therefore, no valid opinion on it."[51] The opinions of those who disagreed with the FDA line, in other words, were invalid.

Other potential witnesses as well felt there was really no problem with meprobamate. Moxness struck out with Don Rockwell at the Langley Porter Neuropsychiatric Institute in San Francisco: "No cases of Meprobamate habituation or addiction have been seen. . . . He believes the drug is infrequently used and poses no special problem."[52] Dr. Maurice Levine in Cincinnati didn't believe there was a problem either.[53] Edward Auer, chair of psychiatry at Saint Louis University, said he had "not had any recent experience with Meprobamate habituation or addiction. He had a case about five or ten years ago who experienced withdrawal symptoms. Dr. Auer believes it is little used at present and probably no further control is warranted."[54]

In the meantime, the FDA lawyers who were to argue the case were pursuing their own line of investigation into the drug. On May 23, John McElroy on the FDA legal staff came to the office of John Merandino of the FDA's Division of Medical Information, "to discuss the need for accumulating information demonstrating the need for placing Meprobamate on the list of 'potentially abusive drugs.'" What could be done? How about reviewing all of the New Drug Applications involving the compound (of which there were 24, given all the forms in which meprobamate had been marketed) and searching for a smoking gun? This would be a big job, Merandino told McElroy. McElroy said he would coordinate a full-court press, in which many FDA staffers from a number of divisions would go through NDAs and comb the literature in order to get something on the drug.[55]

How about suicide? Showing that meprobamate had been heavily involved in suicide would surely show well in court. The Drug Surveillance Branch requested the Adverse Reaction Branch to review all reports on addiction and overdose; to be sure, they were able to scare up 47 reports of attempted suicide with meprobamate. Unfortunately for the agency (fortunately for the public health), "We have no fatalities." Undeterred, they would review death certificates and try to find some indicating fatalities caused by meprobamate.[56] They found almost nothing.

The FDA also beat the bushes among the drug control offices of state mental health agencies, asking if meprobamate abuse had been reported. When the answer was no, the agency lost interest in the testimony. Alfred Murphy, senior food and drug inspector in the Drugs Control Section of the Massachusetts Department of Public Health, was not aware of any meprobamate abuse as a street drug and offered to fetch detailed police journal reports as back up. FDA counsel rejected his testimony on the grounds that the records were "of no value." FDA attorney Axel Kleiboemer, one of the lead lawyers at the hearing, faux-sympathized with Murphy that "it would be too burdensome to expect you to do all this."[57]

Finally, the FDA scratched together whatever witnesses it could and was ready to go to court. The hearings opened on June 14, 1966, in the heat of the Washington summer—high of 87°—with the dramatis personae present in their gray wool business suits. William Brennan, a lawyer from the Federal Trade Commission, served as hearing examiner, advised by pharmacologist Louis Lasagna, who was said often to whisper pharmacological explanations in Brennan's ear when they went off the record.[58] Three attorneys represented Carter-Wallace, and two in-house counsel from the FDA represented the government. Among those present in the courtroom were 13 representatives from Hoffmann-La Roche, which soon would be facing its own hearing over Librium and Valium.[59]

From the get-go it was clear that the FDA was going to suspend the normal rules of assessing benefit and harm in going after meprobamate. Customarily, when regulators evaluate a drug, there is some weighing of advantage and disadvantage: A drug such as penicillin has a few adverse effects, and some patients are allergic to it. Yet on the whole these are offset by its great benefits for the public health in terms of the treatment of infectious illness. This was not the way the FDA chose to go with meprobamate: If there were any absolute risk, any risk at all, the drug must be listed as dangerous. As FDA lawyer Walter Byerley argued at the beginning of the hearings, it didn't really matter if Congress had stipulated "significant" harm as a condition for listing. Harm was harm. "Let's always remember if you have one out of a million, this may be a low percentage, but for that one it is a hundred per cent, so I can't agree that the issue should be 'significant number of individuals were abusing the drug.'"[60]

The evidence presented at the hearing actually favored meprobamate overwhelmingly as a safe and useful drug in the treatment of anxiety and tension. Carter-Wallace had no difficulty compiling a list of distinguished physicians willing to speak up on behalf of the drug, and the parade of experts who argued against its potential for addiction, habituation, suicide, and street use reads like a who's who of American psychopharmacology. Melvin Sabshin, then head of psychiatry at the University of Illinois at Chicago and later medical director of the American Psychiatric Association, said that in the years he had been at the Michael Reese Hospital in Chicago he had never seen a case of meprobamate addiction. There was no abuse, no dependence, no "kick." There had been no attempted suicides, as opposed to 60 attempted suicides on barbiturates. In teaching psychiatry residents at the University of Illinois, "We state meprobamate is an unusually safe drug; it is useful for mild to moderate conditions of anxiety."[61]

Frank Ayd, a Baltimore psychiatrist who figured among the pioneers of psychopharmacology, pooh-poohed the government's whole concept of a "CNS depressant effect" creating a capacity for abuse. He had never seen a case of meprobamate addiction. Most patients had a great fear of addiction, he noted, and were inclined to take less of a drug rather than more. As for suicide, "to kill yourself with a minor or major tranquilizer is an extremely difficult thing."[62]

Herman ("Hy") Denber, in charge of psychiatric research at Manhattan State Hospital in New York, said that meprobamate addiction "must be so rare that it is an interesting finding. . . . I suppose if one is in the practice of medicine long enough . . . one will run into anything." Yet his staff at Manhattan State had never seen it. Denber noted that he had experimented on himself to see if the drug granted a "kick" (it didn't). Did patients increase the dosage with time (which would constitute evidence of habituation)? No. "On the contrary, our problem is to have the patients take the amount prescribed to them. If anything, they will reduce the amount." He had never heard of a patient who'd taken the drug to excess.[63]

Leo Alexander of Boston had first come to public attention as the psychiatric consultant at the Nuremberg trials of Nazi war criminals. By the mid-1960s he had a worldwide reputation as a psychopharmacologist and specialist in somatic treatments. He called meprobamate and chlorpromazine "the two great drugs" that had launched modern psychopharmacology. Outpatient treatment would be impossible without them, he said. "Our whole new look of psychiatry being a clinical science, extramural treatment, is based on the continuance of these drugs. . . . I think to discredit psychopharmacology would be the greatest blow clinical psychiatry could receive."[64]

These were the stakes: Discrediting psychopharmacology by calling a mainstay drug like meprobamate as dangerous as the amphetamines. Many of the 16 other drugs marked for listing under DACA were also anchors of the new psychopharmaceutical treatments that psychiatry—and medicine as a whole—was turning to. What did it matter if one were hypercautious and listed them all as potentially subject to "abuse"? The problem, said Edward Annis, a Miami surgeon and former president of the American Medical Association, is that patients would shy away from drugs considered addictive. He opposed listing meprobamate because "it places a question in the minds of my patients as to whether or not I am giving them a drug that is dangerous." He didn't want meprobamate classed among the "goofballs," a term for amphetamine: "I believe that it will suffer from guilt by association."[65]

Thus, turning patients off a useful drug was one hurtful consequence of listing. Inserting the government in the doctor-patient relationship was another. Said a family doctor from Geneva, Illinois, who was pleased to have an alternative to the barbiturates, "I find that this would impose an undesirable obstacle in the physician-patient relationship as it relates to my practice. These patients are very close to me. They rely on me implicitly to prescribe the necessary and safe drugs. It is a real position of trust, a real personal, very close relationship. This is a rather fragile relationship which can be very easily destroyed, and very easily broken by their finding out that I am prescribing what has been designated as a dangerous drug."[66] (In 1974, some members of the FDA's own Controlled Substances Advisory Committee seconded this logic, arguing that "the weak psychoactive drugs should not be controlled since such controls would discourage physicians prescribing and could lead to the use of more potent and abusable substances. In addition, criminal sanctions would be imposed if these substances were controlled.")[67]

Against quite a lot of testimony that meprobamate was safe and effective, with no more abuse potential than aspirin, the FDA mounted rather a weak case. In fact, as the hearings wore on, the agency actually sent inspectors out to the offices of at least one physician, H. Robert Greenhouse, director of the alcoholism division of the State Department of Mental Health in New Haven, Connecticut, to search his patient records for evidence that might show up contradictions in testimony he gave in August in support of the drug. The FDA had previously sounded Greenhouse out as a government witness, and when Greenhouse appeared on the stand for Carter-Wallace, FDA lawyers confronted him with what he had told the FDA inspector at the time.[68]

The agency could find only a few witnesses whose clinical experience was vast enough to make them credible or whose scientific authority was acknowledged in the field. Carl Essig, at the NIMH's Addiction Research Center in Lexington, Kentucky, had not originally wanted to testify. He told the FDA that meprobamate addiction was not his field, that he had seen only one case in humans, and that the doses used on dogs, in research that formed the basis of his professional expertise, were much higher—20 times higher it later came out—than in humans. Nonetheless, the FDA was able to prevail upon Essig to testify;[69] Essig showed a home movie of dogs having convulsions after being suddenly withdrawn from the drug. This was intended to represent evidence of addictiveness. Reports of the dog film made it into the *New York Times*.[70] In his testimony, Essig concluded that meprobamate was a drug "with a potential for abuse."[71]

The Lexington addiction people considered many drugs capable of abuse. Essig mentioned a host of others he thought addictive, similar to the barbiturates, in particular glutethimide (Doriden), ethchlorvynol (Placidyl), ethinamate (Valmid), chlordiazepoxide (Librium), and diazepam (Valium).[72] All seem to have been effective hypnotics and anxiolytics in the 1950s and early '60s. All save Librium and Valium have since been forgotten, discarded as drugs of "potential abuse" in roughly the same manner as meprobamate.

The agency had two other high cards to play in the hearings. One was John Ewing, head of psychiatry at the University of North Carolina Medical School at Chapel Hill. Virtually alone among academic experts, Ewing considered meprobamate to be a bad drug; he had verified, he said, the existence of a clinical withdrawal syndrome.[73] The coauthor of the paper describing this syndrome, Jefferson Davis Bulla, who was a student at the time, was uneasy about the conclusions that Ewing had drawn from it.[74] Ewing further loses some of his credibility as an expert on addiction in failing to recognize "Desoxyn" as methamphetamine, then commercially available as an antidepressant. He thought it was a "hormone."[75]

The highest FDA card was Jerome Jaffe, psychiatrist and pharmacologist and genuine expert on addiction at Albert Einstein College of Medicine in New York. When sounded out in May 1966, he told the FDA that "he has personally seen one private patient with meprobamate addiction. . . . Dr. Jaffe feels quite strongly that meprobamate is an addicting drug (less so about Librium and Valium); he would be glad to appear as a witness."[76] Jaffe appeared twice at the hearings, the first time in July when he was vague and tentative about meprobamate as similar to the barbiturates.[77] The second time was in September, toward the end of the almost endless hearings, and it was a transformed Jaffe who took the stand, delivering a classroom lecture about addictiveness and its evils.[78] The Carter-Wallace counsel, which up to this point had been vigorous in its objections to various FDA witnesses, sat in silence through this peroration. By contrast, the hearing examiner, William Brennan, gazed in admiration and encouraged Jaffe to go on and on.

Although Brennan strove to preserve the appearance of objectivity, he does seem to have been systematically biased in favor of the government's case. At one point Brennan, exasperated at Carter-Wallace counsel's objections to the admissibility of government evidence, blurted, "Mr. Lang, I'm through arguing rulings," basically an instruction to Lang to sit down and shut up.[79] At another point Brennan actually urged the government counsel to offer an objection to some question of Lang's, a kind of intervention from which judges normally abstain in trials.[80]

Mid-hearings, the Carter-Wallace counsel became aware that things were going badly and said quite matter-of-factly that they intended to bring the case to the Court of Appeals.[81] The deck had been stacked against meprobamate from the very beginning.

The final report of the hearings reads as though it had been written by the FDA's own lawyers. Although the transcript of the hearings has been preserved, Brennan's concluding remarks have vanished. Yet customarily the hearing examiner writes the report, and it is almost certain that Brennan wrote the FDA's resume of the case against meprobamate published in the *Federal Register* in April 1967, in the name of FDA Commissioner James Goddard. The final report basically ignored all the evidence that Carter-Wallace had presented, and inflated the government's highly speculative offerings to the status of certainties.

Meprobamate does have a depressant effect, said the report, and large doses can cause a depression of mood.[82] (Leo Alexander had argued that Deprol, a Wallace combo of meprobamate and benactyzine, acted as an antidepressant.)[83] Meprobamate's withdrawal effects were similar to those of the barbiturates and alcohol, said the report. Could it be abused? Yes. There were three abuse criteria, said the report—overdose, diversion to street use, and self-medication rather than medication under medical supervision—and meprobamate fulfilled all three.

Evidence of harm from overdose? In contrast to countless Carter-Wallace witnesses who had said they'd never seen such a thing, the government's evidence of harm came mainly from anecdotes.[84] One bears in mind that a drug taken by a hundred million patients will produce a variety of unusual effects in occasional individuals. But the report argued that such harm was really quite close to the norm, in the form of people operating motor vehicles under the influence, staggering gaits, slurred speech, and personality changes that led to crime, child abuse, and failed marriages. There had been bits of testimony at the hearings on all these subjects, yet the witnesses' clear consensus was that they were marginal, isolated phenomena. In the report they became inevitable consequences of meprobamate use.

The report dwelt upon meprobamate as a common agent of suicide, which was an almost hallucinatory falsification of the evidence before the hearings. One government expert, Frederic Riederer, a toxicologist who worked for the medical examiner in Philadelphia, had argued that meprobamate was mentioned in drug screens conducted in a number of suicides. Yet on closer inspection it turned out that many of these victims had on board massive amounts of barbiturates, the obvious lethal agent, and that meprobamate turned up positive simply because the victims, under the influence of a psychiatric illness, had been taking it.[85] Many experts dismissed meprobamate as a suicide drug, which did not stop the final report from elevating suicide into an urgent indication for action.

Much was made of the diversion of meprobamate from legitimate medical prescription into illicit use, on the model of the barbiturates and amphetamines. The problem here, from the government's viewpoint, was that there was simply no evidence of the street use of meprobamate; there was no black market in it; the drug was not traded illicitly at bus stops or at student parties. Yet not everyone who took it had a medical prescription; some obtained it from friends; and drug audits at numerous pharmacies seemed unable to account for reductions in the pharmacy's meprobamate stock in terms of prescriptions. The obvious solution said the report was diversion. (This conclusion overlooked sloppy record keeping and pharmacists' indifference to prescriptions in dispensing drugs, both common features of pharmacy practice in the 1950s.[86] Only in June 1957 did the FDA even begin to enforce for "tranquilizers" the prescription requirements of the Durham-Humphrey Act of 1951.[87]) Thus, the abuse case turned on whether you as a patient had a medical prescription for your drug: If not, your use was "abusive."

The FDA case on addictiveness was so thin that the issue should be consigned to the status of an urban myth. Often grasping at straws, the FDA lawyers asked witnesses, how do you know your patients are not going from doctor to doctor, obtaining multiple prescriptions for meprobamate? (This did happen with genuinely addictive drugs.) Many witnesses, knowing their patients well, found this kind of prescription-mongering so unlikely that they were stunned at such a question. In the report, this obscure possibility became raised to a central mechanism of diversion into abusive use.

The report concluded that, even though Congress had not mentioned meprobamate by name, controlling meprobamate certainly accorded with Congress's wishes. The prescribing and dispensing of the drug must immediately be curtailed, and the FDA would shortly recommend to the drug enforcement authorities mechanisms for doing so. It was in May 1966 that the FDA had postponed an initial listing of meprobamate subsequent to hearings. Now, in April 1967, the agency had decided to terminate that suspension ("stay") and to proceed with the original plan of listing the drug. Some time would pass before that actual listing took place but those are details. The essential feature of the ruling was that meprobamate was toast.

The FDA's meprobamate hearings exemplified what can happen when a government agency decides to play hardball and spin the evidence on behalf of a theory that suits its own interests. "They were obviously stacked against Carter-Wallace," said Frank Berger later of the hearings. "The argument with the Food and Drug was primary—that there is no difference between tranquilizers and [barbiturate] sleeping pills. They are all the same."[88]

Why would the FDA have wished to take on meprobamate? It seems likely that, following the new powers they got from DACA in 1965, they wanted a test case to establish their authority over the pharmaceutical industry. Indeed, it may have been the hard-driving new commissioner James Goddard himself behind this effort.[89] Goddard had begun his tenure with a series of "hard-hitting, mean-spirited speeches [against industry]," said William W. Goodrich later, who was at the time the general counsel. "I mean, he in effect called them crooks."[90] Before the FDA took on meprobamate, the agency had never had a real head-to-head fight with a big company.[91] Winning this one established a precedent: The FDA was now a regulatory force to be reckoned with. These years saw a stunning rise in the power of the FDA over the pharmaceutical industry, and the destruction of Carter-Wallace's blockbuster drug was an initial severed head to fling upon the banquet table. Others followed.

The Unhappy Later History of Meprobamate

Carter-Wallace appealed the decision of the Commissioner to the federal Court of Appeals for the Fourth Circuit. In 1969, in *Carter-Wallace v. John W. Gardner, Secretary of HEW,* the Court upheld the decision of the FDA on the grounds that meprobamate had a "depressant effect on the central nervous system" and that this effect gave it a "potential for abuse." Although this proposition was pharmacological hocus-pocus, the Court agreed po-faced with the FDA lawyers that tolerance and withdrawal reactions were major issues. Psychopharmacologists in black robes, the court thought the drug's most likely site of action was "the sub-cortical region."[92] In June 1970, the U.S. Supreme Court refused to review the decision and meprobamate entered the list of dangerous drugs subject to abuse.[93]

The reality was that by this time meprobamate was swamped in the U.S. marketplace by Valium. Both brands of meprobamate—Equanil and Miltown—had gained sales volume from 1956 through 1960, despite competition from 45 other "tranquilizers." Yet from 1960 to 1961 Equanil and Miltown both suffered big drops in sales, "apparently reflect[ing] the entry of Roche's Librium into the tranquilizer competition as a smash success," as the *Pink Sheet* put it.[94] Sales dropped even further following Valium's introduction in 1963. In 1971 Carter-Wallace stopped advertising meprobamate in part because the benzodiazepines had clearly carried the day. It is still unclear whether meprobamate was clinically superior to Librium or Valium, although there are experienced clinicians who believe that it was. Its tight control as a "dangerous drug" meant no one would try to confirm it one way or the other.

The meprobamate story put the FDA in the light of a rising power-hungry empire rather than a saintly guardian of the public trust. But the agency employed large numbers of scientists for whom power was not necessarily the first desideratum. Thus, recriminations within the agency about the crucifying of an important drug began to surface in internal discussions.

In 1969, early in an FDA initiative called the Drug Efficacy Study Implementation (about which much more will be said in Chapter 6), Dorothy Dobbs, by now director of the Division of Neuropharmacologic Drugs, proposed implementing the recommendation of an expert committee that meprobamate was "effective for the relief of anxiety and tension."[95] Already, this was a big volte-face from the FDA's position in the 1966 hearings. Dobbs then rubbed salt into the wounds of the antimeprobamate group by saying there was no need to consider meprobamate a "new drug,"[96] a designation that by this time was being applied retroactively to various pre-1962 medications and meant redoing the entire battery of clinical trials in order gain renewed FDA approval of them. Dobb's recommendation was too much for Goodrich, one of the leaders of the antimeprobamate fight. Have you forgotten the hearings? he asked in a memo. ". . . It would be a serious error to list meprobamate as generally recognized as safe and effective and no longer a new drug. . . . The testimony adduced at the hearing on meprobamate established that its mechanism of action was unknown even to the best experts in the field." There had been concerns about dangers. "The apparent inconsistency would not be readily explainable."[97] The decision to spare meprobamate the new drug route was abandoned, although the drug remained on the market, if with significant warnings about its use.

Internal sniping continued. Early in 1974, Barrett Scoville, deputy director of the FDA's Division of Neuropharmacological Drug Products, observed somewhat triumphantly to the deputy director of the Bureau of Drugs that brief usage of meprobamate was not addicting: "10 weeks of therapy do not appear adequate to produce tolerance and withdrawal symptoms." He then cited studies published by researcher Ronald Lipman and coworkers that "thus strongly suggested that three to four weeks of therapy at approved dosage levels do not produce tolerance." Scoville had discussed this personally with Lipman, who agreed.[98]

Yet the effect of the hearing's condemnation of meprobamate lingered long. In 2002, a group of senators led by Ted Kennedy protested a proposed limiting of the agency's control of pharmaceutical advertising. The senators cited the FDA's watchdog role in protecting the public from "ineffective drugs," and mentioned Deprol, the Carter-Wallace combo of meprobamate and benactyzine, "a tranquilizer promoted for use in depressed patients for whom it had been shown to be ineffective, with serious side effects, including addiction, and risk of suicide."[99] None of these statements was true, but they had entered the received wisdom, becoming part of the pharmacologic folklore of congressional committees.

The entire meprobamate episode was a travesty of science and a triumph of regulatory hubris. In retrospect, meprobamate was probably one of the best drugs in the history of psychiatry. Thomas Ban, founder of the psychopharmacology program at McGill University, later said of meprobamate, "It's a very good drug, easily comparable to the benzodiazepines. I used it well into the '80s. In outpatient psychiatry, it's the best thing that ever happened. It's a very, very important drug."[100]

5
Killer Drugs!

Taking down meprobamate was a real triumph for the Feds, the first time the formerly inert cop agency had stood up against a substantial company. Yet Carter-Wallace was not one of the majors. Hoffmann-La Roche was. In 1960, the American affiliate of this Swiss drug company, its headquarters in Nutley, New Jersey, launched the first of the benzodiazepine series, Librium (chlordiazepoxide). Valium (diazepam) followed 3 years later. These drugs have customarily never been considered part of the first drug set. For one thing, the benzodiazepine period didn't peak until well past the heyday of the first drug set. For another, the "benzos" were not "tranquilizers"; rather, as antianxiety drugs, a different clinical effect was claimed for them. But these terms are really just conventions: Carter-Wallace claimed tybamate (Solacen), meprobamate's sister drug, to be an "antineurotic,"[1] and there is no reason why the benzos should not also have been declared "antineurotics" (but for reasons of commercial competition never were). Whatever their designation, in terms of real-world effectiveness, the benzos have probably been the best drug class in history, for they have few side effects and deliver a significant therapeutic punch in a wide range of illnesses. It was therefore a decision of awesome import that in the 1960s, the Food and Drug Administration decided they must be destroyed.

The Launch of Librium and Valium

The story begins in the late 1950s when Librium was in trials. Girding itself for the imminent FDA ban on its drug iproniazid (Marsilid) because of liver toxicity, Hoffmann-La Roche was keen to find another psychoactive bestseller. Librium was clearly useful for a number of different conditions.

"When did you first use Librium?" a lawyer later asked Dr. Angelo D'Agostino, who in 1959 had been a psychiatric resident in Washington, D.C. "In my capacity as a resident in psychiatry at the D.C. General, which is a municipal hospital," D'Agostino responded. "I would have to treat the acute alcoholics who were brought in by the police, often in rather severe degrees of delirium tremens."

The staff administered Librium intravenously. "It was remarkable in its ability to clear up the hallucinosis. The patients within a matter of minutes would actually be quite clear of the hallucinations that these delirium tremens cases are so classically subject to."

D'Agostino remembered one patient who was brought in. "He was complaining of spiders that were crawling all over him, all over the room, table, chairs, all over the walls and the ceiling.

"I administered 100 milligrams, and we had to see some other patients; we returned in about 15 minutes, and I fully expected that he would be pretty well relieved of his symptoms. He seemed much calmer, but when I asked him about the spiders, he looked around and said, 'Yes, they are pretty much gone. There are still a couple on the ceiling.'"

D'Agostino and the medical student with him went away and returned in another 10 minutes. "I asked him again so I could show the student how it works. And he again looked pretty calm, and was less agitated than he had been.

". . . He looked around again and said, 'Well, they are pretty much gone. I don't feel any anymore, but there are still a couple on the ceiling,' whereupon I looked up, and sure enough there were a couple on the ceiling."[2]

Librium was considered at the time a kind of wonder drug. Muscle spasms, gastrointestinal upset, alcoholic hallucinosis, psychic and somatic anxiety: At a time when many psychiatrists outside institutions were still ensnared in psychoanalysis, Librium was prescribed mainly by family doctors and internists. "Librium has virtually replaced liniment," said one observer of general practice in Manchester, England, in 1972.[3]

Librium, and later Valium, were received with hosannahs. They were thought superior to the antipsychotics (then mainly the phenothiazines) for the treatment of anxiety because they did not produce unwanted movement side effects, such as extrapyramidal syndromes and tardive dyskinesia. And they were deemed superior to the barbiturates because it was much harder (though not impossible) to commit suicide with them. "For the general practitioner the benzodiazepines are almost too good to be true," said Andy Rose, a family doctor in London, in 1983. "They are very safe in overdosage. . . . Long-term administration has never been encouraged, but it seems to produce few serious problems when it occurs."[4]

When Librium first came into use, nobody really knew what it was most useful for. The indications had to be slowly established through trial and error. Before the 1962 Kefauver-Harris Act, the FDA did not require approval of efficacy, and companies didn't have to chisel out the responsive disorders before submitting a New Drug Application. In early trials in South Dakota, Librium seemed effective for "the frustrated farmer's frau syndrome," meaning older South Dakota farmwives of German origin who were worried about menopause. Other physicians thought Librium had about the same range of indications as gin.[5] When in January 1959 researchers Joseph Tobin and Nolan D. C. Lewis began a large Librium trial in New Jersey with 212 outpatients who had a mixture of disorders from schizophrenia on down, they found that it was effective in anxiety: 88 percent of the patients "who experienced free-floating anxiety . . . derived some degree of relief." But Librium also showed efficacy in "phobic reactions," obsessive thinking, and "tension."[6] Such a trial left hanging the big question, What do we actually put on the label? Hoffmann-La Roche ended up flogging it for "anxiety and tension," mainly because these conditions seemed the common denominator of this clinical breadbasket.

Librium was first tried in the United Kingdom by Alec Jenner, then a staff doctor in the outpatients' clinic of the United Sheffield Hospitals and the University of Sheffield. He later said, "The psychiatric outpatients in those days at Sheffield involved absolutely crowds of disturbed people to whom little individual time could possibly have been given by a junior doctor. Here then [with Librium] was a chance to do something for them. . . ." The doctors gave the patients bottles labeled a, b, or c, containing either benzodiazepine, barbiturate, or a placebo. The patients "simply had to say which they found most helpful," usually picking the benzo. In later trials at Sheffield, the benzos gave consistently positive results, particularly in anxiety states. "So we felt delighted that we had found drugs which you could take in very large doses, and we took enormous doses ourselves to see whether they were toxic. They didn't do that much harm. It seemed a wonderful replacement for the barbiturates which were what people were given before."[7]

Moreover, the benzos were not "tranquilizers," Hoffmann-La Roche emphasized. By the early 1960s "tranquilizer" had come to be dissected into major and minor, with the major tranquilizers referring to a drug for "disturbed psychotics . . . and to be regarded in the patient's milieu as a stigma," as Ralph Gerard, from 1955 at the Mental Health Research Institute of the University of Michigan, put it.[8] So Hoffmann-La Roche was careful to distance their new drug from any sort of "tranquilizer" association and from the "equanimity-producing drugs" (meaning meprobamate). Instead, they billed Librium as "in a class by itself, chemically, pharmacologically, and therapeutically."[9] The class later became known as the benzodiazepines.

The uptake of Librium was dramatic. Introduced in March 1960, by October it had already become the "big boom product" of the year.[10] By 1966 in the United States more than 15 million patients had taken it, swallowing more than 6 billion capsules of the drug.[11] It had also become the second-most-prescribed drug for the elderly, following Orinase (an antidiabetic).[12] As Mrs. Mae M. in Johannesburg, Michigan, told the FDA in 1973 about her case of shingles, " . . . The itching about drives you crazy and I guess it's all nerves. I guess it's my punishment for thinking there must be something wrong with nervous people when I was younger." She took Librium for her itching. "I sure wish someone would find a cheap cure for shingles, because the older you are the longer they last." She took two Librium capsules per day for her complaint, never more than that, she said.[13] Elderly people in particular were fond of the absence of significant side effects other than drowsiness. When benzodiazepines in nursing homes later became drastically restricted, psychiatrist Carl Salzman at Harvard found the results "disastrous." It "will make prescribing much more difficult," he said.[14]

In the marketplace, Librium immediately leaped past meprobamate. By 1964 its annual number of prescriptions was almost twice that of the two main meprobamate marketers' (Wyeth's Equanil and Carter Products' Miltown) combined.[15] In 1971 the American Medical Association's Council on Drugs held Librium superior in efficacy to meprobamate,[16] which was really the seal of death for the latter drug. In the United States meprobamate faded to the margin of history.[17]

Yet Librium's career as a blockbuster was relatively short-lived. In 1963, Hoffmann-La Roche launched Valium (diazepam), one of the best-selling drugs in history and emblematic of an era in which nerves were treated with benzos and the primary diagnosis was anxiety rather than depression. By 1970, Valium had begun to diminish the Librium market, causing the first decline in Librium sales. In 1972 over 50 million prescriptions a year were being written for Valium, up from 4 million in 1964.[18] Two years later, the *New York Times* announced in a front-page story that Valium "has become the No. 1 prescribed drug in the United States and perhaps in the world." Last year, the story said, 1 in 10 Americans had taken it.[19] After the Valium patent expired in 1985, it appeared in generic form all over the world under 88 different trade names: Aliseum in Italy, Apollonset in Greece, Betapam in Russia, and so on.[20]

Not wishing to cannibalize the Librium franchise, initially Hoffmann-La Roche indicated Valium for "psychic tension," as well as a "muscle relaxant" (where diazepam indeed performs useful service). Later, the company aimed it at the "easy-weepers" in the depression market.[21] Hoffmann-La Roche also aspired to the huge "stress" market until the FDA said that stress was "not a disease."[22] The indications used in the early controlled trials were all over the map, yet in each of the five trials conducted by 1969, Valium beat the barbiturates: for "functional gastrointestinal disorders," for "anxious outpatients no depression," for "neurotic, psychotic and personality disordered outpatients," and for "anxious neurotic outpatients."[23] Valium had few side effects, was on the whole nonaddictive, and enjoyed staggering popularity.

In 1971, Librium and Valium accounted for $200 million of Hoffmann-La Roche's $280 million sales in the United States. A piece in *Fortune* called Librium and Valium "the greatest commercial successes in the history of prescription drugs."[24]

Hoffmann-La Roche started to get competition in the benzo market. In 1965 Wyeth brought out Serax (oxazepam), "relieving symptoms without producing disruptive psychomotor incoordination" (a snipe at Librium and Valium's tendency to cause mild ataxia in high doses).[25] Hoffmann-La Roche countered in 1970 with Dalmane (flurazepam), billed as a hypnotic rather than an anxiolytic. (The convention developed that some benzos were merely sedative, or "anxiolytic," a term that industry preferred to sedative, which was associated with the barbiturates. Other benzos with a different chemical structure had a more powerful sedative action and were deemed "hypnotic.")[26] Abbott's Tranxene (clorazepate), Hoffmann-La Roche's Klonopin (clonazepam), Wyeth's Ativan (lorazepam), and Upjohn's Halcion (triazolam) all arrived in the United States during the 1970s or early 1980s. In 1977 some 8,000 tons of benzos were consumed in the United States.[27] Upjohn launched its Xanax (alprazolam) in 1981, a drug that had become by 1988 the worldwide number one best seller in psychopharmacology.[28]

Many of these compounds were huge international hits. Lorazepam alone appeared worldwide under 66 different names.[29]

By the early 1990s there were more than one hundred different benzos on world markets.[30] In 2001 around 163,000 kilograms (179 U.S. tons) of diazepam were being produced around the globe, with large amounts of the other classic benzos as well.[31] The benzos were the most successful drug class in history, before the arrival of the SSRIs.

The Benzos as Antidepressants

It is 1966. Paul Feldman, director of research at the Topeka State Hospital, is testifying at the FDA's Librium-Valium hearings.

> *Q: What do you prescribe Librium for?*
>
> *Feldman: We found Librium to be most effective for . . . patients who are hyperactive, tense, anxious.*
>
> *Q: What do you prescribe Valium for?*
>
> *Feldman: [It's] most importantly effective on a number of targets for which Librium had little or no effect.*
>
> *I am thinking of the targets which we usually associate with a degree of depression . . . We found Valium quite useful in the treatment of patients showing disinterest [sic] in their environment, difficulty in being reached, a certain degree of hypoactivity and, of course, tension and anxiety. But primarily it was the sort of symptoms which we frequently associate with mild depression—disinterest in environment, failure to participate in adjunctive therapy. . . .[32]*

It was mainly the family physicians who prescribed the benzos, and it was almost an article of faith among them that Librium, Valium, and related drugs were effective for depression. Indeed, although Hoffmann-La Roche's first ad hyped Librium for "the treatment of common anxieties and tension,"[33] the commonest form of anxiety is mixed anxiety-depression;[34] drugs that treat "anxiety" without touching mood don't exist, and all anxiolytics are simultaneously antidepressants, at least for nonmelancholic depression. "A number of years ago we looked at the prescribing habits of general practitioners," said Manchester psychiatrist Donald W. Johnson at a benzo symposium in England in 1983.

"We found that they used antidepressants and benzodiazepines almost interchangeably." In fact, the longer these patients were depressed, the more likely they were to receive a benzo. Why? It was a matter of compliance. The patients rebelled at the side effects of the tricyclic antidepressants then available and preferred the more comfortable benzos.[35]

In a large international study combining data from 15 centers from Athens to Nagasaki, sponsored by the World Health Organization in 1991–92, it was found that in "current depression" family physicians prescribed "sedatives" (the great majority of which would have been benzos) in 27.6 percent of their patients, antidepressants in 22.2 percent. (Their prescribing for anxiety was remarkably similar: 31.1 percent sedatives, 21.4 percent antidepressants, suggesting that on a worldwide basis, family physicians really saw little difference between depression and anxiety.)[36]

As for psychiatrists themselves, many were still attached to psychodynamic psychotherapy and shunned prescribing benzos. Yet from the very beginning, a core of psychiatrists did use benzos in depression. H. Angus Bowes spoke in 1959 of his premarketing experience with Librium at the Mental Health Center he had just founded in Aberdeen, South Dakota: In "mixed neurotic pictures," Librium's "antidepressant and euphoriant action made unnecessary in many cases the addition of other drugs aimed at the target symptom of depression." As for "occult depression . . . mimick[ing] anything from anxiety to dementia," Bowes gave Librium together with an MAOI and a tricyclic antidepressant: " . . . A dramatic improvement could be seen within hours [as opposed to weeks, which is more normal with these other drug classes]."[37]

The best evidence for the effectiveness of the benzos in mood disorders comes not in undifferentiated "depression," but in nonmelancholia (as opposed to melancholia). This evidence is found in two forms, informed clinical opinion and statistics.

Bernard Carroll, then at the University of Michigan, was well instructed about the treatment of depressive illnesses. He was a member of the FDA's Psychopharmacologic Drugs Advisory Committee in December 1981 as the tricyclic antidepressant dothiepin came up for approval. What clinical population could be mentioned in the label? You can't just "give it an approval as an antidepressant without some further specification," Carroll said. Maybe in outpatients dothiepin could be compared "against not only placebo, but just a regular anxiolytic drug like a benzodiazepine, and we don't know what a drug like diazepam would have done with this population, but I would not be astonished if there would have been significant clinical improvement with diazepam as there was with amitriptyline."[38] (The drug's sponsor had used the TCA amitriptyline as an active control in some outpatient trials.) This is an example of thoughtful opinion, not the same as numbers to be sure, but of some value.

Then there are trials. When Tobin and Lewis described in 1960 the effectiveness of Librium in their New Jersey trial, they noticed the usefulness of Librium in nonmelancholic depression. "The improvement of depression was most consistent when this symptom occurred in conjunction with directly perceived anxiety. . . . The improvement of depression was less pronounced in the presence of severe retardation."[39] Retardation is a hallmark of melancholic depression.

Other scholars drew the results of various trials together and summed them up in "meta-analyses." Several such analyses found differential efficacy of the benzodiazepines in nonmelancholia. In a review of the literature in 1978, psychiatrists Alan Schatzberg and Jonathan Cole at McLean Hospital in Belmont, Massachusetts, concluded that, even though the benzos are not "antidepressants," they are useful in reactive depression and anxiety-depression: " . . . They are not effective in combating symptoms of endogenous depressions. . . . On the other hand, benzodiazepines appear to combat some of the symptoms of nonendogenous depressive illnesses and many of those found in anxiety disorders, including depressed mood."[40] In another kick at this particular can 17 years later, in 1995, three Dutch scholars, in a literature review, concluded that the classical benzos had some efficacy in "minor depression," though were inferior to the tricyclics in "melancholic depression." A newer class of benzos, however, the main representative of which was alprazolam (Xanax), appeared a bit more promising in nonmelancholia.[41] Several kinds of evidence, therefore, suggest an antidepressant role for the benzos in nonmelancholic depression.

One final comment about the benzos as antidepressants: These drugs get really good results when combined with tricyclic antidepressants. This has been known since the early days of psychopharmacology. At a symposium in Los Angeles in 1961, one psychiatrist in the audience volunteered that he found the effectiveness of Librium "tremendously enhanced by the addition of Tofranil [imipramine]." He had thirty patients, some with frank melancholia. "Librium worked well when I added Tofranil, but it did not do it alone. . . . Librium with Tofranil, in my experience, has produced 100 per cent benefit. I don't know why. I have tried countless other drugs, and none of them worked.

As I said, I had about thirty people who are entirely well and useful."[42]
The reader reflects that perhaps Tofranil alone would also have done
the trick. But Tofranil unaided certainly does not produce 100 percent
results in a series of 30 patients. The remark is intriguing.

Forty years later came more solid evidence about adding benzos to
tricyclics. In a meta-analysis in 2002 of nine studies of depression in
which benzos had been added to an antidepressant (8 of the 9 antidepressants were TCAs), investigators found that the combo was better
tolerated by the patients and had a better outcome than the TCA alone.
The authors concluded, "Unless you as a physician are among the few
who never ever prescribe a benzodiazepine, there are good reasons to
consider adding a benzodiazepine . . . to the antidepressant you prescribe
to the next patient you see with major depression. . . ."[43]

In 2007, Thomas Ban, emeritus professor of psychopharmacology
at Vanderbilt University, said on the basis of decades of experience,
"Those benzos which are promoted for 'neurotic depression,' such as
diazepam, a long acting one, and alprazolam [Xanax] a short acting one,
were just as good as the barbiturates, and much better than the amphetamines. But for one or another reason the clinical reality remains in a
miraculous way hidden."[44]

When we start agonizing today about the lack of new antidepressants, let us recall that in the history of psychopharmacology
there were some perfectly serviceable old ones. And the benzos were
probably the most effective and safest class of antidepressant in the
history of psychopharmacology. The loss of the classic benzos, therefore, has been a disaster for public health, for today in the United States
and the United Kingdom these agents are almost never prescribed for
mood disorders; solely, the short-acting benzos are offered as hypnotics
(though they may well treat the underlying anxiety-depression causing
the insomnia).

What brought about the decline of the benzos?

Control

In the years after 1965, when the Drug Abuse Control Act (DACA) was
passed, the FDA mounted a sustained campaign against the benzodiazepines. It was a campaign that would reverberate for decades in dim
apprehensions that the benzos were somehow terribly addictive. At
high doses these drugs do encourage a certain level of dependency, as

do almost all the other drugs used in psychiatry. But following the maxim that anything worth doing is worth overdoing, medicine permitted these drugs to become demonized, rather than balancing justifiable but moderate concerns about dependence against the benzos' great therapeutic benefits.

In DACA in 1965, Congress had followed the barbiturate-amphetamine model: Get rid of drugs that people could use to kill themselves with, that leaked into the streets, and that caused addicts to break into widows' apartments seeking money for a "kick." As we saw in the previous chapter, Congress determined that this model was inappropriate for drugs such as meprobamate, or Librium and Valium, to which patients became attached but which were not really sought on the street or subject to diversion from legal channels. To no avail. The FDA pressed to get them listed under DACA anyway.

On January 18, 1966, Winton Rankin, FDA acting commissioner, announced that Librium and Valium, together with a number of other drugs with a "depressant effect on the central nervous system," would be subject to control as having a "potential for abuse."[45] There had been resistance within the FDA hierarchy to including Librium and Valium in this list. In November 1965, Norman Alberstadt of the Division of Medical Review had told executive officer Julius Hauser that, "The evidence gathered from the scientific literature and from reports recently submitted by the field districts is not sufficient to support a finding that diazepam has a potential for abuse. . . ." Hauser evidently reported to Joe Sadusk, head of the FDA's Bureau of Drugs. That same month, in a memo to the acting commissioner about the drugs to be controlled, Sadusk omitted Valium (though he included Librium).[46] Thus, the decision within the FDA to control Librium and Valium was anything but unanimous.

Hoffmann-La Roche decided to appeal the decision. The stage was set for a replay of the meprobamate hearing: The FDA, a big bureaucracy willing to play hardball in order to win, was intent upon developing evidence of diversion, street abuse, suicide, and convulsions. Hoffmann-La Roche, though a powerhouse of big pharma, had little chance in this kind of game.

A moment of background. Newly aggressive following the Kefauver-Harris Amendments of 1962, the FDA had already started nipping at the company for its plans to advertise Valium for such indications as "nervousness." In the summer of 1963, after Hoffmann-La Roche had submitted its proposed labeling for Valium, Matthew Ellenhorn of the

FDA's Division of New Drugs had summoned Dr. Lee Gordon from the company's headquarters in Nutley, New Jersey, to D.C. for a scolding. "I told the secretary to have Dr. Gordon bring with him what he considers to be the best evidence supporting the labeling claims," said Ellenhorn.[47] When Gordon came down to D.C. a couple of weeks later, he was ready to push back. Ellenhorn noted many inadequacies in Hoffmann-La Roche's trials (that had been conducted in the late 1950s, before the Kefauver-Harris Amendments requiring controls). Gordon replied, "We cannot ignore 200 doctors' work."[48]

Hoffmann-La Roche went right ahead and ran the ads that the FDA had challenged. The company's very first ad for Valium in the *Journal of the American Medical Association* (*JAMA*) on December 21, 1963, claimed that Valium was effective in "forty-four patients with incapacitating symptoms of insomnia, nervousness, agitation, tension, irritability, and associated physical symptoms such as anorexia. . . ."[49] This must have been very irritating to the bureaucrats.

There were further collisions with the company. In the spring of 1964, FDA officers met with Hoffmann-La Roche again, worried about the promotional phrase in Valium ads, "no serious side effects." The protagonists at the meeting quibbled about "serious": "Aren't ataxia and incoordination serious side effects?" asked FDA staffer Maurice Rath at the New Drug Surveillance Branch.[50] Hoffmann-La Roche asked for another meeting. It would be fair to surmise that by the time of the announcement of the hearings in January 1966, the company was being targeted for a humbling.

During this time, the public started to be heard from. Among the many communications pro and con, there was, for example, Ed C. of Los Angeles, who believed that Librium had ruined his life: "My wife has suffered several rages because of careless prescribing; 50 LIBRIUMS at a time, that plus the use of alcohol brings us into the divorce court on March 2 at which time my life will be ruined. I say this because at age 64 I can look forward only to a desolate and lonely existence."[51] One bears in mind that in 1965 alone, 21 million prescriptions had been written for Librium in the United States. Among these patients there would have been many with destroyed lives who blamed the Hoffmann-La Roche drug.

Some of the physicians who wrote in were a bit more skeptical of the need for listing. Dr. H. J. Bulgerin in Eastland, Texas, called the proposed listing "carrying things much too far. Perhaps the motivation under this law is good, but anyone with a little common sense and powers of observation can see over a period of years that these drugs are not nearly as dangerous as some of the so-called experts say. Quit wasting my money and other tax payers' money with your plain outright stupidity."[52]

Hearings were scheduled for August 1966. The FDA's objective was to attach the barbiturate-amphetamine model of the Drug Abuse Control Amendments to Librium and Valium. The agency wanted to list the two benzos as drugs of "potential abuse," and this model was the only legal tool for doing so. The benzodiazepines are indeed capable of inducing dependency after ultra-long use at high doses. Yet no one would break into an apartment for money to buy Librium, which has about the same euphoric effect as a cup of coffee. And Valium was only rarely sold by street dealers. Indeed, dependence was not initially even on the FDA's radar: By October 1964 the agency had eleven reports of side effects in Valium, the commonest being jaundice. Dependence was not among them.[53] So gross was the inappropriateness of pursuing Librium and Valium with the amphetamine-barbiturate model that the Feds must have had something else in mind than simply protecting the public health. And the tenacity with which the career bureaucrats waged the struggle suggests that indeed they did.

In the summer of 1966, the FDA began to get its case in order, beating the bushes for expert witnesses and discovering evidence, much as we saw previously for meprobamate. We shall dwell less long here on the mechanics of drumming up evidence because the agency's technique was already clear. Finding witnesses? Could Charles Llewellen, a psychiatrist at Duke University, help? Some of his patients had continued Valium "without medical advice," but only one had abused it; he was nonetheless willing to testify.[54] Later in July, the FDA asked Henry Verhulst, director of the National Clearinghouse for Poison Control Centers of the Public Health Service, to scour his records for evidence of Librium and Valium in suicide attempts. "There is a possibility that counsel for Hoffman [sic] LaRoche will ask for production of the actual reports for purposes of cross examination," the agency told him. "We would resist any such demand."[55] In other words, if Hoffmann-La Roche lawyers wanted to bring out that benzo traces in suicide victims might not have been the cause of death—and that many depressed people coincidentally took Librium and Valium for symptom relief—the agency would try to thwart this.

On July 29, 1966, John Finlator, director of the FDA's Bureau of Drug Abuse Control, who was marshaling the government case, reported to

Commissioner James Goddard on how things were coming. Splendidly! Several of the medical staff of the government center for addiction in Lexington, Kentucky, were coming up for the hearings or would be deposed. Members of the FDA's Advisory Committee on Abuse of Depressant and Stimulant Drugs would testify. The agency had found 50 death certificates "in which the deaths were attributed to Librium or Valium." The FDA also had "one compilation of terminated Durham-Humphrey prosecutions," pharmacies that had dispensed Librium and Valium in some irregular manner. And they had just heard that "a teacher in Pennsylvania was arrested for molesting two of his male students after having given them a drug." He had procured the drugs from an accountant who had a stock of Librium capsules at home.[56] Surely this would clinch the case.

A month later an embarrassed-sounding Finlator informed Goddard that the evidence of dependence in the FDA case was not actually all that strong. "Because of the dearth of medical experience with respect to dependence and abuses of these drugs, (because of their short existence) we are relying in large measure on instances of gross diversion and street abuse."[57] In retrospect this is incredible: The agency had virtually no evidence of abuse or dependence for Librium, which had been on the market for 6 years, or for Valium, 3 years on the market, and would base their case on a nonevent: diversion to street pushers! If Hoffmann-La Roche's lawyers had been able to discover this letter, the government case would have been laughed out of court. Unfortunately for them, they didn't know it existed.

The Librium-Valium hearings began August 8, 1966 (after two days of prehearings), and concluded November 18. The oral arguments took place in February 1967, and hearing examiner Edgar Buttle, a lawyer for the Federal Trade Commission, rendered his decision that Librium and Valium "have a potential for abuse" on April 7, 1967. Buttle had governed the hearings evenhandedly, at one point rebuking the FDA lawyers, "Your evidence is a whole lot less conclusive than you think it is."[58] Indeed, in Buttle's final opinion he made a display of how unconvincing he found much of the government's case.[59]

As Finlator had forecast, much of the government case hinged on evidence of diversion and street use. FDA counsel said in summing up that we may "deduce from this record of past abuse potential for future greater abuse."[60] This kind of case is easily buttressed by anecdotes and does not entail the relative weighing of instances of "abuse" against the undoubted benefits for public health of this therapeutic class.[61]

Hoffmann-La Roche's lawyers, from the white-shoe Washington firm Clifford and Miller, scorned the FDA's contention that the two drugs produced "euphoria": "I could sit here and eat them by the handful," said Hoffmann-La Roche's lawyer Thomas Finney, "and feed them to the Presiding Officer and Mr. Reilly [FDA lawyer] and say, 'Do you feel anything?' And the only thing you will feel is that when you get enough of it you begin to get the incoordination and drowsiness and ataxia. And good heavens, the same warning is on every over-the-counter antihistamine that is in the drug store."[62]

Street use? Hoffmann-La Roche brought in John E. Storer, chief of the California Bureau of Narcotic Enforcement, who testified about 250 recent "dangerous drug cases," mainly involving barbiturates and amphetamines.

Q: In the years 1965 and 1966 . . . did your Bureau have occasion to investigate any case involving either the drug Librium or Valium?

Storer: No, sir.

Q: During the time you have been Chief of the Bureau of Narcotics has your Bureau ever had occasion to investigate illegal traffic that involved the drug either Librium or Valium?

Storer: To the best of my knowledge we have never had a case involving either Librium or Valium.[63]

The FDA was never able to present convincing evidence of diversion or street use: The drugs were simply not that appealing to those in search of what was referred to at the time as "kicks."[64]

How about addicted patients who refilled their prescriptions countless times? Hoffmann-La Roche established that the refill rate for both drugs was actually quite low. For Librium, the refill rate for the 5 mg tablets was 2.3 times, for other size doses, equal or lower; for Valium, the refill rate for the 5 mg tablets was 2.4 times, that of the other size tablets lower.[65]

Suicide? Arthur McBay, chief of the chemical laboratory of the Massachusetts Department of Public Safety, said he had never seen a fatal dose of Librium or Valium. When there was no autopsy, he pointed out in regard to the government's 50 death certificates, you can't tell whether a death was due to Librium, whatever the certificate said. He went through all the exhibits in which Librium was mentioned in connection with a death: In all but six the Librium level was too low to be fatal and the death was evidently due to other drugs the victim had on board.[66]

As Finney summed up the company's case, he said about the standard of absolute lack of harm that the government was proposing, "If you are going to make your test whether a drug can be used for intentional self-harm I can impeach every classification in the Food, Drug, and Cosmetic Act [of 1938]. . . . How in the name of heaven do you leave iodine on the counter, which is the most potent poison in the pharmacopoeia? If that is the test, how do you leave aspirin on the counter, which can and does today account for more accidental deaths of children than any other thing?" He said that you had to balance risk versus benefit.[67] Later, a Finnish scholar worked out the suicide rate in Finland for 1987–88 by drug class: Barbiturates had 105.3 suicides relative to the amount consumed (defined daily doses), antidepressants 9.6 benzodiazepines 0.3.[68]

Tolerance, in the sense of steadily increasing doses? Alberto Di Mascio, one of the founders of psychopharmacology in the United States and head of the psychopharm service at the Massachusetts Mental Health Center, said that, unlike the barbiturates, he had never seen a case of escalating dosage among patients on Librium or Valium.[69]

A long series of Hoffmann-La Roche witnesses—distinguished scientists and clinicians—said they had never witnessed any of the specters that the FDA had conjured up in its nightmare scenarios of Librium and Valium as equal in harm to the barbiturates and amphetamines. But it did not matter. Buttle found for the FDA, not for the company, on the grounds that "there was medical opinion as to potentiality for abuse." "Under the concepts of administrative law and the Administrative Procedure Act, agency action may be premised on substantial evidence rather than a preponderance of evidence." Yet he pointed out, "There is no doubt that Hoffmann-La Roche has offered perhaps substantial evidence indicative of the nonabuse of Librium and Valium. The evidence concerning abuse is highly conflicting."[70]

Aware perhaps of the tenuousness of the government's case, in 1968 Commissioner Goddard rejected giving Librium and Valium an abuse listing, despite Buttle's recommendation.[71] But at about this time, the FDA lost the authority to decide this issue when its Bureau of Drug Abuse Control was transferred to the Department of Justice (DOJ), becoming the Bureau of Narcotics and Dangerous Drugs, the addiction police. There had been "a high-level battle" over whether the Department of Health, Education, and Welfare (HEW), to which the FDA belonged, or the Department of Justice had the authority to put drugs on the abuse list.[72] The DOJ won, with the stipulation that HEW would provide scientific input. It was not long before observers learned, in May 1969, that the Bureau of Narcotics and Dangerous Drugs would shortly list Librium and Valium as controlled drugs. Meanwhile, still another drug bill was pending, and the DOJ evidently preferred not to take a chance that Congress would somehow falter. The department decided to control the drugs on its own hook rather than include them in the draft bill.[73]

The DOJ's case against Librium and Valium was published on May 21, 1969, in the *Federal Register*, over the signature of John E. Ingersoll, director of the Bureau of Narcotics and Dangerous Drugs.[74] In the department's hands, all the nuances in Buttle's manuscript report vanished. The DOJ made it sound as though Buttle had declared emphatically that the drugs induced "psychic dependence," that euphoria in their use was common, that tolerance in the sense of steadily increasing doses was the inevitable result, that Librium and Valium had created "a hazard to the health of the individual and to the safety of other individuals and the community." Buttle's own report had been far more balanced. These bald assertions were the work of behind-the-scenes DOJ bureaucrats, attempting to lay before the public a devastating case on behalf of control. Exactly as with meprobamate, all of the respondent's evidence was dismissed.

This DOJ report was prefatory to listing. It now would be the cops, not the government doctors, who were making decisions about psychopharmacology.

There is a coda to these events. In February 1971 the Bureau of Narcotics and Dangerous Drugs ordered that Librium and Valium be listed as controlled substances. Hoffmann-La Roche appealed the decision, and in the course of the appeal, a number of documents surfaced that the FDA had not shared with Hoffmann-La Roche in 1966 during the hearings. One document in particular turned out to be even more interesting than was appreciated at the time.

The story is as follows:

In 1966 the FDA's Advisory Committee on Abuse of Depressant and Stimulant Drugs held a meeting on April 25 and 26 at the Crystal Plaza Office Center in Arlington, Virginia. Which drugs should be listed for control? The committee had no problem with listing the barbiturates and some of the classic sedatives such as Sulfonal and Trional. Then the minutes of the meeting state, "The minor tranquilizers and sedatives on the agenda in Appendix 'B' were discussed. The Committee believed that the evidence at present did not justify placing any of them under the controls of the Drug Abuse Amendments."[75] Appendix B, however, was not included with the copy of these minutes preserved in the National Archives.

On the basis of what evidence could the abuse committee have decided that the minor tranquilizers weren't sufficiently problematic to merit control? They doubtless had their own experience, plus the literature. In addition, in August 1965 Dorothy Dobbs at the FDA had written them a letter saying that abuse of Librium was "minimal."[76]

Fast forward to the early 1970s. Hoffmann-La Roche is suing the Department of Health, Education, and Welfare not to list Librium and Valium. The company argues that essential documents had not been produced by the federal government at the 1966 hearings, documents that might have altered the hearings' outcome had they been discovered. Among these documents were the minutes of this advisory committee that the FDA had refused to produce at the time. The court earnestly petitioned the federal government to make these documents available. The Third Circuit Court of Appeals wrote, "At long last, on July 10, 1972, pursuant to our direction, the report was produced and is attached to this opinion as Appendix 'B.'" The FDA evidently claimed originally to have misplaced the report and finally procured a copy of it (albeit still minus the report's Appendix B) "from a member of the advisory committee who had retained possession of the supporting documents." Thus the documentary trail had been quite obscured. (NB: the missing Appendix B to the advisory committee's 1966 report is different from the Appendix B to the court's 1973 opinion.)

The undated one-page report of the advisory committee, as it reached the court from the FDA, said the opposite of what the minutes said the committee had decided. In the one-pager attached to the court's opinion, Librium and Valium were listed among nine drugs that the advisory committee was said to have recommended as having a "potential for abuse." The advisory committee was quoted as saying, "It is our recommendation that such drugs be included in the regulations implementing the drug abuse law."[77] Originally, the advisory committee had recommended the exact opposite.

There are a benign and a malignant explanation of this apparent change of heart: The benign is that the committee simply changed its mind, without recording the change in the minutes, so that the committee chair, University of Michigan pharmacologist Frederick Shideman, faithfully recorded this change of heart in the one-page report; the malignant explanation is that the FDA bureaucrats found the committee's original report impossibly disappointing, and changed the decision themselves, removing the evidentiary trail from documents they shipped over to the Federal Archives. The evidence currently available does not allow us to determine which explanation is correct.

In 1973 the Third Circuit vacated the Bureau of Narcotics and Dangerous Drugs' order to list Librium and Valium, on the grounds that the FDA's nondisclosure of various documents was "so egregious as to have tainted the entire procedure."[78] But it was a short-lived victory for Hoffmann-La Roche. There was more to-ing and fro-ing between the various parties. Meanwhile, in 1970 a new Controlled Substances Act had been passed, setting up different classes ("schedules") of dangerousness for drugs. Finally, in July 1975, the Department of Justice succeeded in placing Librium and Valium on schedule IV (having a lower abuse risk) on the list of controlled substances.[79]

Being listed as potential drugs of abuse represented a substantial setback for these two useful agents. Valium was by this time the largest selling drug on the United States market. In 1974 almost three billion tablets were sold.[80] Medical revulsion was soon to follow.

Dependence and Chronic Use

There is, as we have seen, a basic rule in medicine that anything worth reacting to is worth overreacting to. Many remedies carry the side effect of some habituation, meaning the need to increase the dosage to get the same effect; or of some withdrawal effect, meaning that the symptoms briefly worsen after you discontinue the drug. Few are the meds that entail genuine addictiveness, with its components of drug-seeking behavior and inability to discontinue. Yet many of the drugs that carry these minor side effects also entail large therapeutic benefits; balancing the slight risks against the advantages for the patient is a legitimate medical exercise rather than an inducement to dissolution. The basic problem in the history of American psychopharmacology has always been the magnification of these minor risks beyond their true level, so that a drug class is destroyed once such curses as "dependence" and "abuse" are whispered.

One might respond, But if there's any risk, why shouldn't a drug be controlled, as the 1970 Controlled Substances Act provided for? It doesn't ban the drug; it merely wraps it in safeguards. What's wrong with that? Members of the FDA's own Controlled Substances Advisory Committee (CSAC)—struck in 1973, the successor of the Advisory Committee on Abuse of Depressant and Stimulant Drugs—soon realized there was plenty wrong with it. The logic of control was creating an avalanche of drugs to be listed. At the CSAC's November meeting in 1974, "Several Committee members reiterated the concern expressed at previous CSAC meetings that many physicians may view control of drugs as an 'all or none' process. Therefore, it is possible that controlled drugs may be under-utilized and non-controlled drugs, particularly analgesics, over-utilized. . . . The widespread use of propoxyphene [Lilly's Darvon] lends credence to the hypothesis."[81] The logic of control led to a distortion of rational therapeutics.

Thus, balancing risk and benefit in the benzos was important. Initially, dependence was a nonissue. Said Alec Jenner, the first psychiatrist to try Librium in the United Kingdom, looking back in 1998, "We had no thoughts about them being addictive. . . . I did some good I think by putting people on them, getting them over small patches [of distress]. I did a great deal more harm aggressively taking people off when I thought that we were doing something legally harmful."[82]

In the 1966 hearings the government had tried to make the case that any use was addicting, and this aroused considerable skepticism. But they didn't single out ultra-long-term use because that would have weakened what was essentially a prohibitionist case.[83]

But they should have.

Let's concede that some patients did become dependent on the benzos. As Jonathan Katz, staff psychiatrist at the National Institute on Drug Abuse (NIDA) Addiction Research Center in Baltimore, pointed out in 1990 of the benzodiazepines, " . . . This dependence in itself does not appear to represent a significant risk, since it is not likely to be accompanied by inappropriate patterns of use, such as increasing doses." Nor, he said, were there "adverse clinical effects" associated with dependence, unless the patient stopped suddenly.[84] So under what circumstances did dependence turn into addiction?

It is an old story in psychopharmacology that patients tend to become dependent on effective drugs, especially those designed to relieve anxiety. The tricyclic antidepressants, which have side effects so distracting that patients are usually glad to be off them as soon as possible, are an exception to this. But every other drug class from the barbiturates to the stimulants, the 1950s "tranquilizers," and later the SSRIs, has produced complaints of dependence. Sidney Brandon, psychiatrist at the

University of Leicester, said in 1990, "With every naturally occurring and synthetic agent used to alleviate anxiety the borderline between that use, which enabled the individual to function in otherwise intolerable conditions—the state of forgetful indolence achieved by the lotus eaters—and the deterioration of the addict, has never been easy to draw."[85] So the issue of dependence in the benzos is not entirely straightforward, not as open-and-shut as, say, heroin. Patients do become attached to the drugs. Yet the drugs are highly effective.

How attached?

Alarm was first sounded in the early 1960s that patients might experience marked withdrawal reactions on discontinuation. In 1961 Leo Hollister and colleagues at the Veterans Administration Hospital in Palo Alto, California, said that normal doses of Librium did not produce habituation, but that if patients on ultra-large doses, 8–20 times the usual therapeutic range, were suddenly discontinued, agitation, insomnia, loss of appetite, and nausea might eventuate. The lesson was not that Librium was habituating but that, "If large doses of chlordiazepoxide [Librium] are used, the drug should not be abruptly discontinued."[86] (The federal case in the hearings made a great deal of Hollister's finding and, as we'll see later, Hollister spent years living this down.)[87]

Another alarm went off in 1969 as a group of researchers at the Johns Hopkins University and the University of Pennsylvania, in a study coordinated by the Psychopharmacology Service Center of NIMH, investigated withdrawal reactions in patients on meprobamate (Miltown) and chlordiazepoxide (Librium). Using a placebo control, they found, following sudden discontinuation of chlordiazepoxide, withdrawal reactions after 4 months of use.[88] Returning to this theme again in 1973, they said sudden discontinuation of Librium induced "a minor abstinence syndrome of the barbiturate type." They recommend ending Librium treatment after 4 months.[89]

In the late 1970s there was a quickening of concern about possible benzo dependence, for stories such as this were becoming common: "I've been on one or the other habit forming drugs for at least if not more than 10 years," Herman X, of Darby, Pennsylvania, wrote the FDA in October 1979. The Veterans Administration Clinic in Philadelphia had put him on Valium, Librium, and Verstran (prazepam), at monthly doses of 120, sometimes 240, pills. "This has left me very ill," he said, "and without a job. The reason for writing this letter is for you to know how easy it is to get habit forming drugs."[90] So this issue of benzo addiction is not to be trivialized; it is not the same as taking handfuls of vitamins every day for 10 years. The benzodiazepines have the capacity to become drugs of mass addiction, when taken as Herman X took them.

In 1978 Malcolm Lader at the Institute of Psychiatry in London, the premier British training center, called the benzos "the opium of the masses," and said, "Dependence occurs with the benzodiazepines as with all drugs of this class but it is less severe and less of a hazard than with the barbiturates." High doses were required for the appearance of "marked withdrawal symptoms," he said. Also, "Mild psychological dependence is probably very common but is difficult to document."[91] In 1981 Peter Tyrer and colleagues at several London hospitals decided to withdraw suddenly 40 outpatients who had been on diazepam and lorazepam for 3 to 6 years in order to assess dependence: Of the 22 patients who completed the study, 14 were withdrawn to the beta-blocker propanolol, 8 to placebo. Half of both groups experienced withdrawal symptoms.[92] The lesson was clear: Doctor, if your patient has been on benzos for 3.6 years (the mean in the study) or more, don't withdraw him or her suddenly.

Articles proliferated. Later in 1981, Lader and a coauthor called attention to withdrawal symptoms in long-term use. "Because of the risk of dependence on benzodiazepines these agents should probably not be given as regular daily treatment for chronic anxiety," they concluded.[93]

In 1984 Heather Ashton, senior lecturer in the clinical psychopharmacology unit of the university hospital in Newcastle-upon-Tyne, described twelve patients who had been on benzos for 3 to 22 years and now expressed a wish for help in withdrawing. Many of these long-term users became highly symptomatic as they were slowly weaned onto other drugs or to no drug. Ashton said in the *British Medical Journal*, "The features of benzodiazepine withdrawal appear to constitute a new syndrome."[94]

Benzo Hysteria

These were important scientific contributions that sharpened the clinical focus of benzo use. But they stirred a reflex that is constantly present in the trenches of clinical medicine—a reflex vastly exacerbated by the threat of litigation: Why merely react when you can overreact? A massive overreaction followed these scientific findings, as the benzos became stigmatized as addictive and conducive to habituation and dependency.

The patients' world overreacted. This was part of the general hysteria about addiction from pharmaceuticals that swept American society in the 1970s. Tranquilizers, pep pills, diet pills, and sleeping pills alike became indicted as leading the nation into a swamp of drug dependence.

But after the wide publicity of the FDA hearings and subsequent talk about controlled drugs, Librium and Valium became particularly incriminated as drugs of abuse. Who would want to take a potentially addictive controlled substance? In December 1972, one patient in Chicago wrote to Henry Simmons, Director of the Bureau of Drugs at the FDA, "The legalized abuse of tranquilizers is making this country a nation of cripples. . . . I do know that from the Valium that started my problems to the Mellaril [antipsychotic thioridazine] that made me a lifetime cripple, all these drugs are poison. Far worse than heroin from the standpoint of causing irriversible [sic] lifetime damage."[95] Some years later, "I'm dancing as fast as I can," shrieked one journalist who believed herself addicted to Valium, and warned the nation in 1979 of the drug's effects on her.[96]

When John Hinckley attempted to assassinate President Reagan on March 30, 1981, in Washington, D.C., he wounded several bystanders, who later sued Hinckley's psychiatrist, Dr. John Hopper, Jr., on the grounds that he had prescribed the Valium that motivated Hinckley to perform his crime. "Specifically," said the court, "plaintiffs assert that the prescription of Valium and biofeedback therapy . . . aggravated Hinckley's condition and actually contributed to his dangerous propensity."[97]

So it was not just chronic use; it was any use of these drugs that spelled evil.

When in January 1988 Ricky Jones was confined in a correctional institution in Wisconsin, he complained of stress and was prescribed a tablet of Valium on each of the following two days. When the medication was stopped (as Jones's effort to palm a third tablet was discovered), Jones sued the prison authorities, asserting that "withdrawing his medication caused him to experience withdrawal symptoms and made him 'susceptible' to seizures and extreme emotional distress."[98] The court dismissed the action, but it was only in a media-churned climate that believed anything imaginable of these drugs that such a lawsuit would have been entertained.

Once greeted with enthusiasm in the patients' world as an alternative to the barbiturates, Librium and Valium now seemed like a curse devised by the wicked drug companies to plague the walking wounded.

Politicians jumped to the public's aid. As the Senate debated the narcotics and drug-abuse bill in October 1970 (that became the Controlled Substances Act of 1970), Thomas Dodd of Connecticut proposed to shift the two Hoffmann-La Roche tranquilizers from schedule V, where they had first been tentatively billeted, to schedule IV; it received "unanimous consent" in a vote that took place after 5:30 P.M. with only six senators present, including Dodd. Dodd seemed to have a grudge against Hoffmann-La Roche and throughout the debate on the bill had campaigned against Librium and Valium.[99] Later that week, as the House threatened to drop the two drugs from the bill, Dodd said, "I was shocked and distressed to find that the House conferees bludgeoned the Senate conferees into eliminating these 'killer' drugs. . . . I am using the word 'killer' drugs advisedly and knowing well what the term implies."[100]

Spiro Agnew, vice-president of the United States under Richard Nixon who later resigned in disgrace, excoriated "mood drugs" in 1970 at the National Sheriffs' Association in Hot Springs, Arkansas. "Over one-half million citizens are now dependent on non-narcotic drugs," he told them.[101] For politicians, there clearly was gold in the hills of Librium and Valium.

As pressure against Librium, Valium, and the other benzos now coming onto the market mounted in the 1970s, grandstanding in the Senate became inevitable. In September 1979 Ted Kennedy convened a hearing of the Subcommittee on Health and Scientific Research on "use and misuse of benzodiazepines." It was a wonderful opportunity for alerting voters to the need to seek help if they were eating benzos. In his introductory remarks, Kennedy intoned that "these drugs have produced a nightmare of dependence and addiction, both very difficult to treat and to recover from." "I believe that what we will hear about today," he continued, "is the tip of the iceberg—thousands of Americans are hooked and do not know it." The hearings reprinted all of the anti-Valium articles in the medical literature.[102]

To identify those wicked physicians still prescribing benzodiazepines, in 1990 California congressman Pete Stark proposed a bill mandating all states to adopt multiple-copy prescription programs for schedule II to IV substances[103]—programs already in effect in some states. In 1991 Stark suggested an electronic data transfer program to track physicians prescribing controlled substances. If you as a doctor somehow fell afoul of this EDT tracking, you would end up in the National Practitioner Data Bank that was put into effect in September 1990, which would stay on your record approximately until the sun exploded.[104] Congressman Stark's proposal was never enacted into law but won him much credit as a guardian of the public health.

And abuse? In 1976 the world of psychopharm reeled as the National Institute on Drug Abuse announced that Valium was the "number one" abused drug in emergency rooms across the nation: in NIDA's Drug Abuse Warning Network (DAWN) reports, of the approximately 14,000 incidents of Valium abuse identified nationwide, half involved a suicide attempt! This put Valium right up there alongside alcohol and heroin as one of "the most frequently abused drugs in the United States."[105] The medical world was stunned. Valium was at the time the most prescribed drug in the country, and to think it had been causing such ruination. Who knew?

Few at the time were aware of the deficiencies of these much-cited DAWN data. For one thing, a mention is a mention, not a cause. Consider the case of Mrs. Thekla X of Emerson, New Jersey, who in 1963 was hospitalized at Englewood Hospital for symptoms of "forgetfulness and unsteadiness in her legs." She had recently taken "Librium tranquilizer pills for 7 or 8 days." Her family doctor had informed her that "these symptoms possibly could have been side effects of 'Librium.'" Surely, this was an open-and-shut case. Had the DAWN monitoring system been then in existence, Mrs. X would have received a "mention."

But it turned out that Mrs. X's real problem was "progressively deteriorating cerebral atrophy." She was 72. The neurologist who attended her in hospital told an FDA inspector "emphatically that this drug could not have brought about the described symptoms." "The condition existed before she took the Librium."

"We plan no follow-up," the FDA inspector told the file.[106]

The DAWN system incorporated toxicologists' reports of high Valium levels. How could those err? It was commonly known that toxicologists were far too inclined to put down "Valium" as a cause of overdose or death because it had such a long half-life. Several participants at a roundtable on Valium organized by Leo Hollister in 1976 pointed this out, noting that the other drugs involved in the death might already have cleared. Said David Greenblatt, chief of pharmacology at Massachusetts General Hospital, of the toxicologists in the coroners' offices who conducted the drug screens: "Rather than not state the cause of death they will put down anything. You can't sign a death certificate by saying 'I don't know.'" Hollister added, "They tend to struggle to find some cause. If the drug [Valium] is around they usually attribute it to an overdose in desperation to have some plausible cause of death, when clearly the levels are often within therapeutic ranges."[107]

Also, in the DAWN system, a "responsible reporter" at each facility was charged with recording any mention of any controlled drug in any case, not just the drug taken with suicidal intent or the drug causing the need for admission to the emergency room. Thirty percent of the reporters were head nurses or nursing supervisors, 22 percent were emergency room nurses, 18 percent emergency room ward secretaries, and 11 percent medical records librarians. Rather than making medical judgments about significance, they simply noted whatever was recorded in the chart.[108] Precisely because Valium was so widely used, it appeared frequently in the charts of patients who had attempted suicide with other agents entirely, or who had otherwise come to medical attention.

So inadequate were the DAWN data that in 1978 the Drug Abuse Advisory Committee of the FDA struck a subcommittee on the "effects of scheduling" to consider how the acquisition of data on drugs of abuse might be improved. In 1980 this subcommittee reported back, emphasizing the role of medical examiners and alternative sites to emergency rooms, among other recommendations.[109] In the background was a certain tension between the then relatively liberal FDA drug abuse committee and the grimly repressive Drug Enforcement Agency (DEA). The DAWN data were easily misusable for alarmist purposes, which is exactly how the DEA and NIDA used them.[110]

Finally, inadequate though the DAWN data were, they made clear that street abuse, or nonprescription abuse, was not a significant factor in the benzodiazepines. DAWN data for 1985 show that Valium was number 4 and Librium number 20 on the list of drugs mentioned in emergency-room visits.[111] Where did the patients get the drugs? For Librium, in 65 percent the source was a legal prescription, in 29 percent the source was unknown or no response, in 3 percent the drug was stolen, and in 1 percent a street buy.[112] For Valium, the source was a prescription in 49 percent, unknown in 39 percent, a street buy in 8 percent, and stolen in 3 percent.[113]

Were the "unknowns" just lying about their use of a controlled substance? That would greatly increase alarm about illicit use. It turns out, no. For the tricyclic antidepressant amitriptyline (Elavil), eleventh on the list of emergency-room mentions in 1985 and not a controlled substance, the source was a legal prescription in 65 percent, unknown in 29 percent, stolen in 3 percent, and a street buy in 2 percent—a profile quite comparable to that of Librium and not vastly different from Valium.[114] It is, of course, possible for patients with legitimate prescriptions to abuse drugs, but illicit use—of which so much had been made in this troubled history—was not really an issue.

Decline

At an international level, the 1990s and after saw great growth in the medical use of benzodiazepines. In 1990, France was, according to the insider newsletter *Scrip*, "the largest consumer of benzodiazepines in the world."[115] In France, Valium was injectable and said to be for "major anxiety"—*les grands anxieux*—as opposed to the United States, where, the French believed, people took Valium for "minor anxiety"— *les petits anxieux*.[116] Global manufacture of benzodiazepine-type anxiolytics rose steadily between 1996 and 2002, half of which was diazepam.[117]

Yet in these years the United Kingdom and the United States saw the definitive decline of the benzos for depression and anxiety. This was not a chance event. They were ultimately shoved off stage by the Prozac-style drugs, the SSRIs. Events in the United Kingdom and United States represent Exhibit A for those who believe that the rise and fall of drug classes are more a result of marketing than of science. Yet marketing was not especially significant in this story until after the late 1980s, with the launch of Prozac in the United States in 1988. Initially, the desuetude of the benzos was more a result of medical herd behavior than of cunning pharmaceutical spin.

The Decline of the Benzos: United Kingdom

In the United Kingdom starting in the late 1970s, revulsion mounted among doctors against such terrible drugs. The papers of Tyrer, Ashton, and others, mentioned above, were widely circulated, discussed, and misunderstood, so easy is it to conflate "long-term use" and "all use."

The leaders of the field of psychopharmacology attempted to still the rising fears: The benzodiazepines were actually rather useful drugs and not half as dangerous as thought, they said. As Malcolm Lader at the Institute of Psychiatry in London put it, " . . . Every previous antianxiety/sedative drug has sooner or later been found to induce dependence and . . . withdrawal reactions."[118] So "abuse" and dependence have dogged many psychiatric drug classes, not just the benzos.

Among the leaders in British psychopharmacology, Lader insisted a number of times on the relative safety and effectiveness of the benzos. His 1977 survey in London found "little evidence of 'recreational' use of these drugs. I think that the problems associated with benzodiazepines are going to be related to . . . the high incidence of anxiety in the community rather than abuse due to their euphoric properties."[119] Dependence, he said, did "occur with benzodiazepines as with all drugs of this class but it is less severe and less of a hazard than with the barbiturates. . . . To date, the benzodiazepines seem safe drugs. In overdose they are astonishingly non-toxic." To be sure, it was "often difficult to wean patients" off them. Thus, bottom line for Lader: "Tranquilizers should be reserved for the severely anxious who really need them."[120]

John Marks, a psychiatrist at Girton College in Cambridge and author of a major monograph on the benzos, denied in 1979 that the agents were any more addictive than any other psychotropic drug. ". . . The risk of dependence is low at therapeutic levels," he said, "particularly over relatively short periods of administration."[121] Six years later, in a second edition of his monograph, Marks agreed that more caution was indicated. Yet on a scale of dependence, the benzos fell somewhere between alcohol and "compulsive crossword completion." He said there was no real danger of "withdrawal phenomena"—the core concern in abuse—if used less than a year.[122]

A number of other senior figures in British psychopharmacology, such as Peter Tyrer, then at Mapperley Hospital in Nottingham, and Anthony Clare at the Institute of Psychiatry, contributed to the discussion along the lines of yes, caution indicated, but nonetheless, useful drugs.[123] In 1988 Kevin Power at the University of Stirling in Scotland wrapped up the view of what was really the British psychopharmacology establishment: "The benzodiazepines are one of the most safe and widely used classes of drugs in modern medicine. While they are prone to abuse, this occurs in an exceedingly small minority of cases. Abandoning benzodiazepine use would seem extreme at present."[124]

Did all of this balance and moderation, this clear-eyed assessment of efficacy and side effect, do any good? No. Both sides of the Atlantic saw these brave attempts to hoist the banner of science and common sense. It is dispiriting how little impact these efforts had on the medical profession as a whole, on the media, and on the public.

The high point of benzo prescribing in Great Britain was 1979, with 31 million prescriptions. The decline began just as the Committee on the Review of Medicines issued its "guidelines" in March 1980 suggesting that prescribing of this class be limited to "short-term use."[125]

A series of blows followed. Indeed, "1986 proved to be a bleak year for benzodiazepines in the UK," said psychopharmacologist Ian Hindmarch, then at the University of Leeds, when the government decided to introduce a "'black list' which restricted the prescribing of many derivatives and which effectively stopped any major research on this most useful group of drugs."[126]

The death warrant of the benzos in the United Kingdom was signed 2 years later, in 1988, when the Committee on the Safety of Medicines recommended limiting their prescribing, noting withdrawal symptoms and dependence even after short periods of time. They might be prescribed for a maximum of 4 weeks, and then only for symptoms of "disabling" anxiety or insomnia. Oh yes, and if you prescribe them alone you might precipitate a depressed patient into suicide.[127] So, that was the end of that.

The decline of benzo use in the United Kingdom had been continuous since 1980, and had been almost cut in half by 2001.[128] Irish-American psychopharmacologist David Sheehan, watching from the relative safety of the Institute for Research in Psychiatry in Tampa, Florida, said much later of these events, "What some people in the UK didn't understand was that, outside of this island in the North Atlantic, the rest of the world were watching this and laughing at them and saying, 'They've lost their marbles.' . . . This has got so far out of control that it's comical or actually embarrassing."[129]

The Decline of the Benzos: United States

In the United States, few insiders believed in the benzo-dependence scenario, even those who publicly might have been obliged to mouth minatory platitudes, such as the acerbic Paul Leber, director of the FDA's Neuropharmacology Division. During the public skirmish in the late 1980s over the purported addictiveness of a short-acting benzo called Halcion (triazolam), Leber demonstrated himself in private to be a complete doubter. He told the agency's Psychopharmacologic Drugs Advisory Committee in September 1989, "In the last 150 years since the advent of medicinal chemistry, there have been literally hundreds of drugs used as hypnotics. It is an interesting thing, for anyone who is even a superficial student of the history of pharmacology, that each and every one of these drugs used to induce sleep is a CNS depressant. As such, each and every one of them has been associated with a variety of adverse phenomena that are common to the drugs as a class." They all at some dose, he said, caused intoxication, stupor, "states of dependence, physiologic dependence, therefore, subjecting individuals to withdrawal reactions." Once, he said, it was the barbiturates that got this rap. Now it is the benzodiazepines.[130]

A small band of psychopharmacologists also resisted the conventional wisdom that the benzos were terrible drugs of addiction. Leo Hollister, whose early findings on withdrawal at ultra-high doses had been exploited so baldly at the 1966 hearings, remained a strong advocate of benzo use. In 1977 he convoked a roundtable discussion in Chicago that included a number of senior figures in American psychopharmacology such as Louis Lasagna, at the University of Rochester, and Daniel Freedman, chair of the psychiatry department at the University of Chicago. Hollister said that after his 1961 study of Librium, he thought there would be "a flood of reports of withdrawal reactions from chlordiazepoxide [Librium]. You can virtually count on your fingers the verified reports over the last 15 years."[131]

At the roundtable, Karl Rickels at the University of Pennsylvania, another of the pioneer figures in American psychopharmacology, found Valium such a benign drug that he treated anxious college students with it so they could write their papers. "[They] suddenly begin to realize that they can speak without difficulty. After a few months they don't need Valium anymore."[132]

Rickels continued to plead on behalf of the benzos. In 1981 he called them "remarkably safe substances," and said again in 1987, "All drugs have a number of actions, but until a specific anxiolytic with no side-effects becomes available, the benzos are the most useful for the treatment of anxiety."[133]

The comment was actually a rather fateful one, for in December 1987 the FDA approved Prozac for release, the first of the SSRIs to be launched in the United States. It was the SSRIs that definitively destroyed the benzos in the United States and Great Britain and heightened the shift in the attention of psychiatry from anxiety to "depression."

Yet the destruction of the benzos in the United States began well before that portentous launch. The year 1975, when Librium and Valium were finally listed as controlled substances, represents the high-water mark of the benzos. Thereafter, a continuous and uninterrupted decline set in that may be measured by the annual number of benzodiazepine-related emergency room episodes: 24,000 in 1976, 14,000 in 1985.[134] It is, of course, positive that emergency room visits involving the benzos dropped off. Yet in these visits a benzo was usually not the *reason* for the visit but rather a coincidental finding in a visit motivated by some other substance. Nonetheless, the number of visits gives a measure of frequency of use in the absence of other data in the public domain. The addition of benzodiazepines to the triplicate prescription regulations in New York State in 1989 resulted in a 44 percent reduction in use there over the next 2 years.[135]

Where have we heard this story of decline before? We heard it with, among other drug classes, the barbiturates. Did the barbiturates, too, deserve to die? For surely today they, too, are as dead as Librium and Valium. Was it the danger of death and addiction that pulled down these drug classes, or was it commercial rivalry? Manufacturers of the many new classes of drugs that came along in the 1950s and '60s made sure to point out in their advertising the dangerousness of the barbiturates compared to the sponsors' new products. But these drugs would similarly be trashed by the producers of future generations of pharmaceuticals further down the pipeline. This has much more to do with commercial competition than with science.

The benzos in their turn were scorned in the ads of the competition. "Sidetracked," shouted an ad for the tricyclic antidepressant amitriptyline (Elavil) in *JAMA* in 1968. The ad showed a woman standing forlornly on a rail siding; the text said, "Use of a tranquilizer in treating depression may get the patient nowhere."[136] (Many family docs, who read *JAMA*, thought of the benzos as antidepressants.) So, doctors, if you prescribe benzos, you'll just make your patients worse!

A small band of American academic psychiatrists continued to stick up for the benzos, considerably so after their colleagues had followed the herd to newer drug classes. In 1990, a task force on benzodiazepines, established by the American Psychiatric Association, chaired by Carl Salzman, and including Leo Hollister, Karl Rickels, David Sheehan, and Malcolm Lader, among others, spoke up bravely: "There are no data to suggest that long-term therapeutic use of benzodiazepines by patients commonly leads to dose escalation or to recreational abuse." Dependence was not an issue before 4 months, the report said. "Benzodiazepines . . . are not widely abused drugs," the authors concluded.[137]

Nonetheless, the sedative benzos leaked out of American medicine. By 1990 Valium had sunk to number 47 on a list of most frequently prescribed drugs.[138] American physicians continued to prescribe such benzos as lorazepam for insomnia. But the benzos as antianxiety agents basically went off the boards in the United States.

In 2007, a psychiatrist in a small town in Georgia was giving advice on a psychopharm listserv about what other members of the list might prescribe for insomnia. Finally he came to his own practice. "Me? I prescribe trazodone frequently for my patients and have had good success with many of them." He mentioned other agents that he also offered. Then finally, "I have a couple patients who still take flurazepam [a benzo], having taken it for years and don't want to give it up."[139] Somewhat embarrassed, he had to justify this to his colleagues on the list.

How does it happen that perfectly serviceable drug classes become lost? English psychiatrist Sidney Brandon spoke in 1990 of how one fashionable class of anxiolytics soon succeeds another: "The pattern commonly followed is that the 'new' agent displaces the previously most widely used substance which has been causing increasing alarm. . . ." How does this occur? "Evidence of long-term use, sometimes of escalating dosage, its use as a recreational drug and then finally evidence of addiction . . . mark the progression to the next wonder drug."[140]

This progression is exactly what happened with the benzos. Thomas Ban said, "Habituation and suicide dominated the psychopharmacology picture from the 1960s on. Meprobamate was the beginning of the addiction scare. The suicide alerts. Then Librium claimed that meprobamate was dangerous and addictive. So it happened: the propanediols [meprobamate-style drugs] pushed out the barbiturates; the benzos pushed out the propanediols. These are all political issues."[141]

In diagnosis, following the decline of the benzodiazepines, psychiatric emphasis shifted from anxiety, now associated with the supposedly addictive Librium-Valium drug class, to depression. In treatment, the death of the benzos cleared away an effective class of drugs to make way for an ineffective drug class of antidepressants: the SSRIs.

But why did the spotlight fall on depression?

6

Death Sentences

Of the first drug set of the 1950s, little remains 60 years later. How did it happen that these important agents were relegated to the sidelines? Part of the story is that they were forcefully sidelined, by the very authorities who are supposed to safeguard the public health and ensure that the remedies in the marketplace are optimal. That effort began to gain traction with such events as the 1966 hearings on meprobamate, Librium, and Valium, but the outcomes of those proceedings were small potatoes compared to the results of a larger government initiative that was then just getting underway for a wide variety of medications.

Right up front, the class of drugs now formally called antidepressants triumphed over all other drug classes—and depression over all other competing diagnoses—partly because they were federally mandated through broadly sweeping FDA activities from the late 1960s to the early 1980s. During this period, the FDA came to believe in the purity of the concept of "antidepressants," and the agency was able to impose its views on the pharmaceutical industry, which in turn responded by producing scads of antidepressants for the suffering public. It was also helpful that, in tilting the table toward depression, the agency simultaneously wiped out about half of the existing drugs competing for the neurosis market. This portentous chapter in the history of psychiatry and psychopharmacology is almost unknown. It is called DESI.

The Clouds Gather

In 1997, in an interview with colleagues, J. Richard Crout, who had been director of the FDA's Bureau of Drugs from 1973 to 1982, described

"DESI" as "really a bad, very bureaucratic term." It stands for Drug Efficacy Study Implementation. His colleagues at the interview laughed appreciatively.[1] Indeed, the term itself has a my-eyes-glaze-over quality. Yet the administrative search-and-destroy operation conducted under its aegis carved huge gashes in the American psychopharmacopoeia, as well as setting all players aquiver about drugs for an illness increasingly on the tip of every tongue: "depression."

What was DESI? It was conceived as part of a massive retroactive evaluation of the effectiveness of thousands of drugs that the FDA had previously approved between 1938 and 1962 on the basis of safety alone, in accordance with the federal drug regulations that were in place during those years. This drug evaluation had two phases. The first was the work of the National Academy of Sciences' National Research Council between 1966 and 1969 in which academic experts on panels evaluated most of the drugs marketed in the United States at that time. This is called the NAS/NRC, or the Drug Efficacy Study (DES), phase.[2] The second was the internal efforts of the FDA from 1968 to the early 1980s to implement the panels' recommendations and, as it turns out, to greatly expand their scope. This is called the DESI phase, the implementation of the Drug Efficacy Study.

The legislative thrust behind this effort began in 1960 and 1961. At that time Senator Estes Kefauver of Tennessee, chair of the subcommittee on Antitrust and Monopoly of the Senate Judiciary Committee, led seemingly endless hearings on "administered prices" in the pharmaceutical industry. Kefauver, a left-leaning Democrat, had the idea that the companies were conspiring to keep drug prices up and that government action was needed. His efforts almost certainly would not have been passed into legislation by the Senate or the Congress. But when in December 1961 the thalidomide crisis broke—the discovery that a hypnotic agent then in trials in the United States deformed the limbs of fetuses whose mothers took the drug—Kefauver's efforts were given a new lease on life. The Kefauver-Harris Amendments that Congress passed late in 1962, amending the Food, Drug and Cosmetic Act of 1938, were substantially different from those Kefauver originally had in mind. It was the regulation of drugs, not their pricing, that was to be more extensively controlled, and the FDA was given new power to judge the efficacy of drugs as well as their safety (safety had been mandated in the 1938 act). The Kefauver Harris Amendments stipulated in particular that the FDA was to consider "'substantial evidence,' mean[ing] evidence consisting of adequate and well-controlled investigations, including clinical investigations, by experts . . . to evaluate the effectiveness of the drug involved."[3]

Which drugs, exactly, were to be assessed? During the negotiations surrounding the passage of the act, the Senate version exempted from scrutiny proprietary drugs (that had never had a New Drug Application [NDA]) and currently marketed drugs that had an NDA, as long as the NDA remained unchallenged by the FDA. The agency, however, was impatient with such exemptions, and insisted on its right to bring all post-1938 drugs under review.[4] This was in line with the agency's ongoing desire to expand its power over the drug supply. But other players pushed back, and the Kefauver-Harris Amendments ultimately weaseled on this conflict by saying that "new drugs" would be subject to FDA review. A "new drug" was any drug not already agreed by experts to be effective. Drugs marketed before 1938 were supposedly "grandfathered," or exempt from review, but the agency didn't care for that restriction either.

So what? This is important because an efficacy review would open the door to massive deletions of marketed drugs if "adequate" trials did not show them to be effective. To be sure, there had been in American history previous such deletions, namely the dropping of hundreds of obsolete botanical compounds from the inventories of the "broad line" drug houses in the 1930s and '40s. Indeed, of 900 single chemical entity drugs introduced in the United States between 1941 and 1968, 152 had been deleted.[5] But many of those drugs had been pokey little alkaloids brought to market with relatively little expense and having nothing remotely resembling blockbuster sales. In the synthetic drugs marketed in the 1950s and '60s big bucks were at stake. The sales of agents such as meprobamate had been staggering. Subjecting these products to an efficacy review was a different kettle of fish.

Yet the FDA under George Larrick, commissioner since 1954, was not terribly keen to get going on such a review. Larrick correctly foresaw the enormousness of this project for his then tiny agency. Congress, however, was impatient. Drugs and addictiveness were headline news. In 1963 Hubert Humphrey of Minnesota convened the Subcommittee on Reorganization and International Organizations, falling under the auspices of the Senate's Committee on Government Operations, and set out to find why the government wasn't moving ahead faster on drug safety and efficacy. Committee members put the spotlight on FDA "inadequacies," and in June 1963, Ernest Gruening of Alaska reproached the agency for letting "useless drugs" onto the market: "Physicians continue to use these useless drugs in large numbers."[6] A couple of months later, Lowell Coggeshall, chairman of the Commission on Drug Safety (established in August 1962 by the Pharmaceutical Manufacturers Association following the thalidomide tragedy) and vice-president of the University of Chicago, told the subcommittee that a "supreme court" of drugs was needed to pass on safety and efficacy, and suggested the National Academy of Science's National Research Council.[7] (It must have irked the FDA that he intended to leave them out of the loop entirely.)

In those days industry had been talking about "clinical experience" as acceptable evidence, vastly cheaper than controlled drug trials, because clinical experience in this context basically meant lining up medical friends of the company and encouraging them to say nice things about one's drug. Yet Humphrey was not having any talk of clinical experience. The following year, 1964, he told Larrick that Congress wanted "controlled clinical trials" constituting "scientific proof of efficacy."[8] Larrick responded evasively.[9] The point is important because it was later contended that in 1964 the FDA was indeed prepared to accept "well-documented clinical experience" rather than the evidence of controlled trials.[10]

Despite Larrick's foot-dragging, the FDA bureaucracy was champing at the bit to expand the agency's power. Just as senior administrators were beginning to proceed against meprobamate (see Chapter 4), they thrilled at the prospect of the agency taking control of the entire pharmacopoeia. At a meeting on January 31, 1964, in Larrick's office on surveilling the nation's drug supply for safety and efficacy, the senior leadership tier agreed that the FDA would "make the companies take an inventory, that is, weed out all drugs once marketed but no longer on the market." The agency would compile a master list of all New Drug Applications and centralize all information on them. Companies that didn't go along would have their NDAs canceled.[11]

On February 5, 1964, an officer in the FDA's New Drug Surveillance Branch sent Ralph Smith, who was the agency's acting medical director, a list of psychopharmaceuticals that he thought should be removed from the market in the interest of "safety and/or efficacy." The list tore a huge hole in the current psychopharmacopoeia, and included "all MAO inhibitors," all reserpine derivatives, and a whole slew of antineurotics such as Striatran (emylcamate) and Atarax (hydroxyzine). In addition, the officer felt that phenothiazines should be restricted to use as antipsychotics (as opposed to the myriad indications for which a drug such as chlorpromazine had been prescribed since its appearance on the American market in 1954).[12] Some of the MAO inhibitors survived, but in fact, this memo nicely foreshadowed much of DESI's later outcome.

The NAS/NRC Phase

These internal FDA discussions soon resulted in action. On February 25, 1964, the agency told industry it was going to review every drug covered by an NDA since 1938. The proposed regulation governing this review said that industry would have to submit extensive documentation on effectiveness for all of its drugs and that any drug for which such documentation was not provided would be withdrawn.[13] This was a huge assertion of FDA authority, for many generics and "me-too" drugs, coattailing on a pioneer drug originally marketed under an NDA, had previously not been considered "new," meaning that years of successful use had established their safety and effectiveness, and they did not have NDAs. But the FDA wanted to take a look at them as well, despite their manufacturers' pleas that they were "old" drugs. Congress backed the FDA: In June 1964, Humphrey said that the agency must insist on "controlled clinical studies rather than subjective clinical impressions."[14]

Still, there was a long gap between asking industry to send in documentation and actively deciding which drugs should be scrapped. Larrick shied back from the latter, and it was only with his retirement in December 1965 that the FDA acquired real teeth: In January 1966, James "Go-Go" Goddard became commissioner and the agency resolved to move ahead with a gigantic reevaluation of all drugs marketed after 1938, "new" and "old" alike. In June 1966, Goddard signed a contract with the National Research Council, which is the operating arm of the National Academy of Sciences. For $843,000, the NAS/NRC would have their Division of Medical Sciences conduct this evaluation (dubbed the Drug Efficacy Study) of all drugs marketed between 1938 and 1962, when the new efficacy provisions of the Kefauver-Harris Act kicked in. Thirty panels would be set up, each with six physician members who mainly were academic experts, to evaluate drugs in various medical areas, including psychiatry. The identity of the members was kept secret from the public at the time. Ten young physicians working for the Public Health Service in lieu of military service would do the legwork for the panels in finding scientific articles on efficacy, or the lack thereof, and the expert members of the panels would deliberate about how to classify the drugs according to categories of effectiveness that were determined by the FDA.

The National Academy of Sciences certainly did not see itself setting up a massive drug housecleaning. As R. Keith Cannan, head of the Division of Medical Sciences at NAS/NRC, said in March 1968, "I have heard it said that the recommendations of the Academy will be that such-and-such drug shall be removed from the market. . . . It will be only in that unusual situation in which all claims have been rejected that the Academy's report can be interpreted as a recommendation that the drug should be removed from the market."[15] This opinion in retrospect turned out to be either disingenuous or naïve.

On July 6, 1966, the FDA published a notice in the *Federal Register* telling companies that wanted to keep their drugs on the market to submit evidence of efficacy. As it turned out, 237 firms sent in information on 2,824 drug products, the majority of them prescription drugs but about 15 percent over-the-counter items as well. There was, of course, a lot of overlap among drugs. For example, 140 different preparations containing reserpine were sent in for review.[16] These nearly three thousand drugs represented around 90 percent of the drugs commonly marketed in the United States,[17] and so the NAS/NRC study was by no means a marginal exercise.

The FDA's classification system within which the panels were to rank each drug had the following four categories: effective, probably effective, possibly effective, and ineffective.[18] This sounds quite straightforward, but there were two problems with it:

One, in camera, the FDA developed a different system that used exactly the opposite interpretation of what was meant by the categories of "probably" and "possibly." As Herb Ley, then director of the FDA's Bureau of Medicine, the head office, casually explained to the agency's Advisory Committee on Abuse of Depressant and Stimulant Drugs, the main categories were "effective, possibly ineffective, and probably ineffective."[19] Possibly and probably, therefore, rather than suggesting approval of a drug with minor modifications, were death sentences.

Two, it is evident from some panel members' subsequent reports that the FDA did not share with the panels the consequences of a drug's being found "probably" or "possibly": According to the FDA's classification system, the possiblies would have 6 months to submit new data on efficacy; the probablies a year. If the evidence—in the form of controlled clinical trials—did not come in within that time, *the drug would be withdrawn.*[20] This short deadline—during which companies would need to design, power, conduct, analyze, and report on such trials—was unrealistic. Perhaps if the panels had known of these conditions, the process and outcome of the DES phase would have evolved differently. But only after most of the panels' evaluative work was done did these circumstances become public.

The work of the panels began in the fall of 1966 and was essentially completed by midsummer of 1968. Each panel met every 10 weeks or so, and considered anywhere from 50 to several hundred drugs. The documentation was often inadequate. When in 1971 one panel reconvened to rectify a classification error they had earlier committed (using a category the panels had invented called "yes, but . . ." that was useless to the FDA), panel members got the literature in advance on only two drugs. The chair of the panel told the NRC they would have to make assessments on the basis of their personal experience.[21] Even though the panels theoretically had the option of going to the agency's NDA files for further information, or of applying to the company directly, this almost never happened. (Smith, Kline & French, for example, with 41 dosage forms before the panels, was asked only two questions, both trivial.)[22] So what the panels relied on, basically, was the literature that the young doctors from the Public Health Service had managed to cobble together for them—which rarely contained proper statistical studies because there were so few at the time—plus their personal experience. FDA staffers later complained privately "that the panels' reports are frequently vague and self-contradictory, and that when hard documentation is lacking, they fall back . . . on the catch-all phrase 'informed opinion of the panel.'"[23]

There was one more intriguing wrinkle: the extent to which the Public Health Service doctors themselves came up with many panel recommendations, especially the fateful less-than-effectives. Joseph Cooper, chair of political science at Howard University and a consummate agency insider, later said, "There is a great mystery which surrounds the NAS/NRC methodology. The FDA itself was not fully aware . . . of the roles played by the young Public Health officers assigned by the FDA to the panels. To what extent did they write up the assessments of the 'probably effective' or 'possibly effective'? How much was delegated to them and how much sagacity was invested by busy panelists in these people? No one really knows. Perhaps the story will come out one day."[24]

On balance, the whole panel approach had some serious flaws. The "consensus" approach to science often produces horse-trading rather than scientific truths (just imagine a consensus panel deciding the speed of light). The acerbic William Wardell, pharmacologist at the University of Rochester, later said of the panels, ". . . Committees of experts may not be in a position to make decisions that are appropriate for individual physicians and individual patients (and in any case experts can, and often do, disagree violently among themselves). In the light of this it would seem questionable for such panel decisions to be binding on all physicians and all patients."[25]

As for disagreements among experts, years later Louis Lasagna, who like Wardell did not suffer fools gladly, did several mock-DES studies, using five internists and five pharmacologists (all of whom were at Hopkins), plus a number of former members of the actual DES panel in that area, depending on the drug. Their scores for Ritalin (methylphenidate), for example, were all over the map. "For seven of the 22 items, there was either at least one doctor who checked 'uncertain,' while at least one other checked 'strongly approve' or 'strongly disapprove,' or at least one physician who checked 'mildly approve' while another checked 'mildly disapprove.'"[26] An average of the scores would have been as useless as an average of proposed speeds of light.

Lasagna noted of the real DES panels, the "extraordinary degree of naiveté on the parts of the experts who constituted the panels."[27] So alarmed did the Drug Research Board of NAS/NRC become about the apparent cluelessness of the experts that in October 1970, it convened a special committee to consider the "probably" and "possibly" ratings. Said the *Pink Sheet*, the pharmaceutical insider newsletter, " . . . Some of the discussion at the Board meeting reflected the doubts that are being expressed in industry and in drug investigational circles on whether all panels—and their memberships—were fully aware of the 'consequences of their actions' when they sat in judgment on the efficacy of the pre-1962 drugs." The *Pink Sheet* continued, "There is a strong suspicion that at least some members of the NAS/NRC panels fell back on 'probably' and 'possibly' as the type of 'weasel words' which all MDs are prone to use, without a clear understanding of the legal effect that would be generated by use of the key words in the efficacy review."[28]

Was a rigorous application of the DES classification system distorted or undermined by committee politics? The word "Probably," said William Barclay, a vice-president of the American Medical Association who had served on one panel, was often the result of a compromise on the panel. "If all but one member of the panel found the drug effective, you compromise and find it 'probably effective.' You know how committees work."[29] Yes, indeed. But given the stakes, a modus less indulgent of these academic mannerisms might have been found.

The psychiatry panel had its own challenges. Head of the panel was the impish Daniel X. Freedman, who had just left Yale to become chair of psychiatry at Chicago and who would shortly take over editorship of the prestigious *Archives of General Psychiatry*. Coauthor of a well-known textbook, *The Theory and Practice of Psychiatry*, Freedman was among the stars of the discipline. He was described as "kind, very gentle, and extremely supportive."[30] The five other members of the panel included Jonathan Cole at Tufts University, who had been chief of the Psychopharmacology Service Center at the National Institute of Mental Health (and who had given grants for drug trials to the four other members of the panel); David Engelhardt, an internist who worked with psychiatric patients at Downstate Medical Center in Brooklyn of the State University of New York; Leo Hollister of the Veterans Administration hospital in Palo Alto, California, who was one of the senior figures in American psychopharmacology in those years; Sidney Merlis at the Central Islip State Hospital in Long Island; and Karl Rickels of the University of Pennsylvania, a veteran drug trialist. The panel was heavy on the academic side of psychopharmacology, light on the community side, a possible handicap in their evaluation of drugs used in outpatient psychiatry and family medicine.[31]

The panel had "quite a few meetings," according to Sidney Merlis, "in some building in Washington and we would have our homework assigned to us and we would do it and come back again. And there would be some correspondence between us and the chairman and he eventually, as I recall, ended up writing the summary reports of each of the drugs involved."

Merlis also recalled that Frances Kelsey, the FDA administrator who had kept the drug thalidomide off the American market (though not, alas, away from the patients who took it in medical trials), also attended some of the meetings.

The material the psychiatry panel had to go on was, in Merlis's words, "the medical literature that existed, which was relatively sparse, some data from the FDA, some data from the drug company, and a lot of anecdotal data from members of the committee." Another panel member, Jonathan Cole, recalled in a later interview how surprised the members were at the companies' lack of knowledge about their own drugs. "We were a bit irked at them for not documenting these indications more."[32]

Merlis was clear that the FDA in no sense gave the panel instructions on such matters as combination drugs (two different agents in a drug at a fixed ratio).[33] Nor did panel members have any contact with industry.

Asked about the consequences of giving a drug the recommendation of "possibly" or "probably" effective, some panel members thought nothing dire would occur. Said Leo Hollister in 1972, " . . . I had the distinct feeling that we viewed the ratings of 'possibly' and 'probably' effective in a positive rather than a negative light. Such a rating meant to us that the drug might very well be effective in some situations, but that the evidence presented in support of its indication didn't allow a more conclusive judgment. It did *not* mean, as so many make it seem, probably *in*effective."[34]

Freedman's own conception was that ratings of "probably" and "possibly" would, at most, prompt further studies.[35] Thus at the time, the panel evidently had no inkling of the draconian application that the FDA had in mind for these "gray" ratings.

How did things go on the psychiatry panel? Freedman was unhappy at many outcomes, he said afterward. "The final report, to my mind, was pushed. I would have preferred waiting a year or two longer. You couldn't because industry had to know, but I was very leery of a panel of experts at the very start. . . ." Freedman was sympathetic in particular to combos, many of which the various panels, and then the FDA, slaughtered mercilessly: "There are aspects of medical practice which explain why it is convenient to have something in one package to give to patients, rather than 10 pills."[36] In 1969, after the NAS/NRC phase was essentially over, Freedman told Congress, "There are some very good (psychotropic) drugs backed up by very little objective data," implying that he was unhappy with the tendency to judge the drugs in terms of the quality of the evidence rather than the quality of the drug.[37]

Of the drugs the psychiatry panel assessed, how many were later withdrawn from the market during the DESI phase? We look first at drugs containing a single active ingredient:

Of the 18 antineurotic, or meprobamate-style, drugs, 67 percent were later withdrawn.[38] Hard hit were such chemical classes as the carbamates, with emylcamate (Striatran) and hydroxyphenamate (Listica) taken off the market; likewise the diphenylmethane derivatives, with benactyzine (a tranquilizer ingredient of the meprobamate combo Deprol) and captodiame (Ayerst's Suvren) withdrawn. Mephenesin, the drug that launched the tranquilizers, went down the tubes. Of the antineurotics, meprobamate was the main member to survive the two-thirds purge.

Of 12 antipsychotics the panel considered, only 2 were later removed from market, doubtless a reflection of the panel's own experiences in treating serious illness. The 2 were mepazine (Warner-Chilcott's Pacatal), which psychiatrist Donald Klein once called "distinguished for being the only phenothiazine that just didn't work."[39] The second was azacyclonal, a diphenylmethane derivative that Merrell marketed as Frenquel. New York psychiatrist and veteran psychopharmacologist William Karliner had dismissed it saying, "It has failed to benefit any of my patients."[40] The panel's calls on the antipsychotics were thus probably pretty good, because the phenothiazines in general were seen as effective drugs and the members' own clinical experience came into play.

Yet in the phenothiazines the panel made one huge change, removing the anxiety and depression indications. From the launch of chlorpromazine in 1954 on, the phenothiazines had been widely used as anxiolytics. The panel's main evidence for this sweeping change was "clinical experience."[41] Jon Cole later said of this decision, "We felt they probably worked but we weren't sure that it was appropriate to use them [for anxiety] because of the side effects. And we may have been wrong in that, but that was, I think, probably our position."[42] Rightly or wrongly, the prescribing of chlorpromazine-style drugs for psychoneurotic illness came to an end. Henceforth the phenothiazines would be accepted almost exclusively only for psychosis. Smith, Kline & French got a deferment and continued to advertise chlorpromazine for "chronic neurotic anxiety," noting that DESI finds it only "possibly" effective; so "possibly" was pitched to the public as "not too bad," whereas the FDA meant by it "possibly not too good."[43]

Then the psychiatry panel looked at a mixed bag of agents.

All three barbiturates that the panel examined—secobarbital, talbutal, and butabarbital—stayed on the market. The panel didn't look at the other members of this class, many of which had been marketed before 1938. Jon Cole said that the FDA's view of what constituted an "old drug" was "one that was on a 3x5 card in a card box kept by Ralph Smith of the FDA." The psychiatry panel didn't consider the "drugs that he thought had been in use and effective for a long period of time." Hence, the barbiturates, at that point, did not come under scrutiny.[44]

Of the nine stimulants the panel considered as mood-changers and not as appetite suppressants, eight remained on the market (pipradrol, marketed in the United States as Meratran, drew a "possibly" and was gone by 1974).[45] This assessment corresponded to the balance of opinion in psychopharmacology in those years that believed the stimulants effective in mild depression.

The panel looked at three monoamine oxidase inhibitors (MAOIs), two of which ultimately survived DESI scrutiny and stayed on the market but only for highly circumscribed indications: tranylcypromine (Parnate) and phenelzine (Nardil). Pfizer withdrew nialamide (Niamid) in 1974 after the panel gave it a "possibly." Two tricyclic antidepressants the panel examined—imipramine (Tofranil) and amitriptyline (Elavil)—passed with flying colors.

Most of the wreckage wrought by the psychiatry panel—and by the later DESI exercise as a whole—was in the combination drugs, a mainstay of American family medicine, representing over half the pharmaceutical products sold nationwide.[46] In psychopharmacology, typical combos involved a tranquilizer such as meprobamate plus an anticholinergic (acetylcholine blocker), or a barbiturate sedative and an anticholinergic. They were usually prescribed not by psychiatrists but by internists and family physicians for nervous stomachs and nervous bowels, or a tranquilizer plus a heart drug for nervous hearts. The FDA's Advisory Committee on Abuse of Depressant and Stimulant Drugs had just cleared the combos of involvement in drug abuse, and there was actually no pressing policy reason for abolishing them.[47]

Of the seven combo antineurotics the panel examined, five were later withdrawn. One of these was Enarax, a combo of hydroxyzine (an antianxiety drug) and oxyphencyclimine (an anticholinergic agent), which Pfizer had marketed for the treatment of peptic ulcer disease. Anxiety was thought (probably incorrectly) a cause of ulcers, and the anticholinergic reduced the ulceration by slowing the secretion of stomach acid. The drug had been quite successful, but the NAS/NRC gastrointestinal panel gave it only a "probably" on peptic ulcer, and the psychiatry panel, somewhat over their heads with this drug used mainly in family medicine, said they didn't really know. They didn't agree with the package statement that hydroxyzine was a useful anxiolytic, and thought its effect mainly sedative.[48] There was then much toing and fro-ing between Pfizer and the FDA, leading to the ultimate withdrawal of Enarax in 1983.

Wallace Labs' Deprol and Ayerst's PMB survived the psychiatry panel's combo purge of the antineurotics. Deprol, marketed in 1957, contained meprobamate and benactyzine, PMB meprobamate and estrogen. The panel gave the Deprol combo only a "possibly," convinced that meprobamate was a useful antidepressant but dubious of the validity of mixing it with another weakly antidepressant drug.[49] (Benactyzine was in fact a very active anticholinergic that desynchronized the electroencephalograph.) Wallace then asked Karl Rickels to undertake a controlled trial of the combo, which was positive.[50] The FDA let Deprol stay on the market with a black-box warning that an NAS/NRC review had rated it only "possibly."

All three of the combo antipsychotics the psychiatry panel evaluated were subsequently withdrawn, as were the three barbiturate combos and four of the five stimulant combos. Smith, Kline & French's Eskatrol Spansules (dextroamphetamine and prochlorperazine), which had been on the market since 1959, survived DESI but not later addictiveness concerns.[51]

Why did this wreckage ultimately occur among the combos? It was partly due to a hostility at the FDA that Louis Lasagna called "out of touch, at the very least, with a significant segment of medical practice."[52] It was also due to expediency. Although the anticombo theme had been building in American pharmacology throughout the 1960s, it became a rigid doctrine because the agency because simply couldn't cope with the avalanche of NAS/NRC recommendations now descending on it, plus the appeals of the companies, the requests for hearings, and the whole administrative traffic this enormous review had generated. As Herb Ley, who succeeded James Goddard as FDA commissioner from mid-1968 through late 1969, said somewhat incautiously about "a mixture of two agents," in front of a microphone at a meeting in 1971, "The FDA's reaction at that time was one of, I would say, expediency. It was felt that if some major change were not instituted, the whole hearing procedure and the regulatory response on this NAS/NRC review would be delayed, probably for decades."[53] Thus the psychiatry panel's recommended dumping of what had been a highly useful drug class was possibly initiated, and certainly endorsed, by an agency that had simply bitten off more than it could chew, and had no qualms about pulling the plug on the class for reasons of bureaucratic convenience.

In sum, of the 60 psychopharmacological drugs commonly used in psychiatry, internal medicine, and family medicine in the 1950s and the early 1960s, the psychiatry panel of the NAS/NRC review caused 45 percent to be withdrawn. That is almost half of the total formulary. To be sure, the single-agent drugs were treated more gingerly: Only 34 percent of them were withdrawn as a result of regulatory action in the following decade. Eighty-five percent of the combos were removed from the market, wiping out a drug class that had stood physicians and patients in good stead for many years.[54]

Gotcha!

This brings us to DESI, which the FDA used greatly to enlarge its control over the American pharmaceutical industry and the drug supply. To cope with the mass of NAS/NRC reports, in 1968 the agency set up a DESI Task Force within the Office of Director of the Bureau of Drugs; the task force started with 5 professional and support staff, but quickly expanded to a team of 50 people.[55]

At first, the pharmaceutical industry was shocked at seeing many profitable agents threatened with disappearance on the grounds that panels of academic experts, more out of personal experience than scientific evidence, thought them unworthy. The quality of the drugs in question seemed to have little to do with it. Herb Ley later said, " . . . The issue is not whether the drug is effective" but whether there are controlled trials "to support the claims made for the product." Lasagna expostulated that most of the antibiotics had had no controlled trials and still were effective.[56]

The agency first reached out its big paw in February 1968, revoking many of the "not-new drug" letters it had issued between 1938 and 1962, generally in cases in which the agency had received a supplementary request from a pharmaceutical company for a me-too drug already covered by the NDA of a pioneer drug, and in which "the drug was generally recognized as safe under the approved labeling." Those pre–Kefauver-Harris letters, of course, did not cover efficacy, and now they were revoked.[57] This edict evoked great consternation among industry.

Originally, industry had the right to request hearings, on the model of the meprobamate and Librium-Valium hearings of 1966. But by 1968 this right was beginning to be eroded, with the suggestion that if you, as a manufacturer, made too much trouble, your drug's NDA would simply be withdrawn.[58] Those manufacturers who still persisted in confronting FDA decisions faced an uphill battle. In October 1969 the Upjohn Company challenged the DESI decision to withdraw a profitable antibiotic combo marketed under the name Panalba. Upjohn lost in court, and the Panalba decision gave the FDA the right to decide whether a company's evidence even justified a hearing. If the evidence was not in the form of a controlled trial—not the clinical impressions the agency had previously accepted—the hearing would be denied. On May 8, 1970, the FDA announced that henceforth only clinical trials would be acceptable in fulfillment of the Kefauver-Harris request for "adequate and well-controlled investigations."[59] This edict, upheld by a Supreme Court decision in June 1973, made the placebo-controlled clinical trial the gold standard for the evaluation of all drugs that had ever been on the American market. Early in the 1970s, in DESI appeals, this requirement was expanded from one trial to two.[60] And it was pointless to appeal:[61] By 1984 only five hearings had been granted.[62] The FDA's power over the existing drug supply was by that point absolute.

In getting to that end, however, the FDA had to take other steps toward centralizing agency control over pharmaceuticals. One of those steps was abolishing the "grandfather clause" and making all drugs, whenever they had been launched, "new drugs." During the 1962 legislative wrangling that led to the Kefauver-Harris Amendments, the agency had successfully lobbied against grandfathering post-1938 drugs and exempting them from efficacy review. But by at least 1968 voices within the FDA—notably that of the aggressive counsel William Goodrich—were arguing against grandfathering on a broader scale.[63] It was in 1974 that the agency decided to end all pleas for exemption on the grounds that one's drug had appeared before 1938; put another way, the FDA started requiring NDAs for any prescription drug, no matter how long it had been out in the market, for which there was any question of efficacy for any indication.[64] Louis Lasagna, now at the University of Rochester, said that the FDA's view that old and new drugs must be judged by the same standards, "smacks of pathological even-handedness. . . . Old drugs . . . have one advantage over new drugs—a track record. A drug that has been taken by many thousands or millions of patients and prescribed by doctors for years is hardly in the same position as one that has not." "Is it desirable," he asked, "to have time-tested remedies taken off the market because the manufacturer is unwilling or unable to perform new trials?"[65]

Between October 1967 and April 1969, the NAS/NRC panels had forwarded to the FDA 2,824 reports on 4,349 drugs.[66] Processing these was now a major bureaucratic headache. Yet the exercise was not unwelcome because at the end of DESI, the agency's size and powers had grown enormously. By October 1976, the staff within the Bureau of Drugs ("BuDrugs") devoted to DESI had increased to 437, up from 5 in 1968. An earlier legal decision had set up an exact timetable and the agency was now pouring out rulings.[67] The 6-month deadline for companies to submit additional trial data for the possiblies (i.e., the FDA's possibly ineffective) had been recognized as unrealistic and companies now had to negotiate on an individual basis with "BuDrugs" for extensions,[68] thus prolonging the DESI process for a decade.

What is interesting for our story is that, among its various rulings, the agency belched forth pronouncements about drugs that the psychiatry panel of NAS/NRC had never considered. In April 1971, for example, the agency found the reserpine derivative deserpidine probably effective for some indications, possibly for others, including "mild anxiety states,"[69] but ended up withdrawing its previously approved NDA. The NAS/NRC psychiatry panel had never considered deserpidine, which Abbott marketed as Harmonyl with the hook, "Are your hypertensives troubled with lethargy?" The agency decision here was not on the basis of the psychiatry panel's recommendations, and so arbitrarily withdrawing an existing NDA represented a gratuitous extension of Food and Drug's bureaucratic authority.

The psychiatry panel never considered chlordiazepoxide (Librium); nor for that matter did they pass judgment on any other benzodiazepines because most postdated the 1962 cutoff date for the DES review. Yet in 1972, the FDA of its own hook labeled Librax, a combo of chlordiazepoxide and clidinium bromide (an anticholinergic) that Hoffmann-La Roche had brought out in 1965 for anxiety and gastric distress, only a "possibly" and withdrew its approved NDA, on the logic that Librax was in a NAS/NRC-reviewed category.[70] So if any NAS/NRC panel had even considered a drug class, the agency bureaucrats felt free on their own to withdraw members of that class.

One final example: In 1959 Hoffmann-La Roche introduced isocarboxazid (Marplan), an MAOI, as a "mood regulator." Various clinicians thought quite highly of it, and Jon Cole said, "That's the only time I've ever used what I guess might be insider knowledge to think about [buying stock in] a drug."[71] The NAS/NRC psychiatry panel did not review isocarboxazid. In April 1975, the FDA asked its Psychopharmacological Agents Advisory Subcommittee whether it should include isocarboxazid in a review, given that it was wrestling with two other members of the MAOI drug class—Nardil and Parnate—that the NAS/NRC psychiatry panel had considered. What the subcommittee responded is unclear.[72] In October 1976, the FDA withdrew the approval of isocarboxazid's NDA, claiming "that substantial evidence of effectiveness of the drug is lacking." There were, to be sure, eight controlled studies, four of which showed some effect, but four did not.[73] (The underpowered studies of those days often showed no effect over placebo, but this is simply because too few patients were included in the trial to show small but important differences, i.e., less than penicillin-scale.)[74] This was setting the bar very high. If the American pharmacopoeia had been subjected to such rigor across the board, the nation would have been left treating itself with mint tea. (And nothing approaching this requirement was ever applied to any SSRI, or Prozac-style drug; see Chapter 8.)

The FDA subsequently, in 1979, reversed itself on Marplan, allowing it to stay on the market with a warning showing "probably" effective.[75] The FDA-mandated black-box label on the drug said, "Based on a review of this drug by the National Academy of Sciences-National Research Council and/or other information, FDA has classified the indications as follows. . . ."[76] But this was flummery. The agency regulators themselves, like restless cowboys, were wandering about the herd, picking out drugs that struck their fancy, and withdrawing NDAs.

Under the cover of DESI, agency administrators went to the psychopharmacological drug stock and began removing items that seemed to them, as individuals, questionable. All of this occurred without legal protection for industry, now unable to appeal save with evidence of new, expensive controlled trials.

If these drugs were so important, why didn't industry spring for clinical trials that might have established their efficacy? The answer is that the patents were running out, or had run out. Why spend money on expensive new trials when generic competition would merely piggyback on the trials and carve up the market as soon as the patent expired? In general, industry preferred to move on rather than to fight rear-guard actions that would not increase shareholder value.

Yet many of the products that DESI scythed away were effective drugs, and even after being forgotten, they did not lose their efficacy. Of Alertonic, a combo that the William Merrell Company introduced in 1957 containing pipradrol with vitamins and minerals and scorned by the psychiatry panel as "ineffective," Jon Cole later said, "It's a lifesaving drug, because it kept [nursing home] people from getting venous thrombosis."[77] This is worth something.

In DESI as a whole, the FDA removed many more drugs that it ever let on. In an unpublished assessment in 1978, Robert Temple, then acting director of the FDA's Office of Drug Research, said that only 12 percent of the drugs the panels reviewed were found effective for all indications and another 47 percent found effective for some of the claimed indications. That is 59 percent of the total drug supply in 1968 that somehow survived.

Yet here is the problematic aspect: Of the remaining 41 percent originally considered "ineffective," "possibly," or "probably," only an eighth ultimately won upgrades to "effective." Many of those original possiblies and probablies resulted, as we have seen, from panel dynamics rather than from evidence of a genuine lack of efficacy. Yet few of the less-than-effective drugs were ever rescued. As Temple put it, "The 18 years of effort to upgrade less than effective products by the sponsors have resulted in a total, as of January [1984], of 214 upgradings, about 15% of the nearly 1400 products that were considered less than effective."[78] To my knowledge this statistic was never made public. It is a testimony to the sacking of the nation's drug supply that nearly half of it was eliminated by a bureaucratic machine running out of control. Psychopharmacology was no less affected than other areas of the drug supply.

Industry found the highhandedness and inflexibility of the agency maddening. Of the 11 "Federal Register" notices that Smith, Kline & French received, only 1 drug was deemed effective, 4 or 5 ineffective; the rest were "probablies" and "possiblies." One of the company's executives said in 1971 that they thought there had been an error, "but we have met with a nondecision, with no reaction whatever over a period of 5 months." The company thought studies were unnecessary, a point that the review officers at the agency agreed with. But these review officers were unwilling to take the company's case "upstairs" because they knew what the FDA leadership wanted. Said the executive, "What is at issue is the inflexibility further down the line where nobody really wants to take all that upstairs in the system and fight it out for you because, after all, if you will just do the studies they [the reviewers] will be better off."[79]

Many physicians as well were upset at this bureaucratic highhandedness, because it denied them drugs with which they and their patients had long felt comfortable. One outraged Texas internist expostulated to his congressman, John Young, about "the dangerous legal implications to the physician who prescribes medications listed by the FDA as 'possibly' or 'probably' effective. From my personal experience, John, after 32 years of practice, I can *personally* verify that some drugs listed as 'possibly' or 'probably' effective are *very definitely useful* in the treatment of the disease . . . for which they are indicated. It is time you men of Congress demand that H.E.W. departments cease legislation by edict and regulation—a function limited by law to Congress only."[80] There were many such protests from across the country.

Was the Food and Drug Administration's DESI merely bureaucratic overkill, or was it part of a larger effort on the part of the agency to aggrandize its own power? A good deal of evidence points to the latter.

For one thing, the FDA saw a need to strengthen its bureaucratic reach. In these years, industry's acceptance of FDA control was often begrudging and conditional. There was a sense among insiders that if the companies decided massively to reject FDA authority, they could get away with it. Nobody would ever say something like this publicly. Yet when Robert Tutag, president of a small pharmaceutical firm, the S. J. Tutag Company in Detroit, came to Washington for a conference in 1973 with the FDA about other companies' unfair competition in marketing generic chlorpromazine for non-DESI indications, there was a hint of threat at the table. Said Tutag, according to a memorandum of the conference, " . . . If a positive reaction is not taken against the illegal marketing of a unique product such as chlorpromazine, this would encourage industry to proliferate the marketing of drugs under DESI review . . . since industry would feel FDA is not vigorously enforcing DESI provisions for marketing." Tutag said it would be tempting to market such drugs as chlordiazepoxide (Hoffman-La Roche's Librium) and imipramine (Geigy's Tofranil) outside of FDA control. This, he pointed out, "would increase FDA's regulatory problems. Ultimately, FDA would lose control of the marketing of generic drugs across the board."

Present on the FDA side at the meeting were Albert Lavender, head of the DESI Regulatory Control Staff, the unit responsible for dealing with industry, and Theodore Byers, director of the Office of Compliance. Byers rather lamely explained to Tutag that up to now the FDA had directed its compliance efforts toward the "ineffective" drugs rather than toward the dodgy "possibly" (and very profitable) indications that otherwise effective drugs such as chlorpromazine had received. Tutag told Byers there was big money at stake here: " . . . Most firms would be willing to trade off an ineffective drug . . . for an effective, high market volume item such as hydrochlorothiazide [a popular diuretic]."[81] In clear text: Companies would take the hit on drugs classed "ineffective" as long as they could continue to market profitable "possiblies" and "probablies," given that the FDA wasn't cracking down on the latter. Bottom line: We in industry are capable of defying you if commercial considerations drive us to it.

So talk of the FDA's "imperial" ambition was not just metaphorical. In the early 1970s the agency's authority over this teeming, restless pharmaceutical industry, experiencing historic growth of billions of dollars, was still tentative. But that was going to change. Any agency official who chanced to glance at this memo would have muttered, "Tutag, baby, it ain't gonna happen."

Within the FDA itself, this sense of muscle flexing was almost palpable. The mood was, We're going to show industry who's boss! As Lavender preened to his fellow regulators several months after the Tutag conference: "This policy in dealing with industry has given the program a credibility of handling DESI compliance matters in a no nonsense manner, which approach has proven very successful." He continued, "It is our view that this undertaking has had a greater compliance impact on the regulated industry than any other program in the history of the Food and Drug Administration."[82]

It was not lost on others that DESI represented a signal opportunity to expand FDA power. Members of Congress were suspicious. "My dear Charles," Durward Hall, a congressman from Missouri, wrote then FDA Commissioner Charles Edwards in December 1972, " . . . I'm concerned that you might be overstepping your bounds, and limiting the capability of physicians by fiat and decree rather than following legislative intent." Hall wished Edwards season's greetings: "May you have fruition of your dreams."[83]

In power over industry, control of the "labeling," a drug's uses, was crucial. Before 1962, the FDA did not control the indications listed on the label, because its prime mission was checking for safety, not efficacy, and labeling is an efficacy issue. After Kefauver-Harris, the FDA acquired control over a drug's uses. Alexander Schmidt, FDA commissioner between 1973 and 1976, the height of the DES implementation years, later said, "One of the things I tried to do was to change the agency in such a way that I could stay at its head. . . . FDA had the labeling regulations and, of all of the tools FDA has, one of the most valuable is the labeling regs. The use of those regs became a very fine art. And the people who were sophisticated and good enough to understand the use of the labeling regs, fended off any challenge to the agency's authority to declare what was a proper or an improper label."

"What sort of challenge?" an interviewer asked him. Such as maybe sharing labeling authority with the *United States Pharmacopoeia* (an independent, nonprofit organization that sets standards for all medications)?

Schmidt replied, "To give up to them the authority to label . . . would be giving away the ship."[84]

There was a deliberateness about the FDA's imperial growth. Clark Havighurst, law professor at Duke and director of the university's committee on legal issues in health care, called attention at a conference in 1971 to the agency's decision to muscle-flex. "There is in the legislation no direction to the agency that it must proceed against all 2800 pre-1962 drugs, and indeed the agency waited from 1962 to 1966 before doing anything at all. The law says only that the FDA *has the authority* to disapprove a drug if it finds substantial evidence of efficacy to be lacking."[85]

What forces at the FDA might have driven this activism, at the beginning of the agency's phenomenal growth during the DESI period? First, the agency's lawyers were behind this great leap forward. The senior legal leadership—not necessarily Kennedyesque New Frontier types—breathed the dynamism of the 1960s and its optimism about the ability of government to take on big jobs. As general counsel William Goodrich later said, "I know when I was there it was a can-do organization. . . . Everything that came along nobody else would do it. We would end up doing it."[86] Goodrich had at the time a reputation for relentless activism. As the *Pink Sheet* put it in 1970, "Goodrich has developed quite a reputation in his own right for extending the boundaries of FDA regulatory controls by the creative development of new legal approaches."[87] Goodrich's successor as general counsel, Peter Barton Hutt, also aggressively helped expand the agency in the 1970s. Thus, DESI seems to have stemmed from *un excès de zèle* of its lawyer-leadership for inside-the-Beltway power games.

There was also something restlessly expansive about the medical leadership of the agency. Regulatory scholar Paul Quirk attributed this drive for control over the pharmaceutical industry to the predominance of physicians within FDA leadership and reviewing teams. Filled with a sense of mission about public health, said Quirk, "the agency has often been willing to ignore or evade the apparent limitations on its legal authority." Many of the agency's actions, such as postapproval monitoring, occurred "without much support in the words of the statute or the legislative history."[88] This is certainly true of DESI, whose originators grabbed the ball and ran with it.

It is difficult to tease out imperial ambitions from a legitimate concern for the public health. FDA administrators do not earn large salaries, and many are motivated by genuine idealism. Yet idealism is woven of many strands, and the closer to the Beltway one gets, the more numerous become those strands. But however idealistic the motives of some, DESI had a negative impact on psychotherapeutics and thus subtracted from the public health rather than adding to it.

Epilogue

How did the first drug set do in terms of the NAS/NRC evaluation and the FDA's subsequent implementation? Not very well. We've already touched on the outcome of some of them, but let's review the results more closely.

Mephenesin, Frank Berger's baby, was toast. Launched in 1954, it was considered in 1968 by various panels to be "obsolete," of too brief duration, and "clinically ineffective." In a perfect world, there would have been curiosity about the mechanism of action of this drug that could give peace if only briefly to spastic twitching and tics. It was withdrawn in 1970.[89]

As for meprobamate, psychiatry's first blockbuster drug, the FDA had tried to sink it on the grounds of potential addictiveness in the 1966 hearings (Chapter 4), but the drug staggered on in appeals until, losing those, it was listed in 1970 as a controlled and dangerous substance subject to abuse. It made it through the DESI process with its wings further clipped. The evidence of its effectiveness in anxiety-tension was overwhelming. But all other indications (e.g., mood disorders) were removed from the label, which was also toned down.[90] Meprobamate was rapidly losing ground to Librium and Valium anyway.

Methylphenidate (Ritalin), launched in 1955 as an antidepressant and then later the drug of choice for attention deficit hyperactivity disorder (ADHD), was scratched as an antidepressant, though evidence in favor of that indication was impressive. It remained on the market for narcolepsy and hyperactivity in children.[91]

Iproniazid (Marsilid), launched in 1957 as the first of the inhibitors of monoamine oxidase, had already been withdrawn by the time of DESI, in what was probably an unbalanced weighing of its risk of liver toxicity versus its benefit. It was a highly effective antidepressant in some ill-defined subpopulation. Among the later MAOIs, the psychiatry panel found nialamide (Pfizer's Niamid), launched in 1959, "possibly effective" for depression and everything else; it was withdrawn in 1974.[92] Phenelzine (Warner-Chilcott's Nardil), also approved in 1959, made it through the DESI process more or less intact, though it got a prominent warning about hypertensive crises (the "cheese effect") that would have scared many prescribers away.[93] It's still on the market today.

For another MAOI—Smith, Kline & French's tranylcypromine (Parnate), launched in the United States in 1961, the psychiatry panel gave it a "probably," though they evidently didn't realize that in FDA-speak that was a death sentence. The agency was prepared to shut down this highly useful agent for serious depression, but the company did more trials and finally got it through. Bizarrely, today the FDA insists that Parnate is not to be used for melancholia, whereas historically the NAS/NRC psychiatry panel thought it was "probably" useful precisely for "severe" depressions that did not respond to ECT.[94]

Thus, of the MAOIs on the market by 1961, two did not survive the regulatory process and three others, including Hoffmann-La Roche's Marplan (isocarboxazid), came through somehow askew. This was not a triumph for American drug regulation.

What else? Imipramine, the first of the tricyclic antidepressants, launched on the U.S. market in 1959, got thumbs up for depression without any problem, as did the TCA amitriptyline. The antimanic drug lithium was not marketed until 1970 and was not considered by the NAS/NRC panel.

Finally, in terms of the first drug set, the phenothiazine antipsychotics lost the depression and anxiety indications, a highly questionable decision in view of yards of research that showed them useful in serious depression and anxiety. The psychiatry panel gave chlorpromazine a "probably" for "involutional psychoses" (meaning depression in midlife),[95] doubtless believing they were displaying a thoughtful awareness of nuance, unaware that they had just given this drug class the kiss of death for use in depressive disorders, in which the phenothiazines have in fact considerable effectiveness. Chlorpromazine and its cousins remained on the market mainly for psychosis and mania.

The DESI exercise thus had a devastating impact on the first drug set, discarding indications of demonstrated validity and weakening, often on specious grounds, important drug classes by withdrawing them from the market or by black-boxing them into desuetude. DESI was a poster-person example of bureaucratic meddling in relationships based on trust: that of medical practitioners in life-restoring medications; that of patients in the confidence that their physicians will prescribe safe and effective drugs. In subjecting the practice of psychiatry to the oversight, first of federal regulators, later, of federal drug cops, the FDA achieved the antithesis of its supposed mission of safeguarding the public health.

DESI had important consequences for the subsequent history of psychopharmacology. In the 1970s and after, emphasis in drug development was to drift ever more toward "antidepressant drugs." Indeed, from the 1990s on, psychopharmacology was dominated by the theme of depression and its vanquishment. This evolution proved portentous for psychiatry and psychopharmacology as the depression theme drowned out every other save psychosis. This started with DESI.

So keen was the FDA to limit the label of drugs to indications sanctioned by the NAS/NRC panels, that the bureaucrats increasingly saw "depression" as the one indication that seemed solid amidst the tossing overboard of "nervousness," "hysteria," and the like. A DESI ruling of August 26, 1970, was headed "Antidepressant Drugs." The agency was prepared to accept the TCAs imipramine (Tofranil) and amitriptyline (Elavil) for the relief of depression, mainly of the endogenous variety, and for no other indication. The notice continued, in bureaucratic boilerplate, "If the article [drug] is labeled or advertised for use in any condition other than those provided for in this announcement, it may be regarded as an unapproved new drug subject to regulatory proceedings. . . ."[96] This meant that the FDA would register imipramine-style drugs only for depression, nothing else. Control of the label, in this case, turned out to mean control of the field, which increasingly became the "antidepressant" field.

Many years after these events, Jon Cole said that DESI had indeed helped anchor concepts such as "antipsychotic" and "antidepressant," as though such drugs represented magic bullets against the diseases of "psychosis" and "depression," and as though these were illness entities as rock-solid as mumps and measles. "The studies [later drug trials] were done with those ideas in mind and therefore the only good evidence was for these actions, and these names [antipsychotic, antidepressant] were given, and in fact I have so far never seen a published study . . . of an antipsychotic versus placebo in depression that wasn't positive. . . . I think most of these drugs work across a spectrum of cases and are not anywhere near as specific as the nomenclature . . . suggests they are."[97]

Thus with DESI the concept of the "tranquilizer," the drug that worked across a spectrum of nervous illnesses, was definitively dead. Henceforth, magic bullets would match disease labels: There would be only anxiolytics for anxiety, antidepressants for depression, and antipsychotics for what everybody was calling "schizophrenia."

7

"The Plague of Affective Disorders"

Frank Berger said of the 1970s, when he was on staff in the department of psychiatry at the University of Louisville, "My feeling was that most people we saw had really no psychiatric disorders. They were people, in my opinion, with problems of living, people who did not get on with their spouses, did not get on with their children, did not get on with their boss, and had not been taught, had not been educated, had not been prepared to handle all these crises of life. So they got stressed, broke down, and had to see a doctor, and the doctor did not know what to do. So he put one of the psychiatric names on them."[1]

But some of Berger's patients in Louisville had real illnesses, not just problems in living. If they're going to be medicated properly, they need a proper diagnosis. What does Nature recognize?

There is melancholic illness, a biological disorder characterized by high levels of cortisol, slowed thinking and movement, and almost delusive ideas about what a terrible person one is and how worthless one's life has been; over the years it has been called various terms, among them "endogenous depression." Beneath this clear and relatively homogeneous entity of melancholia, there is everything else, a kind of nonmelancholic market basket, in which we find people with a depressive personality style (constitutional depression); people who are depressed because they have been dumped by a lover or have experienced some other life setback (reactive depression); and people who are depressed and anxious at the same time (mixed anxiety-depression). It's important to sort out correctly the contents of this basket of nonmelancholia because it could affect the treatment.[2]

This need to have a correct diagnosis before beginning treatment has been recognized for many years in psychiatry. As Henry Wetherill, a psychiatrist at the Pennsylvania Hospital in Philadelphia, said in 1889, "It should always be the aim of the practitioner to have a scientific motive for every dose prescribed, as it is far safer and more honest to leave Nature to struggle single handed with the malady than to medicate haphazard."[3]

In the days of psychoanalysis, patients exhibiting some aspect of the nonmelancholic market basket would have received a diagnosis of "psychoneurosis." Those with more serious symptoms were frequently packed off to mental institutions where they were treated with a variety of therapeutic approaches, including whatever medications were available at that time. Their diagnoses ranged from madness to melancholia.

Before 1950, the diagnosis didn't matter that much because the available drugs were relatively nonspecific. Barbiturates calmed just about everyone, whatever their diagnosis, and stimulants gingered them up. Then with the profusion of effective new drugs hitting the marketplace in the 1950s and '60s, it did start to matter what one prescribed. As psychiatrists Donald Goodwin and Samuel Guze at Washington University ("Wash U") in St. Louis said in 1974, "With the discovery of relatively specific drug therapies, diagnosis had become *practical*. With the availability of lithium and neuroleptic drugs, distinguishing between mania and schizophrenia—once an interesting academic exercise—might now determine how a patient was treated."[4]

Meanwhile, in the early 1970s the American Psychiatric Association (APA) decided that a new set of psychiatric diagnoses, or nosology, was needed. This led to a revision of their *Diagnostic and Statistical Manual of Mental Disorders*, the first edition of which, subsequently baptized *DSM-I*, had appeared in 1952. There had been a second edition (*DSM-II*) in 1968, even more skewed toward psychoanalysis than the first. The third edition, *DSM-III*, would appear in 1980.

DSM-III is the key to understanding why the diagnosis of depression has become so common in our own time. It was not merely due to the wicked pharmaceutical industry, flinging unwanted compounds at us for depression. As we have seen, industry was forced by the Food and Drug Administration in the DESI exercise to produce "antidepressants," because no other drugs would somehow pass muster at the regulators'. But in addition, the psychiatric profession forced the diagnosis of depression upon itself. And they did so by coining a term, "major depression," that was so broadly defined as to be applicable to almost any conceivable set of symptoms, including the market basket of non-melancholia—precisely what Frank Berger saw in Louisville. Major depression served the then-nascent field of biological psychiatry in the way that psychoneurosis had once served psychoanalysis. And drugs supposedly specific for depression focused the optic: If all you have are antidepressants (given that by the early 1970s the benzodiazepines had been declared terribly addictive), everything you see looks like depression. If all you have is a hammer, everything looks like a nail.

Let's take as an example a group of patients who for the most part may have had nothing at all but seemed to be just crying out for a "depression" diagnosis. Dr. Daniel Greenwald at the Carrier Clinic in New Jersey will help us. Around 1978, as the drafting of *DSM-III* was lurching into its final stages, he told psychiatrist Robert Spitzer, director of the project, that "the most important problem I had with DSM-II is not addressed by DSM-III at all. It concerns a condition I can describe as follows: The patients are mostly women between the ages of 18 and 35. . . ." What was the problem with them?

> They have no true process [schizophrenic] thought disorders, although their thinking shows much distortion and irrationality. . . . Many have delusions and a few have had hallucinations. The delusions are often those of wish-fulfillment, disappointment or abandonment. Affect is responsive to the environment. It is not flat. It is often disproportionate, histrionic or manipulating and may, therefore, be considered inappropriate in duration or amount; but affect is not flat and is not inappropriate in the way of the silly giggle or the nervous laugh of the simple schizophrenic. . . . They are often autistic in that they cannot act in response to the desires of others; yet they have tremendous dependency needs and respond quickly to criticism, disappointment, frustration or abandonment by meaningful others. They show a great deal of concern with issues of separation and closeness. They may show great anger for loved ones who disappoint them.

Any other characteristics of these women, Dr. Greenwald?

"Most [of these female] patients have premorbid histories involving exaggerated dependency needs or histrionic character structures. They have been gregarious in the past and thrived on the company of others. Many have tempestuous interpersonal relationships, poor impulse control and poor ability to tolerate frustrations. . . . They are sometimes called manic depressed." Yet treating them with lithium, said Dr. Greenwald, often produced "ambiguous results." He didn't like the diagnosis "schizo-affective" for them: "This term is at best a horrible misnomer, since they are neither schizophrenic nor do they have an effective [*sic*] disorder." Dr. Greenwald thought "hysterical psychosis" the best diagnosis, yet the condition "is not even listed in the [draft] DSM-III." Therefore, "A clinician who thinks the condition is hysterical psychosis must call it 'other.'"[5]

Why "must"? No treatment without a diagnosis, remember? And since 1952 psychiatry has derived its diagnoses from the homegrown American *DSM* system, whose classification of diseases has uses in psychiatric epidemiology, in basic and clinical mental health research, and in clinical practice, where it is intended to enable practitioners to identify a condition, determine treatment for it, and claim reimbursement from health insurance carriers for that treatment. In all of its uses, the manual is supposed to enable consistent communication among various professionals by establishing a standardized diagnostic nomenclature. But earlier editions of the *DSM*, with their psychoanalytic emphasis, made it difficult to match diagnosis to treatment, to match psychobabble to a scientific description of symptoms (called psychopathology). Dr. Greenwald's letter reflects not only a rather scornful view of his female patients, but a longing for a label that will let him treat rationally women who fear disappointment in love and abandonment, their reactions displaying the full range of dysphoria and anxiety.

The actual *DSM-III* that appeared in 1980 would solve Dr. Greenwald's problems: These women 18–35 with their delusive life hopes and fears of instability in partnership would likely receive the diagnosis "major depression." It was an epochal achievement of sorts, because it further pathologized a large segment of the population once considered merely "neurotic," and mandated their later treatment with the fashionable new Prozac-style antidepressants. How did this happen?

Spitzer

Ultimately, several agendas informed the development of the *DSM-III*— among them, as just suggested, the need for greater reliability and consistency of diagnostic terminology and the need for better diagnoses to help psychiatrists choose among the new drugs flooding the market. But at the outset the main reason the APA decided it was time to update

DSM-II was benumbingly bureaucratic: American medicine wanted to get in step with the *International Classification of Diseases* published by the World Health Organization; a new edition, the ninth, known as *ICD-9*, was coming up, and American psychiatric diagnosis had to be adjusted to fit the psychiatric diagnoses in *ICD-9*.[6] The APA leadership envisioned a document that just trimmed *DSM-II* at the edges, paying a bit more attention to the classification of conditions associated with "the aged, children and mental retardation," or bringing U.S. classification into line with *ICD-9* without letting the foreign document override in any way "national concerns."[7] In 1973, the APA bureaucrats turned to Bob Spitzer to help them handle this task.

Robert Spitzer, 41 in 1973, grew up in White Plains, New York, and graduated MD from New York University School of Medicine in 1957. After training in psychiatry at the New York State Psychiatric Institute, and in psychoanalysis (which he came to hate), in 1961 Spitzer joined the Biometrics Department of PI, as the Psychiatric Institute is called. Psychologist Joseph Zubin was chair of Psychometrics at PI and was well known as a developer of scales for measuring various psychological qualities. Said Spitzer later, "Joe Zubin . . . created a department where the atmosphere was, anything that's valid, you have to be able to measure it, that was the zeitgeist. Within that zeitgeist I flourished."[8] In 1976 Spitzer became chief of psychiatric research within the Biometrics Research Department.

Spitzer had served as a consultant to *DSM-II* in 1968. He emerged again on the radar of the APA leadership as he campaigned in 1973 to have homosexuality removed from the psychiatric diagnoses. He was full of energy and enthusiasm, with a ready ironical sense of humor that made it easier, perhaps, for others to accept the steely determination with which, at the end of the day, he moved forward his own conceptions for the *DSM-III*.

A tiny point: What Spitzer was being asked to craft was a statistical classification, not a "nosology." There's a difference. As Julius (Jan) Hoenig, a thoughtful theorist of psychiatry who emigrated from Czechoslovakia in the late 1930s, bringing the traditional European understanding of psychopathology with him, said in 1981, a nosology uses science to arrive at diagnoses; it is concerned with validity. In the 1890s, German psychiatrist Emil Kraepelin produced a nosology, a system of diagnoses based on the nosological principle of disease course and outcome. A statistical classification, by contrast, is based on consensus. Hoenig: "It must therefore be atheoretical, and must represent a widely negotiated agreement between its future users."[9] In 1973 the American Psychiatric Association executives who called upon Spitzer had very much a statistical classification in mind, because anything based on theory would have torn the profession apart. In psychiatry in those days, as reflected in the APA's membership, there were predominantly two conflicting doctrines: psychoanalysis, a theory of mental symptoms based on unconscious conflict, and biological psychiatry, a theory of mental symptoms based on brain chemistry. So Spitzer was supposed to just trim a bit here and there from the *DSM-II* without offending either camp and to create an American equivalent of the *ICD-9* with minor revisions.[10]

When APA recruited Spitzer, they evidently had little idea what they were getting into. They did not anticipate that he would, as he put it later, "totally ignore the *ICD-9*"[11] and instead start fresh by developing the wholly new classification system that would become the *DSM-III*. By the time APA leadership realized the extent of his mission, he had recruited such a huge following of enthusiastic members in support of his enterprise and impatient with psychoanalysis that it was too late for APA to do much about it.

In 1974 Spitzer struck a task force to guide him in this effort. It created a kind of St. Louis–New York axis. Spitzer later said, "The two universities that had a major influence in *DSM-III* were PI and Wash U, there's no question about that."[12] Washington University in St. Louis, with its genetically oriented department of psychiatry, was one of the birthing sites of biological psychiatry in the United States. The New York State Psychiatric Institute was the other. So the alliance between the two in the core membership of the task force forecast the direction that *DSM-III* would take, even though Spitzer resolutely insisted throughout (to ward off the analysts) that the orientation of the document was "atheoretical." Its conceptualization was in fact resolutely rooted in the Wash U–PI perspective and encompassed work initiated at the St. Louis school. For years, Sam Guze (pronounced Guzé) and a colleague at Wash U, Eli Robins, had been trying to establish new criteria for making reliable psychiatric diagnoses, saying in 1970 that on the basis of mainly clinical features (plus family history), good-prognosis schizophrenia could be separated from poor-prognosis schizophrenia.[13] In 1972 the Wash U school accelerated the new ferment in psychiatric diagnosis with the so-called Feighner criteria, named after John Feighner, a senior resident at the time, who was first author of an article about diagnosis that represented the collective thinking of the three principal figures at Wash U: Guze, Robins, and George Winokur. The Feighner criteria laid out the group's conception of an ideal classification, along with "diagnostic criteria" that a patient must evidence in order to qualify for a given diagnosis (for depression, for example, you'd have to be sad, plus have five of eight given symptoms, plus be ill for at least a month).[14] Spitzer joined this effort in the early 1970s and became quite close to the Wash U group, staying at Eli Robins's home when he went down to St. Louis. The summit of this collaboration occurred in 1978, just as the final drafting of *DSM-III* was in full swing, and became known as the Research Diagnostic Criteria (RDC).[15]

With his boyish energy and often naïve assessment of human relations, Spitzer saw the clinicians at Wash U almost as special chums, soul mates to help him against the bad guys. In 1979, as he and the task force were swept up in a virtual firestorm about some of the ideas in the *DSM-III* draft, he prepared a "confidential" version of a possible introduction to the manual and sent it to "Fellow Deans of the Invisible College (Drs. Eli Robins, Lee Robins [Eli's wife and a noted epidemiologist in her own right], Sam Guze, Gerald Klerman, George Winokur)." Of those on this list, only Gerry Klerman, then at Cornell, was not affiliated with Washington University. The memo began, "Buddies! Enclosed is a draft of the introduction to DSM-III. . . . What is your reaction to the whole shebang? If you have any suggestions for changes—I must know immediately."[16] Spitzer apparently had no awareness at this point that Eli Robins was furious with him for hogging the spotlight. The St. Louis school considered themselves the true architects of *DSM-III*.[17] But however credit is apportioned for beginning a complete overhaul of psychiatric diagnosis, credit for finishing it indisputably goes to Spitzer.

Among Wash U alumni and staffers on Spitzer's task force were Robert Woodruff (replaced by Paula Clayton after he committed suicide), Donald Goodwin, and, indirectly, Nancy Andreasen (a Winokur student at the University of Iowa). Among representatives from PI were Donald Klein, Rachel Gittelman, and Jean Endicott. The task force had, to be sure, other members as well, but it was these two core groups who exchanged most frenetically suggestions for new diagnoses among themselves. Under the direction of the task force, a number of advisory committees, with members from various institutions nationwide, were formed to consider everything from organic mental disorders to impulse control disorders. Spitzer was a member of every advisory committee and basically functioned as the spider at the center of the web.

In any event, when it came to making key decisions—about whether a given diagnosis would be included in the manual, what that diagnosis would be called, what its specific diagnostic criteria would be, in what disease category it would be classified, and so on—the deciding players were the six or seven core members of the task force rather than the members of the advisory committees.

Over the next 6 years, with a combination of iron will and urbane wit, Spitzer guided the task force to a dramatic recasting of the entire panoply of psychiatric diagnoses. At its organizational meeting in New York in September 1974, the task force decided that major surgery was called for: abolishing the distinction between "neurosis" and "psychosis" as a basis of classification, getting rid of the term "functional" for schizophrenia and affective disorders on the grounds that they are "no longer seen as purely psychogenic," and ensuring that classification would be conducted strictly without regard to "etiology," a death thrust against psychoanalysis, which propounded a clear etiology of illness—unconscious conflict.[18]

Spitzer could be headstrong and authoritarian about putting through his own ideas. Nonetheless, the guiding principle in constituting the new classification was inclusiveness. As their work got underway, the task force was fully aware of the massive resistance that awaited them from various quarters, and so the fruit of their efforts, *DSM-III*, was not really a scientific document but a *political* one. Spitzer: "If any group of clinicians had a diagnosis that they thought was very important, with a few exceptions, we would include it. That's the only way to make it acceptable to everyone. If we had just said, 'okay, the Washington U group only recognizes 16 categories, so we'll have 16 categories in *DSM-III*,' that would have been ridiculous. So we had to decide at every point: What do we do with the analysts who want 'narcissistic'? What do we do with the veterans who want 'PTSD?' And the solution was 'we'll include it.'"[19] (This is not the way science is normally done: scientists do not vote on what they think the atomic weight of the elements should be.)

The particular challenge that faced the task force, however, lay not in what was once called "madness" but in the lesser afflictions of daily life: what we have been calling here the nonmelancholic market basket, once referred to by the psychoanalysts as the "neuroses." As Spitzer told the APA in a "progress report" in March 1976, "A criticism of *DSM-I* and *II* was they were only useful for inpatients and irrelevant for outpatients with milder disorders. In *DSM-III* the attempt will be made to accept the challenge of classifying patients with mild conditions."[20] These less-than-psychotic mild conditions included the mood and anxiety disorders. This was a challenge that the World Health Organization had already taken on in *ICD-9* in 1975, distinguishing among a whole slew of "nervous disorders,"[21] but *ICD-9* was another world for American psychiatry, and the correspondence of the *DSM* drafters in the archives of the American Psychiatric Association rarely refers to it.

Let's concentrate on depression. The members of the task force were coming from a long tradition of "two depressions": serious melancholia versus nonmelancholic dysphoria and unhappiness. Continuing this tradition seemed relatively straightforward, but instead the tradition derailed and the two depressions became collapsed into one.

The Triumph of Major Depression

The qualifier "major" seems to surface in psychiatry for the first time in 1968 with the *DSM-II*, which referred to mood disorders as "major affective disorders (affective psychoses)."[22] There was really only one such major affective disorder, Kraepelin's manic-depressive illness, that included all depressions and mania. *DSM-II* then had a separate category for "depressive neurosis." So "major" began its grip on life as a synonym for psychosis, which meant not necessarily hallucinations and delusions but serious mental illness.

It was Bob Spitzer himself who coined the term "major depression."[23] He did so in 1975 as he, Jean Endicott, and Eli Robins beavered away at the research diagnostic criteria. It was at Spitzer's suggestion that "major depressive disorder" was inserted into the RDC classification. The diagnostic criteria for it—the "Chinese menu" approach[24]—asked for five of eight of a list of depressive symptoms, a concept borrowed from the Feighner criteria of 1972. (There were also in the RDC a number of subtypes of major depressive disorder plus a "minor depressive disorder," because it was only in the context of minor that major made sense.)[25]

In August 1975, Spitzer imported major depression to *DSM-III* as the task force completed the first draft of the classification.[26] In the mood disorders section of the draft, there was a listing for "major mood disorders" and one for "minor mood disorders." Each listing—major and minor—included a unipolar depression and a bipolar depression, the latter a concept that had first surfaced in the work of German nosologist Karl Leonhard in 1957,[27] and it had been repeated several times in the work of others. The task force now accepted it as given, and it was retained throughout the *DSM-III* process.

So, in the summer of 1975 this seemed quite straightforward: We'll have basically four kinds of depression: major and minor, bipolar and unipolar, and that's that. It was the term "major unipolar depression," rather than "major depression," that suggested serious illness. Don Klein said they had decided to use "unipolar" rather than "endogenous" (the old-fashioned term for melancholic depression, coined in 1920) "because unipolar doesn't suggest etiology as much as the older term, endogenous, does."[28] As for diagnostic criteria, the task force simply took over those of the St. Louis school.[29]

But what followed over the next few years was a sequence of name changes that was dizzying. Spitzer didn't like the major versus minor distinction, and in the next draft of *DSM-III* in March 1976 it was gone.[30] So was the term "depression," replaced by "depressive disorder." The task force needed something to indicate severity, so they built in a scale from 1 to 3, mild to severe, that could be put into the code for the diagnosis. In addition, they added a listing for "intermittent" affective disorders, which included intermittent depression and intermittent hypomania. Intermittent was really a euphemism for "chronic," but at this point they shied away from that term.

A few months later, in August 1976, the task force incorporated one other interesting feature: Outside of the affective disorders section they put in a section on reactive disorders, among which were "posttraumatic disorder" and "adjustment disorder." One of the adjustment disorders featured "depressed mood."[31] The premise was that, unlike serious disorders that were "autonomous" of external events, adjustment disorder remitted after an external stressor ceased. So you as a physician could code either low severity or adjustment problems and neither the patients nor the insurance companies would know that you considered your patient's problems "minor."

There were no more changes for the time being to the affective disorders section, as the task force wrestled with other areas of the classification. But there was trouble on the horizon. As soon as the psychoanalysts whiffed that the task force was ditching their beloved diagnosis "neurotic depression," they screamed. In November 1976 Spitzer told his fellow classification "mavens," as he often called them, that at a recent meeting of the APA's District Branches, during the Q and A, neurotic depression turned out to be "the toughest question of all."[32]

In May 1977, the annual meeting of the American Psychiatric Association convened in Toronto; a draft of the proposals of the task force was shown around. The analysts were said to be "upset to find the work progressing so far and are upset about the apparent lack of input from psychoanalysts." The APA Board of Trustees gave Spitzer a gentle nudge that the analysts had to be pieced off.[33] And in the next draft of the classification in January 1978, chronic replaced intermittent; and the chronic depressions were made to sound more like personality disorders than mainline affective illnesses.[34] This corresponded to the analytic view of depression as a kind of character disorder treatable only through lifelong psychotherapy. (Chronic depressive disorder in the drafts of *DSM-III* was regarded as equivalent to "neurasthenic neurosis" in *DSM-II*.)[35]

In the meantime, it was actually in June 1977 that major depression made its reappearance. On June 6, Spitzer attended a meeting of the Council on Clinical Classification, responsible for realigning diagnosis in all of American medicine with the *ICD* system of the World Health Organization. There was to be a special U.S. edition of this worldwide manual, entitled *ICD-9-CM*. Spitzer attempted to get the council to incorporate the *DSM-III* terminology into the special edition, with great success on the whole, he reported to the other diagnosis mavens. Yet there was one little problem. The *ICD* types didn't like the task force's "depressive disorder" (which had entered the draft *DSM-III* in August 1975 as "major unipolar depressive disorder"), because *ICD* had appropriated the term for some other purpose entirely. So what to call "depressive disorder"? Said Spitzer, "The only way that I could remedy this situation is to use a term that we had used almost two years ago: Major Depressive Disorder. The objection to that term when it was originally presented was that it was accompanied by the term Minor Depressive Disorder, and many clinicians were concerned that insurance payment would not be given to a category called Minor."[36] Spitzer was now boosting major depression as a stand-alone concept, on the grounds that the research diagnostic criteria of the St. Louis school also used it. (Yes, but they used it with minor.)

The next change in the affective disorders section of the task force's classification, in January 1978, therefore included "major depression" among the episodic mood disorders; the chronic mood disorders, as we have seen, were converted into character afflictions.[37] Note the legerdemain: Major depression was the only real depression; chronic depression a mere character disorder. This fig leaf for the analysts soon vanished, but for the time being they were mollified. And Spitzer recalls major depression as having been uncontroversial among task force members.[38] This was the real beginning of "major depression" in American, and ultimately world, psychiatry.

Some task force members soon realized, however, that major required minor as a counter-pendant. Other kibitzers saw the problem as well. In March 1978, John Racy, a psychiatrist at the University of Rochester, proposed adding "minor depressive disorder" to the classification "to fill what appears to be a hiatus in the depressive continuum. It described the very large group currently labeled as Neurotic Depression." Racy continued, "As the DSM-III proposal presently stands, the only place where this [neurotic depression] group of patients can be put is either under Chronic Depressive Disorder or under Atypical Depressive Disorder [which entered the classification as a residual catchall in March 1977].[39] While this can be justified in some instances, the majority are not chronic. When one considers the very large size of this group, to call it atypical is simply inaccurate. Anything that is common is not atypical." Nor did Racy like shoveling neurotic depression into the adjustment reaction bucket because not all such patients were reacting to stress. There must be a minor depression.[40]

Spitzer exploded at hearing this. "I must admit to some sadness and despair in reviewing your suggestions for the inclusion of a minor depressive category. . . . The very first (or nearly first) proposal in DSM-III for classification of Affective Disorders divided them into major and minor forms. I was severely clobbered by clinicians who said that this would be inviting disaster in so far as third party payment would be concerned."[41]

Spitzer cleverly extracted himself from the growing pressure to include minor. In July 1978, he wrote the "affective disorder mavens": "Having just returned from California (the state that leads the nation), I am now convinced that our latest renaming proposal—to change Chronic Depressive Disorder to Chronic Minor Depressive Disorder— is doomed to fail, and rightfully so. . . . This diagnostic entity can be devastating, and the term 'Minor' certainly does not suggest this.

"I believe that what is needed is drastic surgery for many of the diagnostic terms in the entire section. Assuming that you are sitting down, let us proceed."

Spitzer proposed renaming major depressive disorder "major depression." (He said, in a big fib, that "my own preference would be for Melancholia," but that ICD-9-CM said that they were "stuck with Major

Depressive something." It was Spitzer who put major depressive disorder into *ICD-9-CM!*)

The big change, however, came now: "Instead of Chronic Minor Depressive Disorder, I suggest Dysthymia." *Thymic* meant mood, and *dis* was clear; Spitzer, unaware of the long history of dysthymia in psychiatry, had found the term in a psychiatric dictionary. "For research investigators, there is no big problem in using clumsy terms such as Chronic Minor Affective Disorder. On the other hand, for the clinician and medical student or psychiatric resident, we are obligated to coin terms that are simple as well as descriptive."[42] Thus, major acquired its counter-pendant not in minor but in "dysthymic." But in making dysthymia a synonym for chronic, *the implication was that all episodic (acute) depressive disorders were major depression.*[43]

Meanwhile, in the *DSM* field trials, Spitzer had asked participants to recode in *DSM-III* categories the 912 patients who had received the *DSM-II* diagnosis of "depressive neurosis." Of these 912, 36 percent were recoded to major depression, 36 percent to chronic depressive disorder, and 13 percent to adjustment disorder with depressed mood. The category "neurotic depression" was therefore highly heterogeneous, Spitzer said, and needed to be abolished.[44]

The analysts, whose resistance had been steadily building, finally burst like a steam pipe. They simply could not abide the abolition of "neurotic depression." In early March 1979, a regional branch of the American Psychiatric Association, Area III, which centered in Washington, D.C., planned to bring the draft *DSM-III* to the floor of the upcoming annual May meeting of the APA and persuade the membership to vote it down.[45] Spitzer had to do something "'cause the whole thing would have been stopped at that point. It was absolutely necessary."[46] There was no time to call a meeting of the task force. The APA would be meeting in 2 months' time. So he called a corridor meeting at PI of Don Klein, Mike Sheehy, and Ed Sachar (director of PI who wasn't even on the task force). "We agreed to change 'chronic depressive disorder' to 'dysthymia.'" This, of course, was a decision that Spitzer had proposed months ago, but only now was it ratified by a kind of kitchen cabinet. More importantly, they would insert the words "neurotic depression" next to "dysthymia," thus buying peace with the analysts.[47] This historic capitulation was referred to as "the Neurotic Peace Treaty."

At that hallway meeting, Klein was not in fact in agreement with its outcome and sent a memo to the task force that was simply livid: "I think that Dr. Spitzer's suggestion fails on every count. First, it is clearly a response to political pressure, rather than a conceptual advance . . . embarrassingly transparent." "To respond to this sort of unscientific and illogical, but sociologically understandable, pressure in the fashion that Dr. Spitzer suggests is unworthy of scientists who are attempting to advance our field via clarification and reliable definition."[48]

What Does It Matter?

What did it matter if the term "depressive neurosis" was inserted next to dysthymia in *DSM-III*? It mattered because it suggested that dysthymia was really a psychoanalytic matter that should be treated with psychotherapy, whereas major depression required pharmacotherapy. That was the optics. In clinical terms, major depression and dysthymia were actually not all that different. The *Manual*, when it was published, said that dysthymia, though longer in duration, was less severe than major depression, but that it was pretty much the clinician's judgment call to decide which to apply to particular patients. To qualify for dysthymia, one must experience, for most or all of the past 2 years, 3 of a possible 13 symptoms, which themselves largely overlapped with the 4 of 8 required for major depression, whose duration must be at least 2 weeks.[49] The differences between each diagnosis' symptoms are so thin, however, that rather than being two very different measures of severity, major depression and dysthymia had ended up as fraternal twins.[50] But one twin carried an "I'm for drug therapy" sign, the other "I'm for psychotherapy." In a field on its way to becoming the highest prescribing specialty in medicine, it was clear which twin would be the more popular.[51]

Indeed, the appealing aspect of major depression from the viewpoint of many psychiatrists schooled in psychopharmacology was that it cried out for drug treatment. As Arthur Rifkin at PI, agonizing in March 1978 about the term "chronic" in the *DSM-III* draft, wrote to Spitzer, "I [am] concerned about the present classification leading the clinician to avoid drug treatment because the patient's depression is long standing and therefore chronic and therefore characteralogical [sic] and therefore not responsive to drugs."[52] Major depression was an open-sesame for psychopharmacology, in contrast to the psychotherapeutic approaches that had dominated American psychiatry for the previous half-century.

Thus, with *DSM-III* major depression was the only real depression left standing, and it was diagnosed twice as often as dysthymia in the years to come.[53] It would be the diagnosis of the future, as a number of insiders realized gloomily at the time. In February 1979, Barney Carroll at the University of Michigan urged Spitzer to distinguish among severe and nonsevere depression in some meaningful way. "I am sincerely suggesting these changes to you with the greatest possible sense of urgency. I honestly believe that you will be buying yourself (and the rest of us) a lot of grief if you allow the unitary category of major depressive disorder to remain. I have no doubt that there *are* two distinct types of 'depression' and that it is essential for clinicians to make the distinctions. . . ."[54]

Klein foresaw that the loose definition of depression in *DSM-III*, with the Chinese menu list of symptoms, would expand the diagnosis of depression enormously. In early March 1979 he told Spitzer, "I think you are indeed leaning over backwards to insure that the affective disorders will be more frequently diagnosed."[55] The judgment turned out to be prescient. In 1984 Klein snapped at Spitzer, "One of the more irritating consequences of DSM-III has been the plague of affective disorders that have descended upon us."[56] The incidence of major depression in the United States more than doubled in the 1990s, rising from 3.3 per 100 adult population in 1991–92 to 7.1 percent in 2001–2. The authors of the study from which these statistics emerged professed themselves perplexed about the causes.[57] In 2005 one authority estimated that depression would ultimately hit half of the population.[58]

Wow! Half the population! Do these people all really have a terrible affective illness called major depression? Or is major depression a disease that doesn't exist as the *DSM-III* and later editions of the manual have defined it?

Depression, anxiety, and other mental symptoms are real. They exist. But fever or coughing up sputum are real too, and yet we don't have diseases called "fever" or "horking and gobbing." The task of nosology is to bring psychiatric symptoms together into diseases that really do exist, such as melancholia, now a well-recognized entity: Melancholia brings together the symptoms and findings of mental and physical slowing, high cortisol, and terrible feelings of personal worthlessness and sinfulness. But major depression is not like that. You can have a couple of symptoms on a list of eight or so and still qualify for the diagnosis, but the particular symptoms Mr. X has may well differ from those Ms. Y has. Do they both have the same disease, major depression? Probably not.

It's important to sort symptoms into syndromes, or diseases, as they exist in Nature. What symptoms usually hang together? This is not just an academic exercise because these clusters of symptoms may be differentially treatment-responsive: Melancholia may respond beautifully to one treatment, such as the tricyclic antidepressants or convulsive therapy, whereas another well-defined syndrome—or assortment of symptoms—may respond to another. For example, one particular sorting of symptoms involves leaden fatigue, a compulsive appetite, hypersomnia, and poor stress coping. This is called atypical depression, and, unlike melancholia, it responds well to the monoamine oxidase inhibitors.

But major depression does not respond well to anything because it is so heterogeneous, containing within it a number of different syndromes. As Gordon Parker, the pioneering Australian psychopathologist who introduced the distinction between melancholia and nonmelancholia, observed in 2006, "Viewing [major depression] as an entity—rather than the pseudoentity that it is—risks homogenizing myriad depressive disorders and so clouding assessment of etiological factors and treatment efficacy. . . . There are substantive risks to viewing major depression as an entity, and with such a 'diagnosis' *alone* dictating treatment decisions."[59]

Bottom line: Major depression doesn't exist in Nature. A political process in psychiatry created it. This cautions us that we must be on our guard.

Psychiatrist Max Fink and I interviewed Bob Spitzer in March 2007. Now a bearded patriarch rather than the eager 40-something of *DSM* days, as Spitzer looks back the principal impression he gives of the *DSM* project is its political rather than its scientific nature.

Not by way of confrontation, but just to refresh his memory, we show Spitzer a copy of a letter that Don Klein wrote him in April 1978 and that we found in the archives of the American Psychiatric Association. Klein had been trying to get into *DSM-III* a favorite diagnosis of "hysteroid dysphoria" (which in fact reached *DSM-IV* in 1994 as "atypical depression"). Spitzer urged Klein to wait a bit, and Klein responded,

> I think your suggestion that we wait for DSM IV should be reconsidered. You and I have agreed that there are a number

of categories included in DSM III in which we have little
confidence concerning their reality but feel that at least
this will afford the field an opportunity to decide whether
they are there or not. I think the same logic applies to Hysteroid
Dysphoria.[60]

Shorter: There were categories in which you had little confidence?

*Spitzer: I think he's talking about "borderline" and "narcissistic"
[personality disorders]. He's saying, "You let in those categories that the
analysts want, when they don't have any evidence. Why don't you let
hysteroid dysphoria come in?"*

Fink: And why was it not let in?

Spitzer: Because there didn't seem to be enough to back it up.

Fink: But why not accept his plea?

Shorter: I mean, you're letting in all these analytic categories.

*Spitzer: Yes, but you have a whole analytic community. There's Don Klein
and maybe one or two of his people.*

Shorter: So he wasn't powerful enough?

*Spitzer: Well, who was it said, "How many troops does the Pope have?"
(Laughter)*

Fink: Oh, that's wonderful.

*Shorter: So this is really a very political process. Don just didn't have the
troops on his side.*

*Spitzer: And I didn't give in just because he wanted it, that's no reason to
have it in.*

*Shorter: But you gave in on the analytic categories because they wanted it,
otherwise the whole thing would have been shot down.*

*Spitzer: It would have been shot down, yes. Do you think I did the wrong
thing?[61]*

History has yet to judge whether Spitzer did the right thing in sub-
stituting political considerations for scientific ones. Perhaps the historic
achievement of getting *DSM-III* through a hidebound organization

then dominated by the followers of Freud does overshadow the need to have an evidence-based classification of diseases.

Yet the consequences of these compromises have been considerable. The prescription of antidepressants began a historic rise, increasing from 17.9 percent of all office visits to psychiatrists in 1980, the year of the *DSM-III's* publication, to 30.4 percent in 1989.[62] The antidepressants prescribed during most of that period would have been primarily the monoamine oxidase inhibitors and the tricyclics.

But major depression was a diagnosis that cried out for a drug class of its own. After 1989, with the Prozac-style SSRIs, the wish was granted. As Ross Baldessarini, a leading psychopharmacologist at McLean Hospital in a suburb of Boston, put it much later, "The whole pharmaceutical industry is premised on broad definitions that allow big markets. It's hard to reverse that trend. For example, some people have argued that the SSRIs could just as well have been developed as antianxiety drugs and nobody would have known the difference."[63] The big disease categories, in other words, were so heterogeneous as to be meaningless. Depression, anxiety, what's the difference? One size truly did fit all.

Said Gordon Parker in 2005, "Not only has major depression become the biggest game in town, it has become the 'only game.'"[64] Depression has become as common as the common cold. It starts early in life. "Babies can be depressed," says Dr. Jess Shatkin at New York University's Child Study Center. "We think maybe one in 40 or so."[65] Just imagine: Of a hundred babies lying in a hospital maternity ward, two require treatment with Prozac.

How about adults?

Depression lurks at every corner, such as after redoing your kitchen, for example. In 2007 the *New York Times*, in a story entitled "The New Kitchen Is Done. So Why Can't I Be Happy?" reported on the "House of Blues": "After renovating her California home, Anne Toth said she 'felt empty.' She missed the excitement of construction and began to focus on tiny flaws like the slightly off-kilter kitchen tiles." A photograph showed a supposedly depressed Ms. Toth fingering the maddening tiles. The story quoted Kevin White, a psychologist in Providence, Rhode Island, who said that "acute depression can follow the end of any major project." Indeed, he had felt it several times himself.[66] Is this depression a clinical illness involving a diminished sense of self-worth, slowed thinking and movement, and an urge to do away with oneself that has resounded across the ages, making the "blues" once an urgent indication for admission to a mental hospital?

No, it is not. In fact, it is nothing. But it shows the complete bankruptcy of the mood disorders in psychiatry today.

Coda

There is now much ferment in psychiatry about the inadequacies of the current incarnation of the *DSM* system, *DSM-IV*, published in 1994. Thoughtful psychiatrists are asking how to get into future editions of the *Manual* diagnoses that really cut Nature at the joints, rather than being political artifacts.

As Max Fink and I were leaving Bob Spitzer's home on that day in March 2007, Max asked, how does one approach the *DSM* drafters and show them your scientific evidence on behalf of diagnosis X or Y?

> *Spitzer: I think if it comes primarily from you and not a larger group, it's unlikely anything is going to happen.*
>
> *Fink: Nothing?*
>
> *Spitzer: Changes generally come when there's a big group—PTSD, or borderline, where there's a whole bunch of people who want it, or ADD [attention deficit disorder].*
>
> *Shorter: So what Max has to do is organize a lobby, basically.*
>
> *Spitzer: You have to have a lobby, that's how. You have to have troops.*
>
> *Fink: So it's not a matter of . . .*
>
> *Spitzer: Having the data? No.*
>
> *Fink: It's nothing to do with science then, and nothing to do with evidence?*

Spitzer nodded.[67]

8
Losing Ground

By the year 2000, antidepressants had beaten out all other drug classes used in psychiatry, as well as all drug classes of any kind in medicine. With the exception of nonsteroidal antiinflammatory agents, antidepressants were prescribed more often than any other kind of drug. A survey of the National Center for Health Statistics of the U.S. government found that in 2003–4, antidepressants were prescribed at the rate of 310 per 1,000 patients. NSAIDs, to be sure, came in at 390 per 1,000. But every other drug class used in medicine was way down the list: antiasthmatics 278 per 1,000, antihypertension drugs 242, and vitamins and minerals 173.[1] How could depression, once an obscure and unusual disease, have taken over virtually the entire practice of medicine?

That Pesky Serotonin

In Sweden in the early 1950s, Arvid Carlsson, a recent MD from Lund and graduate student in pharmacology, needed a thesis topic. He chose one of the least exciting subjects in the field: calcium metabolism. He sent a draft of the thesis to one of the experts in the subject, asking him to be a member of his jury. The great man refused, "No, this is no good."

So Carlsson went to one of the noted Swedish research scientists, Sune Bergström, who later received a Nobel Prize for his discoveries involving the prostaglandins, and asked him to read the draft. "It's OK," said Bergström.

Carlsson then applied for an assistant professorship and didn't get it, so underwhelmed was everyone by his work. "What you are doing," said the thesis jury, "is no good for a pharmacologist. This is not centrally located in pharmacology."

Carlsson later said, "I was already a pharmacologist. What could I do?"

So Carlsson went back to Bergström and said, "I have to switch. I want to go to a lab that is a pharmacology lab, that is chemically oriented and it should really be at the top level." Bergström had a great network of contacts, so he wrote to a friend of his, the chemist Bernhard Witkop at the National Institutes of Health in Bethesda. Witkop gave Bergström's letter to Sid Udenfriend at the Heart Institute, and Udenfriend "in turn handed it over to his boss, [Bernard] Brodie. That's how I came to Brodie. And it just so happened that a few months before I came, they had made this breakthrough discovery researching the depletion of the serotonin store. That's how the whole thing started."[2]

It was Carlsson, in at the beginning of the first drug set in the 1950s, who ratcheted up interest in drugs that inhibited the reuptake of serotonin, the Prozac-style drugs, that dominated American psychiatry in the last two decades of the twentieth century. Carlsson won a Nobel Prize in 2000 for his discoveries in the area of dopamine. He is an eminently scientific figure, but the science that he generated ended up in the perversion of therapeutics that is the last chapter of our story: the mania for selective serotonin reuptake inhibitors, or SSRIs, that pushed every other class of drug for mood disorders from view while being themselves not terribly effective as antidepressants.

The Powder Trail to the SSRIs

There is nothing new about the idea that certain drugs inhibit the reuptake of serotonin; antihistamines, on the market since the mid-1940s, do the same thing. It was Swiss-born pharmacologist and later Nobel Prize winner Daniel Bovet, then at the Pasteur Institute in Paris, who synthesized pyrilamine; he joined two phenyl rings with a carbon-amino bridge, creating the first antihistamine for the French drug firm Rhône-Poulenc in 1944; in 1948 Merck marketed it in the United States as Neo-Antergan. One could actually say that the SSRIs are just the latest generation of antihistamines.

Rhône-Poulenc, in search of further antihistamines, also took the old phenothiazine molecule from the late-nineteenth century and added an amine side chain. A version their chemist Paul Charpentier synthesized in 1944, called promethazine (and marketed as Phenergan), turned out to have powerful antihistamine properties and to be somewhat psychoactive as well (it was a precursor of the antipsychotic drug chlorpromazine). Drugs for runny noses were fabulous! But meanwhile, an idle curiosity about antihistamines as psychoactive lingered. In 1949 an American chemist synthesized phenyltoloxamine dihydrogen citrate that Bristol labs brought out in 1952 as "Bristamin," an over-the-counter antihistamine. Then as interest in the psychoactive properties of antihistamines quickened, the company reintroduced Bristamin several years later at a higher dosage as a prescription-only tranquilizer, calling it "PRN," a medical acronym for "pro re nata," or as circumstances may require.[3]

Also in 1949, Schering Labs, realizing that a land-office business was building in antihistamines, brought out chlorpheniramine, marketing it as Chlor-Trimeton. This was a profitable business, so when chlorpheniramine turned out to have antipanic qualities, Schering had no interest in pursuing that indication.[4] In the meantime, at the Brodie lab, the advent of the spectrophotofluorimeter in 1955 made it possible to measure the presence of serotonin in nervous tissue,[5] and word started to get around that chlorpheniramine inhibited the reuptake of serotonin.

This is where Arvid Carlsson comes in. After returning to Sweden in 1956 from the Brodie lab, he bought a spectrophotofluorimeter. As an associate professor in the department of pharmacology at Lund, Carlsson was interested in measuring the presence of such monoamine neurotransmitters as serotonin, dopamine, and norepinephrine in nervous tissue. In 1960 he caused a bit of a stir at a conference in London with photographs that showed vesicles of dopamine in neurons, although the Brits—still involved in theories about electrical neurotransmission—for the most part pooh-poohed the finding.[6]

In the meantime, other researchers had been calling attention to the possible role of serotonin in depression. In 1963, Alec Coppen and associates at the Neuropsychiatric Research Unit of the Medical Research Council in Carshalton, England, determined that adding tryptophan, a serotonin precursor, considerably increased the antidepressant effectiveness of the MAOI tranylcypromine (Parnate).[7] This was an early biochemical link of serotonin to depression in humans.

Alongside such Swedish researchers as the histologist Nils-Ake Hillarp, Carlsson continued to beaver away at making neurotransmitters visible under the spectrophotofluorimeter using "histochemical" techniques.[8] When Paul Kielholz and Walther Pöldinger at the Basel University Psychiatric Clinic published an article in 1968 showing that drugs like desipramine (secondary amines) had a strong component of psychomotor activation, and drugs like amitriptyline (tertiary amines) were more calming,[9] it directed Carlsson's attention toward differences in brain effects between the two types of drugs.[10] (A "tertiary" amine has two methyl groups [CH_3] attached to the nitrogen on the side chain; a "secondary" amine has one. Tertiary amine drugs often metabolize in the body to secondary amines.) Might there be differences in the neurotransmitters involved?

In 1959 Carlsson accepted an appointment at the University of Gothenburg, and in 1969 he conducted a simple experiment. He and his associates gave to mice a chemical that depleted the brain of serotonin and norepinephrine; then they noted which tricyclic antidepressants better protected the neurons against this depletion, the secondary or the tertiary. They saw that the tertiary amines, such as imipramine and amitriptyline, did a better job of inhibiting the reduction of norepinephrine in the brain, and the secondary amines, such as desipramine and protriptyline, better inhibited the depletion of serotonin.[11]

This finding meant that if you thought keeping up brain stores of serotonin was important in the treatment of depression, you could give patients a drug that better inhibited the reuptake of serotonin than of norepinephrine, causing it to persist in the synapse between the neurons and increase its effectiveness. An accompanying article of the Carlsson group cast doubt on the hypothesis that the tricyclic antidepressants, or "thymoleptics" as some people were still calling them, were effective mainly by inhibiting the reuptake of norephinephrine.[12] Increasingly, a smoking gun was pointing at serotonin in depression. But how to prevent its reuptake with a patentable compound? Maybe an antihistamine could be the basis of an innovative new agent that would have patent protection?

In the same year, 1969, Carlsson and Margit Lindqvist said that the antihistamine chlorpheniramine "proved remarkably potent on central 5-hydroxytryptamine [serotonin] neurons." "In fact it compares favourably with imipramine and amitriptyline with respect to actions on both 5-HT [serotonin] and noradrenaline [norepinephrine] neurons. It appears worth while to study the possible antidepressant properties of this and related agents in man."[13] This was the birthing hour of the SSRIs.[14]

Let's go back one step: In 1961 Carlsson had begun consulting for the drug firm A. B. Hässle, which was owned by the Astra group. The firm's dynamic research director, the pharmacist Ivan Öestholm, had hired the Swiss medicinal chemist Hans Corrodi, who also was cross-appointed in the pharmacology department at Gothenburg. The three men became a team dedicated to putting into practice Carlsson's insight that drug discovery should proceed on the basis of scientific principles. In 1968, guided by Carlsson's "serotonin hypothesis" of depression, the three of them decided to go after depression as an indication for drug discovery. They used Schering Lab's brompheniramine as a basis, which was chlorpheniramine but with a bromine atom instead of a chlorine on one of the rings. With this platform compound, Corrodi synthesized a number of molecules having a carbon bridge different from that of the pheniramines. In 1969 he devised one that did well in animal pharmacology, and in April 1971 they applied for a Swedish patent, a date that makes clear that the molecule they decided to put into development, which they called zimelidine (later zimeldine), was the first SSRI.[15] In the spring of 1971 the whole project was moved from Gothenburg to Astra's headquarters at Södertälje outside of Stockholm.[16]

In 1981 zimeldine was approved in Sweden and elsewhere in Europe, and marketed as Zelmid, "the new, specific 5-HT reuptake inhibitor for the treatment of depression," said the ad copy, referring to the biochemical shorthand for serotonin.[17] There was a lot of evidence that zimeldine was just as effective as amitriptyline, the most popular of the tricyclic antidepressants, yet with fewer side effects.[18] The side effects of the tricyclics, of which so much was subsequently made by competing groups of drug manufacturers, were generally minor, consisting of such "anticholinergic" symptoms as dry mouth, blurred vision, and constipation, yet vexatious to patients. As Arthur Prange at the University of North Carolina in Chapel Hill said in late 1981, "Some of them [patients on imipramine] will have some side effects, but compared to the symptoms of depression it is really [just] a nuisance."[19] In unusual cases, the TCAs can also have major cardiac side effects.

Over the 10-plus years between its synthesis and launch, zimeldine was tested extensively in animal and clinical trials, which makes all the more puzzling what happened next. Within a year of its launch, Zelmid turned out to have some major side effects. Carlsson recalls that some "flu-like illnesses" were seen in the trials, but, despite his admonition to take them seriously and convene "an advisory group to handle this," the company didn't react in a timely way.[20]

Meanwhile, Merck had bought the license from Astra to market zimeldine in the United States and guided the drug through phase III trials (the large-scale trials that culminate the investigation process). Said psychopharmacologist Leslie Iversen, who had just started working for Merck, "They were overjoyed because clearly the drug was working as well as amitriptyline, and it was far less toxic. They were over the moon. They were having a party to celebrate the loading of the truck that was going to go down to Washington with the registration file in it." The file was 200 volumes long. "If it had gone through, zimeldine would have been registered probably a year before Prozac in the States."[21]

But no sooner had the truck left the dock than toxicity reports started coming in. In August 1983, a couple of Swedish pharmacologists, Kjell Strandberg and Bengt-Erik Wilholm, dropped by the office of Bob Temple, who was then acting director of the Office of New Drug Evaluation at the FDA, and briefed him on Zelmid; a month later Temple told the Neuropharmacological Drug Products Division about the rash of "adverse reaction reports": "What was particularly striking was an apparent hypersensitivity syndrome consisting initially of headache, nausea, and vomiting, followed by fever, intense muscle pain, joint pain . . ." and liver problems. The Swedish visitors told Temple about "a total of 35 cases of zimelidine syndrome," apparently in Sweden alone. "It is obvious that the side effect picture needs careful evaluation before we consider approval."[22] In fact, it never came to that because as Temple was writing those lines, Astra had pulled the drug. At the time of its withdrawal in September 1983, there had been numerous cases of a demyelinating neurological condition called Guillain-Barré syndrome, and many reports of liver dysfunction and "flu-like illnesses." Indeed, in one trial, of 14 patients treated with Zelmid for over a week, 7 developed some kind of "toxic syndrome."[23]

In an interview, Carlsson was asked if he favored the decision to withdraw the drug. No, he didn't. "The clinical effect was so striking, the therapeutic effect, that if you made a calculation of the number of suicides that were prevented, there would be a lot more than these other cases, that after all weren't lethal either, all of them recovered."[24]

One has the feeling with Zelmid, a feeling not suscitated by any of the other SSRIs, that perhaps here something was lost. After its withdrawal, Swedish clinicians continued to prescribe it; in 1988, in a reanalysis of earlier trial data, Danish psychiatrist Per Bech concluded that it was superior to the tricyclics as an antimelancholic.[25] It is ironical that zimeldine, one of the two of the SSRIs ever to be withdrawn, is the only one of the class that cries out for a second look.[26]

The Flight Groups

Animated by Carlsson's serotonin research, in the early 1970s a wave of drugs inhibiting the reuptake of serotonin went into development. There were two flight groups: a middle group launched primarily in Europe in the mid-1980s, and a late flight group, the real blockbusters, launched primarily in the United States in the late 1980s and early '90s.

The middle flight group included fluvoxamine, which never made it to the United States as an antidepressant (but rather as an agent for obsessive-compulsive disorder), and indalpine, which never reached the United States at all. Company publicity for both glommed onto the "serotonin reuptake inhibition" angle from the get-go.

Fluvoxamine was developed in the early 1970s by Philips-Duphar, a Dutch subsidiary of Brussels-based Solvay.[27] Patented in 1975, the drug was first launched in Switzerland in 1983 as Floxyfral, in the United Kingdom in 1987 as Faverin, and later in the United States in 1995 as Luvox, a "highly effective 5 HT re-uptake inhibitor," for obsessive-compulsive disorder. Chemically, Luvox bore nothing in common with Zelmid, was not an antihistamine, and was trumpeted as a serotonin "reuptake inhibitor" only because that was one of its several effects. So from the very beginning, this notion of a highly specific class of SSRIs (the acronym had not yet been invented) was as much a marketing as a scientific concept. In fact, the original generic name was "myroxim," but fluvoxamine made it sound more "amine-like."

The other mid-flight SSRI, indalpine, had a short life. Gérard Le Fur, at Mar-Pha Société d'Etudes et d'Exploitation de Marques in Paris, developed the drug, filing for a patent in 1976.[28] Fournier Frères-Pharmuka brought it to market as Upstène in 1983 as "the first specific inhibitor of serotonin reuptake," a claim many of the manufacturers made. It was withdrawn 2 years later because of severe side effects, such as agranulocytosis (a deficiency of a kind of white cell needed to fight infection). Indalpine was an antihistamine, though in structure quite different from either zimeldine or fluvoxamine. And it did have a powerful effect on the reuptake of serotonin.

The American Flight Group of SSRIs

The last flight group of SSRIs were the American blockbusters. With the exception of the antibiotics, this is probably the most successful single drug class in history, and had a profound worldwide influence upon the therapeutics of psychiatric illness. Fluoxetine, Eli Lilly's Prozac, was first in the flight group, marketed in the United States in 1988, followed by citalopram (Lundbeck's Cipramil), whose Danish launch was in 1989 (although its American launch by Forest Laboratories under the trade name Celexa did not occur until 1998); then came sertraline, Pfizer's Zoloft, floated in the United States in 1992, after which came paroxetine, which SmithKline Beecham brought out as Paxil in 1993.

Even though Lundbeck came later to market with citalopram, they were the second company after Hässle to begin development of an SSRI, and got a jump start simply because Carlsson happened to visit Lundbeck's Copenhagen offices and put the idea in their heads. Lundbeck's medicinal chemist Klaus Bogeso, a noted "drug hunter," started in 1971 with a compound the firm had earlier synthesized called talopram that inhibited the reuptake of norepinephrine; Bogeso tweaked it a bit, and 55 versions later got citalopram, which inhibited the reuptake of serotonin.[29] It had the classic structure of an antihistamine. Lundbeck's subsidiary Kefalas patented it in 1977. Two years after the agent's launch in Denmark in 1989, Lundbeck brought it out in Switzerland, claiming it was "the first of a new chemical class of highly potent and selective serotonin re-uptake inhibitors."[30] It was nonetheless the last of the SSRIs to become a blockbuster in the United States following its launch there as Celexa 9 years later.

In February 1973, half a year before the publication of the Swedish patent for zimeldine, a team of scientists of the Eli Lilly company in Indianapolis led by chemist Bryan Molloy made the first sample of Prozac (fluoxetine) using as a base the antihistamine diphenhydramine (Benadryl);[31] it had the standard antihistamine structure of two phenyl rings connected by a carbon bridge. Like the other SSRIs, Prozac was scarcely innovative. The principle of uptake inhibition had long been known, and Prozac's main advantage was said to be that, like the other SSRIs, you couldn't commit suicide with it.[32] (This view may have been erroneous, though.)[33] The company got a German patent on fluoxetine in 1975 and a United States patent in 1982.

Fluoxetine had a rocky set of clinical trials. As André Uzan, a Parisian neuroscientist, pointed out in 1981, "If a number of agents recently proposed as inhibitors of the reuptake of serotonin have not been adopted for clinical use, in some of them, such as fluoxetine, it's because of their not inconsiderable side effects."[34] The concerns about central nervous system side effects, such as anxiety, nervousness, insomnia, fatigue, and tremor, and gastrointestinal adverse effects such as nausea and diarrhea, almost dissuaded Lilly from developing fluoxetine for depression.[35]

At a conference in England Alec Coppen suggested to them, "Why don't you try Prozac on depression?" As Arvid Carlsson, who was there, remembered the exchange, "The Lilly man who was on top at this meeting, in his concluding remarks said, 'and I can tell Dr. Coppen we are not going to try Prozac on depression.'"[36]

At some point Lilly clearly must have had a change of heart. During the trials, in order to wrestle with the agent's adverse effects, chloral hydrate and the benzodiazepines were often co-prescribed to patients (meaning that the trial data themselves were as much a measure of benzo and chloral efficacy as fluoxetine efficacy).[37] For all the side effects they experienced, the patients themselves in a number of the trials were apparently not very sick with depression; in fact many were not patients at all but individuals in the community recruited through newspaper advertisements ("Do you feel crummy? Call us.")[38]

One would have to say, on the basis of its development, that fluoxetine was not a promising drug.[39] Nonetheless, it was first launched in Belgium in 1986, then reached the U.S. market in 1988 with the claim that it was "the first highly specific, highly potent blocker of serotonin uptake."[40]

In 1992, Pfizer brought out sertraline as Zoloft, the second big SSRI blockbuster to hit the U.S. market. Kenneth Koe, a Pfizer pharmacologist, had been toying with the idea of enhancing the potency of a norepinephrine reuptake blocker and in 1977 asked their chemist Willard Welch to try to convert Pfizer's tametraline into a serotonin agent;[41] 2 years later he succeeded and named the successful compound sertraline.[42] Sertraline is an antihistamine and has the "bicyclic" structure characteristic of the others. But the trials were conducted sloppily, starting patients out at high doses and not training properly the investigators running the multicenter studies. As with other drugs, the patients tended to be recruited in newspaper ads ("symptomatic volunteers"), and it is unclear what condition, if anything, they really had.[43] Here again, insiders found themselves asking, is this really an antidepressant?

The third U.S. blockbuster among the SSRIs was paroxetine, marketed as Paxil. Paroxetine was synthesized in 1974 by the Danish-Swedish company Ferrosan with research labs in Soborg, Denmark. But the small firm was unable to develop the drug itself, and so in 1980 it licensed the paroxetine technology to the British company Beecham.[44]

In the early 1980s, under a cooperative agreement between Beecham and SmithKline (as Smith, Kline & French was now known), chemists working for both firms sought a process that would let them mass-produce paroxetine; in 1985 it became clear that the agent existed in two forms, one of which was a "hemihydrate" (a technical term referring to the ratio of water in the structure), and that this form should be commercially developed. In May 1985, SmithKline began clinical trials while Beecham filed for a British patent. In 1989, now merged, SmithKline Beecham developed paroxetine hemihydrate as an antidepressant with the brand name Paxil (Seroxat in the United Kingdom). Interestingly, it was claimed that the first trials conducted with the nonhemihydrate form in Europe in the early 1980s were failures.[45] It was not a promising drug.

When SmithKline Beecham launched Paxil in 1993, the company marketed it not merely as a drug that acted on the serotonin system but as an "SSRI." This brilliant acronym was a commercial invention of the company's, though apparently they did not at first appreciate the force of the coinage, and "SSRI" appeared only in the fine print.[46]

Safety was to be the marketing hook for paroxetine, playing off the supposed dangerousness of the competing tricyclics. But in 2004, by which time the company had become GlaxoSmithKline, the agent's safety record was on the line, as indeed was that of the other SSRIs. One patient, Pamela Wild, who had attempted suicide after taking Paxil, told the psychopharmacology advisory committee of the FDA, "I was told not to worry, the only way to die from this drug was to fill a tub with Paxil and water and drown in it."[47] In a sea of competitors that also vaunt their safety, this is not necessarily a winning strategy.

In the 1980s, however, such safety concerns, much less questions of efficacy, were far from the public radar, for none of the SSRIs had yet obtained approval from the Food and Drug Administration to land in the American market. Beginning in 1985, the NDA process would start for the late-flight group: Lilly's fluoxetine, followed some years later by Pfizer's sertraline, SmithKline Beecham's paroxetine, and Lundbeck-Forest's citalopram. All were poor antidepressants, though of course flogged frenetically for that indication. That was the rising buzzword of the era, as "major depression" started to climb ever upward in the nation. How were the SSRIs able to catch and ride that wave? Savvy marketing helped them do it. So did the *DSM-III*. And so did the FDA.

"We Can't Be Solomon in Those Kinds of Things"

From the 1950s to the 1970s, the FDA had been so hostile to industry as almost to constitute a rogue agency, sometimes regulating against the interests of public health and often in favor of its own imperial ambitions. Then early in the 1980s a different wind started to blow in the corridors of power of the FDA's Parklawn Building on Fishers Lane in Rockville, Maryland, at least in psychopharmaceuticals, as Robert Temple and Paul Leber ascended to positions of leadership.

Temple had earned a BA from Harvard College in 1963, graduated MD from New York University School of Medicine in 1967, and then completed training in internal medical and clinical pharmacology at Columbia Presbyterian Hospital in 1969. Joining the FDA in 1972, he advanced through various posts in the Bureau of Drugs and Division of Cardio-Renal Drug Products, becoming in 1982 acting director of the Office of Drug Research and Review. He was among the top power brokers at the Bureau of Drugs (which later became the Office of Drug Evaluation).

Paul Leber had an extraordinarily wide background. When he joined the FDA in 1979 as acting group leader in Psychopharmacology Unit II, he was 42 years old. He had spent most of his life studying. Born in Brooklyn, he had an undergraduate degree from Hamilton College in Clinton, New York, and in 1963 had graduated in medicine from NYU. Leber had trained in internal medicine for 3 years, in pathology for 3 years, and in psychiatry, at the Westchester Division of New York Hospital-Cornell Medical Center in White Plains, New York, from 1974 to 1977. He taught psychiatry at NYU School of Medicine for 2 years, and when he left for the FDA in 1979, they were said in New York to be delighted to get rid of him because of abrasive aspects of his personality that were occasionally visible. Jon Cole later said, "I've heard a lot of complaints about Paul Leber. That's an interesting story. . . . When Leber was announced as the new head of the FDA neuropharmacology branch, screams arose from people at New York University, where he came from. Terrible appointment, awful person. On and on. I mean, it was really character assassination and I never understood the basis of it because as far as I could tell Paul did a very nice job . . . I enjoyed talking to him, and I never saw whatever it was that drove people crazy at NYU."[48] So Leber was a man who had hooks, in a way.

Both Temple and Leber were bright, curious, and articulate men, quite different in manner from the technocrats whose hands previously had been on psychopharm. They were full of wry observations and thoughtful asides in their correspondence and participation at meetings, hitherto a no-no in the ascetic prose exchanges of the bureaucrats. On one occasion, Leber distinguished, in a discussion of how to measure bulimia, between regulatory knowledge versus speculative knowledge: ". . . There are areas that we can delve into reasonably for drug regulatory purposes and those which are more speculative, City of God–City of Man type of separation in an Augustinian sense."[49] One had the impression almost of attending a high-level academic seminar on psychopharmacology. It was a refreshing wind.

It is clear from the verbatim transcripts of the FDA's Psychopharmacologic Drugs Advisory Committee (PDAC), the panel of outside experts convened to advise the agency on all matters relating to psychotropic medications, including some NDAs, that Leber was well-spoken and quick on his feet, able to argue almost any committee member under the table. It is noteworthy that after Leber spoke, the subject was usually considered settled and advisory committee members did not continue to carp. The FDA heads of other drug advisory committees do not seem to have dominated their panels in a similar manner. So Leber's personality and wit gave the PDAC proceedings a rather special stamp. But members could also be railroaded. And with the approval of some of the SSRIs, one has the feeling that this is what happened.

In the background of these events was the steady torrent of DESI-mandated antidepressants pouring onto the American market in the 1980s. As the benzodiazepines came increasingly under attack because of presumptive addictiveness, the accent in industry swung ever more away from anxiety and toward depression. Lederle came out with the tricyclic antidepressant amoxapine (Asendin) in 1980; Ciba launched the tetracyclic antidepressant maprotiline (Ludiomil) in the United States 1981, and Mead Johnson brought out an American edition of the bicyclic antidepressant trazodone (Desyrel) in 1982. None of them was a blockbuster and all now largely forgotten.

As the popularity of "antidepressants" started to gain wind, there was uneasiness in scientific circles. At a PDAC meeting in 1983, the Hungarian-born chair of psychiatry at the University of Pittsburgh, Thomas Detre, said, "It would be nice to abolish the label antidepressant. I am a little worried, it sounds like antibiotic. In the first place, the specificity is in serious question. Secondly, in some studies they are barely distinguishable from placebo. . . . This whole antidepressant category is somehow not right."

Paul Leber replied to Detre, in essence: Just try it. "As a practical matter I wanted to point something out. A lot of the things we would like to be able to do we cannot do. Firms that have long-standing indications for various claims are unlikely to want to give them up voluntarily. . . . You could not make them part with it easily, certainly not with the resources we have."[50] How interesting that no industry-accommodating rhetoric of this kind was ever hinted during the brutal DESI years. But then, it was a new era at the FDA now. Despite the flutterings of doubt that some on the PDAC, like Detre, expressed, the concept of antidepressant had by now entrenched itself deep within the United States pharmaceutical scene. We needed only some blockbuster antidepressants to give it substance.

From 1981, when he became acting director of the Division of Neuropharmacology at the FDA, until January 1999, when he resigned from the agency, Leber was the gatekeeper of American psychopharmacology. As such he was, next to Bob Spitzer, one of the most important people in psychiatry in the United States, for it was, basically, Leber who decided what drugs gained approval, and for what indications.

On this latter point there would be no confusion: Leber strongly supported *DSM-III* indications for various psychiatric disorders. In 1980, just after the appearance of the APA's new *Manual*, Leber said to the PDAC, ". . . You don't want to be in the position of what Humpty-Dumpty said to Alice. Every time I use a word, I know exactly what I mean. But no one else does. I think the issue here is to get a common definition so that when we get finished with the study, and you report the results, and you say it applies to the general population. We say, well, these were, at least by the *DSM III* criteria, the patients that we studied."[51] There was some resistance to the imposition of these new *DSM* criteria within the FDA; yet Leber prevailed, and in the years to come antidepressants were tested according to the criteria of major depression—despite his own personal leanings on the matter, as we shall soon see.

Early on, it became apparent that Leber had certain operating rules, which he never wrote down on paper but may be inferred from watching him in action over the years. One was a hard-nosed commitment to data in approving drugs. "If you can't prove it, you can't claim it," was his view;[52] in other words, all claims for indications must be backed up by placebo-controlled trials. For assessing drug safety, Leber used to cite the "Temple Rule," which was, in fact, his own rule, that in a trial ". . . roughly between 50 and 100 patients [must be studied] for six months

to a year."[53] (This was much larger than the trials of the 1960s and produced data less vulnerable to "type II error," the inability to discriminate
in an underpowered trial.)

Leber's second operating rule was a low tolerance for the kind of
cant that was then increasingly infecting academic psychopharmacology. He had little patience for the argument that "addictiveness" must
disqualify a drug. In 1982, showing perhaps just a touch of abrasive-
ness, he challenged one member of the advisory committee who feared
that the benzodiazepine alprazolam (Xanax) might be addictive,
"I would ask you, what is the evidence, aside from the fact we haven't
tested for it, that this drug actually is capable of inducing dependence
of serious concern, serious enough to block its approval on the basis of
efficacy. . . . I mean, what is the evidence. What you really seem to be
saying is that there is a risk, and we haven't stated the risk."[54]

On another occasion, Leber expressed impatience with the chatter
about "internal cognitive structures"—and "reuptake inhibition"—intended to explain the mechanism of drugs' action. He snapped at the
PDAC, "It probably isn't so important to understand the mechanism
by which the drug has worked. I would challenge any of you to really
know . . . how drugs really work. We'll acknowledge that we don't
know that."[55] What mattered were the numbers on efficacy and safety.

Yet his operating rule number three was the need for speed in getting drugs to market, without endless agonizing about safety. This, too,
was quite unlike the old obstructionist agency of DESI and the Librium-Valium hearings. In a PDAC meeting in 1981, soon after he had
taken over the director's post, Leber hinted at what his thinking was
going to be: When a drug was being approved, he said, there was a
tension between "examin[ing] a drug in all the possible conditions of
strata of use [age groups, gender, race, etc.] and keep[ing] it off the
market . . . or, if you will, current realities, and at the same time, speedy
drug approval, and I think those are the two competing things." The
committee had just considered the antidepressant nomifensine the previous day, in trials of about 160 subjects. Leber continued, "It is clear
that we were limited in the kind of inferences we could make to labeling because we hadn't examined the whole domain of clinical use.
Well, why hadn't we? Because it would be too expensive, too costly, too
time consuming, and I would think against the spirit of deregulation
that probably is going on."[56] These are not the utterances of someone
who plans to long hold up a drug because of concern about every last
subpopulation that it might be put into.

Throughout his tenure at FDA, Leber maintained the primacy of not overagonizing in considering drugs for approval. In 1989, at a meeting considering the TCA clomipramine for obsessive-compulsive disorder, he returned to this theme: "That is something about the reality of the world that we have to look at. Drugs will be marketed before we know everything about them. If you want to wait for the time when you know everything about them, you will not get them marketed. I do not want to sound cavalier about it. I hate to put people at risk but I do not think there is any way to speed drugs to market and, at the same time, know everything."[57] (Leber also thought that it was very easy to overinform the public about potential drug risks.)[58]

Leber's operating rule number four, at least in the first several years of his tenure, was insisting on the existence of two depressions: melancholic and nonmelancholic, although he used various terms for them. Drugs that worked for the one might not be effective for the other. In 1982, talking about the trials supporting the use of alprazolam (Xanax) as an antidepressant, he said, "There is probably a point where it is clearly an antidepressant, and [then] it crosses over, it becomes less and less effective in the collection [of] patients called depressed where you can't call it an antidepressant anymore." He added, "What does it mean to say a patient is severely depressed? Each of us might say terrible anguish, terrible suicidality? If you were doing that, these patients rated very, very low in many scales—that's why they're out-patients."[59]

Later that day, the discussion switched over to bupropion (Wellbutrin), another antidepressant. Again, the problem was, can you infer from outpatient data antidepressant activity in inpatients and vice-versa (outpatients being easier to recruit in trials)? "I mean, is that what we are getting at? That if you have good results as an antidepressant in an in-patient setting with severely ill patients that you can say it is an antidepressant willy-nilly. . . ."

Magda Campbell, a New York City psychiatrist: Well, there is a difference in severity.

Leber: Is that the only difference?[60]

On other occasions, Leber clearly articulated the difference between the two depressions rather than merely quizzing the committee Socratically about them. In 1983: "It seems to me that in the few years I have been coming to these days [PDAC meetings] that some days we require a drug be worked up in what I will call endogenomorphic depression [endogenous depression], to steal from Don Klein, in hospitalized patients and then we will say it is an antidepressant. On other occasions we will rely upon studies done with patients who are dysphoric, who may have a mixture of anxiety and depression. . . . We generally end up saying the drug is an antidepressant."[61] Given the official FDA policy of accepting only *DSM* indications, this is a stunning admission: that a single term, "major depression," harbors two conditions as different from each other as measles and tuberculosis.

Finally, in this list of operating rules that may be inferred from Leber's remarks in thousands of pages of committee transcripts, he thought that drugs should be compared only to placebos, and that comparisons with the standard remedy in the field were to be discouraged. It is this preference, which he did not originate but insisted on fiercely during his 20 years at the helm, that has had such devastating consequences for U.S. psychopharmacology, because it rules out therapeutic progress, and may indeed be a recipe for a regression of efficacy in pharmaceuticals: If you compare only against placebo, you have no idea whether the drug in question is an improvement upon predecessors or not.

It wasn't Leber who brought to FDA the doctrine of no active comparators. Previously, the agency's view of the need for active comparators in a trial had been all over the map, but there certainly was a group discouraging them and calling for placebo-only. In 1968, explaining the agency's view of the NAS/NRC study then still going on, regulations expert Julius Hauser said the FDA did "not intend to determine comparative efficacy." Would a less effective drug have to be removed from the market? Hauser: "If a drug is a useful drug in the sense that its effectiveness and potential benefits outweigh its hazards, its marketing may be continued."[62] In private, the agency was on occasion actively hostile to manufacturers who wanted to make a comparative claim in their advertising. In 1972, agency counsel Peter Hutt told Commissioner Charles Edwards that if the manufacturer of an existing drug claims that it works, for example, "twice as fast as a competitive drug . . . the drug is to be classified as a 'new drug.' . . . "[63] This was the equivalent of dropping the atom bomb, for reclassification as a new drug meant expensive new trials and an uncertain decision about approval. Edwards told outsiders that Congress had never granted the FDA authority "to deny approval of a new drug application for a drug that, although shown to be effective, is relatively less effective than alternative drugs"; he said the agency would not refuse "to approve an NDA for that reason, and does not propose to do so in the future."[64]

Yet in the 1960s and early '70s, a number of agency officers did indeed believe they were charged with ensuring comparative efficacy. There clearly was no central agency doctrine in effect on this subject. In the area of antibiotics, Joe Sadusk, director of the FDA's Bureau of Drugs, told a Pfizer executive, "In our opinion, we may require the labeling of a drug to bear accurate statements of comparative effectiveness and comparative safety whenever such information is available." Pfizer was not entitled to make a broad claim. "We believe the law allows us . . . to remind the physician that penicillin is still the drug of first choice in [gonococcal urethritis]."[65] In 1970 Lou Lasagna said, ". . . When [now former FDA Commissioner] Jim Goddard discusses [comparative efficacy] in public these days, he says that a drug should not be allowed on the market unless it is better than the ones it would be competing with."[66] Marion Finkel, Bureau of Drugs deputy director, sent in 1971 a memo to staffers in drug-approvals mandating them to consider "relative effectiveness." According to the Pharmaceutical Manufacturers Association (PMA), this memo "caused furor both inside the agency and in the drug industry." The memo was ultimately rescinded.[67]

One final example of the agency's lack of clarity on relative effectiveness before Paul Leber took over the Neuropharm Division: In August 1974 staffers in the FDA Office of Scientific Evaluation were agonizing about whether to approve the antipsychotic drug pimozide. Studies had been ambivalent. The clincher in sending out the nonapprovable letter was this: "Discussions at Rounds were held about . . . the fact that pimozide apparently has more side effects than some of the presently marketed antipsychotics, e.g., chlorpromazine and thioridazine. The firm agrees that there is inadequate evidence to support the use of the drug in acute schizophrenia. Dr. Leventhal questioned whether a drug with questionable efficacy should be studied further. . . ."[68] This was a comparative deliberation, without doubt.

Thus, when Leber took command of "Psychopharmacology Unit II" in 1979, the situation about comparative efficacy at the FDA was anything but clear. He proceeded to implement his own policy, and it was very clear indeed: Comparative studies were to be discouraged; only placebo data would be considered for purposes of the well-controlled studies that the Kefauver-Harris Amendments demanded. "We have a hierarchy of clinical trials," he told the PDAC in 1983, just after becoming director of the Neuropharmacological Drug Products Division, "and the hierarchy is mine. It is not an official position of the Agency. . . . My own personal view is that if you want to know whether something works or not, placebo is the way to find out." Was Drug A better than Drug B? "We can't be Solomon in those kinds of things."[69]

Leber started specifically asking companies not to send in comparative data. In 1981 Barney Carroll of the University of Michigan and a member of the PDAC asked the representatives of Marion Laboratories, who had submitted a New Drug Application for the TCA dothiepin, what happened to the comparative data on amitriptyline, also a TCA, in studies the company had conducted?

Marion representative: "The data that we presented basically represents what we were requested to prepare by Food and Drug. We were requested specifically not to do the other analyses, that it was not asked for."

Another Marion representative: "In earlier versions, we had done all three comparisons [dothiepin, amitriptyline, placebo], and at a subsequent meeting here in FDA, they asked us only to do the two. So we stopped doing all three."

Carroll kept boring in: What did the earlier data show? The company admitted that their drug, dothiepin, had not beaten the comparator amitriptyline. The PDAC chairman, John Kane, cut the discussion off.[70]

Over time, the Leber doctrine sharpened: Data from trials were really just to establish if a therapeutic effect existed, not how large that effect was, meaning just how useful a drug would be to clinicians compared to other drugs. In a submission for haloperidol decanoate, a long-lasting version of the popular antipsychotic Haldol, Leber said that clearly the drug had efficacy. "Now, again this brings up the old issue of size of treatment effect versus the existence of a treatment effect. And for purposes of approval we rely on the existence, the hypothesis testing whether or not it is there."[71] On another occasion he said that normally at the FDA, ". . . We shun considerations of the size of treatment effects. In the first place, we do not think they are measurable in any real sense. You get an average effect but it is hard to say for whom and what it means."[72] From the viewpoint of a doctor thinking about prescribing a drug, this verges on regulatory nihilism.

But what if a sponsor really wanted to do a study with an active comparator? Impossible? No, but Leber's conditions were pretty severe. You'd have to compare your drug, the market leader, and the placebo at three different doses,[73] making for a nine-arm study, a very expensive proposition at, say, 50 patients per arm. And then risk that your drug might lose against the comparator! In psychopharmacology, few such studies were ever submitted to the FDA.

This absolutism about not accepting comparative data softened a bit over the years, but only to the extent of using information on an active comparator to ensure that the trial was "sensitive," and not to compare the efficacy of the two drugs.[74] Sensitive in this context means that you have a patient population capable of responding to the drug, in other words, capable of showing a difference. If the patients respond to the comparator but not to your drug, you know the trial was sensitive (but that's not a reason for nonapproval); if the patients respond to neither, you have a "failed" trial, not two unsuccessful drugs. In FDA jargon, such failed trials were often called "nonsensitive," not failed. Leber once said, "The words failed and negative are thrown around. They don't have an official meaning for us."[75]

Showing differences wasn't the agency's job. It was not that all had won and all must have prizes, for many drugs were sent to the back of the class, but usually for errors in trial design. If you designed your trial right, your drug would pass regardless how inert it was (as long as it beat placebo, even by only a small amount). In 2001, 2 years after Leber left the agency, Thomas Laughren, head of the psychiatry drugs group of the Neuropharmacological Drug Products Division, said, "Showing superiority to an active drug . . . is very difficult and it cannot be expected that a new treatment will be superior to standard therapy."[76]

This refusal to compare directly two drugs in order to see which is better created a kind of Alice-in-Wonderland situation. At a PDAC meeting to consider an intramuscular form of Lilly's new "second-generation" antipsychotic olanzapine (Zyprexa), Michael Grundman, a neurologist at the University of California at San Diego, said, "I guess really the critical question for us to grapple with is whether or not we think this is any worse than what clinicians are already doing with haloperidol and lorazepam," referring to an older, "first-generation" antipsychotic and a benzodiazepine, respectively.

Abby Fyer, a psychiatrist at Columbia University, scolded, "It is not going to say in the labeling we are letting you do this because we think what you might do is worse."[77] This was the ultimate logic of not comparing drugs directly against one another: The labeling would give no guidance. You as a clinician would therefore be at the mercy of the drug reps dropping by to give you the real scoop on the competition.

The SSRIs at Food and Drug Administration

In this atmosphere of the noncomparison of drugs, and the inability to track progress or regression in therapeutic efficacy, the SSRIs arrived at the FDA beginning in the early 1980s. First to go before the agency with a New Drug Application was Solvay with fluvoxamine (Luvox), from the mid-flight group of SSRIs. The experience was definitely not typical, defying Leber's speed-of-approval rule: Solvay applied in 1983 for a depression indication, and 11 years later, in December 1994, finally received FDA approval, not for depression, but for obsessive-compulsive disorder. The long delay was a comedy of errors as first one thing, then another went wrong, and the agency strewed the path of the Belgian company with thorns. Also, the inexperience of a European company with the distinctive American regulatory environment might have played a role. Still, there were warning flags raised about this first SSRI to gain approval.

The first warning flag: John Greist at the University of Wisconsin, presenting on behalf of Solvay, told the PDAC in response to a question about the drug's side effects, "Inhibited orgasm was one that, over the long term, got to be problematic." Almost a fifth of the men in the trials experienced "delayed ejaculation."[78]

The second flag: In the trials, fluvoxamine failed to beat an active comparator, the TCA clomipramine. Was this a problem? Not at all, said Leber. ". . . A single point of comparison is always risky because you really don't know what the dose-response relationships are in that trial. . . . I think we ought to at least recognize that a couple of slides don't allow us to adequately assess it."[79]

The third flag: under the influence of fluvoxamine (Luvox), an alarming number of patients seemed to become agitated. Andrew Mosholder was the chief FDA officer to review a later Luvox New Drug Application in 1996 for treatment of obsessive-compulsive disorder in children. Mosholder found that in the adult trials, 2 percent of the patients became agitated (versus 1 percent on placebo), but in the pediatric trials, 12 percent of the children on the drug experienced agitation (versus 3 percent on placebo). Were children at special risk from this first SSRI to present for approval? Apparently, yes, but Mosholder was prevented by FDA superiors from giving this information to the relevant advisory committee meeting at the time.[80] This information didn't become public until much later, in 2004 congressional hearings that were convened to investigate antidepressant use in children. But it was known at the

FDA even during the drug's initial, 11-year approval process for adult use, representing one of the first puzzling signs that with the SSRIs, the FDA was willing to overlook significant data.

The next drug to pass initial Food and Drug surveillance was fluoxetine (Prozac), from the late-flight group of SSRIs. Lilly was not particularly thrilled about the drug, and Dorothy Dobbs, a former FDA official but now part of Lilly's office of regulatory affairs, told the FDA in June 1982 in the run-up leading to a New Drug Application, "There is nothing discernibly unique about either the side effect profile or the improvement seen with fluoxetine or the other study drugs."[81] The company regarded Prozac as pretty much of a muchness. With reason: In six of eight studies presented to the FDA, Prozac failed convincingly to beat placebo. And in four of those six there was really no difference.[82] In the October 1985 PDAC meeting, member Ching-piao Chien of the University of California, Los Angeles said, "So, suppose all eight people publish their papers, that would end up like a disaster."[83] There was no evidence at all that Prozac had any efficacy in hospitalized patients, who usually are the most depressed.[84] And FDA reviewer Hillary Lee raised the possibility that "it is not clear that it [fluoxetine] is effective."[85]

A quarter of the patients in the trials became agitated or anxious, "which is not a small incidence," as Chien put it.[86]

Leber himself was quite dubious of much of Lilly's presentation. "One of the things I find most distressing, for a disinterested and dispassionate assessment of data, is the throwing together and the obfuscation of what is, in fact, the data bases we're looking at? Anybody who chooses, after the fact, can look through yesterday's headlines and prove that, in fact, nothing happened that did, and everything happened that didn't. . . . And I think that your presentation—my concern is that I don't even know what the company's stand is."[87]

It took the FDA another 2 years to approve Prozac, which they did only in December 1987. So nobody could argue that the agency somehow greased the skids for Lilly to accelerate the approval of their drug, as precious patent minutes ticked.

Yet there are aspects of the FDA's—and Paul Leber's—subsequent relations with Lilly that caused comment. At the 1985 PDAC meeting, Leber had quite presciently remarked, "We're going to miss things [side effects]. I guarantee, or at least I'm willing to place a bet with anyone, that fluoxetine, if marketed, will have reports of adverse events we have never seen. Some of them may be due to the drug, some of them may not be due to the drug, but they're going to be out there."[88]

In fact, by 1990 Prozac was back in the dock under accusations of causing suicide. To this day, it has not been established if these accusations have merit. Yet Leber certainly didn't believe them, and trivialized them.

> While we are at it, it shows you how times change. When we first looked at fluoxetine, the great sword of Damocles that hung over us was the issue of zimeldine with ascending paralysis [Guillain-Barré] and its flu-like syndrome. Now with several years under our belt [with fluoxetine], I guess we have accepted one or two cases and . . . that has gone to sleep. Now with fluoxetine being pegged . . . for possibly inducing the strange subset of ideational behavior about suicide, . . . this question comes up. This [fluoxetine] seems to be remarkably clean as antidepressants or, in fact, all drugs go for its safety base.[89]

The judgment of Prozac's remarkable cleanliness goes against the misgivings expressed in FDA internal correspondence at the time. A "summary basis of approval" for fluoxetine, composed in October 1988, a few months after Lilly had been authorized to market the drug, said, "The sponsor [Lilly] has agreed to explore existing databases to further assess the relationship of agitation . . . at baseline to outcome." This was virtually the sole caveat.[90] So, some assessors at the agency were worried: Agitation is a virtual synonym for akathisia, a state of mental unrest leading to physical restlessness, and researchers who fear the possible tendency of Prozac and the other SSRIs to induce suicidality invoke akathisia as the mechanism.[91]

It has been charged that during the suicidality debate, Leber's relations with Lilly were suspiciously close. At one point, internal company correspondence refers to him as "our defender."[92] Yet that could be in reference to the assault by the vehemently antidrug Scientologists under which Lilly then groaned.[93] In fact, the evidence for a possible Leber "sellout" to industry is poor, and certainly the heartburn that he caused Lilly when the company tried to market a combo antipsychotic-antidepressant for psychotic depression speaks against it. According to Alexander Glassman at the New York State Psychiatric Institute, who had insider knowledge of events, "Paul said, 'You know what, you guys . . . try and find every new indication.' [Yet] these are all depressions, they're all the same, but when you break it up into a new kind of depression, then you can advertise it, and then you sell more if you can say agitated depressions, and retarded depressions, and smoking depressions." Glassman added that Lilly "got enormous grief" from Leber.[94]

Then, there is the curious rapidity with which Leber positively shoehorned the next two SSRI blockbusters through FDA approval. In April 1988, Pfizer filed the NDA for sertraline (Zoloft). The drug had not done badly in the trials, according to the data that the company submitted with the NDA—beating placebo in 4 out of 5 treatment "arms" (trials with adequate dosing compared to placebo)[95]—but terribly in some of the trials whose data the company didn't submit.[96] (In one trial postlaunch, over a 10-month period, exercise beat Zoloft for antidepressant efficacy.)[97] Nonetheless, Pfizer's sertraline data available at the time of the NDA's review were considered so weak that just after the PDAC meeting, one FDA staffer, Martin Brecher, told a representative of SmithKline Beecham, which was just about to offer paroxetine (Paxil) for approval, that he, Brecher, would "have been embarrassed having to present sertraline."[98] Leber himself had doubts, and in an internal memo said, "In recommending [approval], I have considered the fact that the evidence marshaled to support [Zoloft's] efficacy as an antidepressant is not as consistent or robust as one might prefer it to be."[99]

Yet Leber militated strongly within the PDAC for a positive vote. Was Zoloft not as effective as other drugs? "I think it should be understood," he said, "that all comparisons are probably odious. . . . I think you have to understand that when we face an application, from a regulatory perspective, we are asked to face what the law requires us to do. We are obliged to approve an NDA unless our review finds that the drug is unsafe for use."[100] So there: The FDA had no choice. The law required approval.

The FDA refused to present to the PDAC the negative results of Pfizer's inpatient trials on sertraline.[101] What was the story? Leber told the committee that if this were an academic seminar, we could hem and haw all day about the design of drug trials. But this was the real world of regulation. "For example, that patients who are in-hospital show a response has not been documented. But you have to ask the question what does it mean not to document that? . . . What inference can you draw from small studies which fail to show that? In a regulatory sense, it is distinct from other general senses." This last sentence is as close as I have ever seen to an admission by the agency that they are playing a kind of little private game distinct from the rules of evidence and common sense in the real world.

PDAC member Javier Escobar at the University of Connecticut asked Leber, "Has it happened that an antidepressant is approved without evidence of inpatient efficacy?"

Leber: Yes.

Escobar: It has?

Leber: Many times.[102]

Escobar found this a bit of a problem. ". . . What often happens is that once one of these agents is approved on the basis of outpatient data, then when you begin using it in the traditional psychiatric populations you may find some surprises. So my concern about consistency in outpatient and inpatient data is because I have a feeling that these populations are very different."[103]

But what did efficacy mean, anyway? Leber proceeded to trash the whole notion: "I have no idea what constitutes proof of efficacy, except on the basis of what we, as a Committee, agree on as an as *ad hoc* case as there needs to be. You can be guided by the past but the inference is an abstraction—what is an antidepressant?" We might, he said, look at some of the various rating scales, "but that is tradition. That is not truth."[104] Later on he said it was just too difficult to gather data on inpatients (remember that most outpatients were recruited in newspaper ads), and that electroconvulsive treatment was probably the best remedy for inpatients anyway![105]

Leber said it was not the drug but the trials that had failed. "If we have studies such as those that failed to find a difference . . . between an active drug and placebo, we do not have assay sensitivity in that trial. Generally, as an Agency . . . we have tended to take such studies and treat them as uninformative. They do not tell you much."[106] This really involved almost bending over backward in order to avoid saying anything negative about sertraline. This was the new FDA: When drugs fail, it is the trial not the drug that is at fault.

It continued to bother the committee that Zoloft seemed to have so little efficacy, so Leber finally said he had figured out what the real "treatment effect" of the drug actually was in outpatients (as opposed to the p value of statistical significance that was normally used in seeing whether a drug beat placebo, a value that measures the presence of a treatment effect rather than its size: a p value of statistical significance will almost always be positive in a large trial even if the treatment effect is very small). "Just for kicks, this morning I ran a few of these using a program I got from a colleague, Dr. [Jeffrey] Lieberman. . . ." The results came out as "a modest to minimal treatment effect size . . . So they are not big treatment effect sizes, make no and's, if's or but's about it, even defined that way. It is a tough problem."[107]

Yes, indeed. It was a tough problem that sertraline was simply not very effective. Yet Leber recommended its approval and the drug was dumped on an unsuspecting population on the basis that it "gets depressed patients back into the mainstream": the first ad showed a sad-looking young woman who then, under the influence of Zoloft, was now happily embracing her husband, her children, telephoning animatedly, and jogging."[108]

The last of the blockbuster SSRIs to pass through the FDA during this period was SmithKline Beecham's paroxetine (Paxil), the New Drug Application for which was submitted in November 1989. (I am excluding further discussion of the last blockbuster, Lundbeck-Forest's citalopram [Celexa], on the grounds that it was approved much later, in 1998, long after this period in question.) It is unnecessary to tarry long here, because the reader already has a good idea what to expect: Paroxetine failed in 45 percent of its trials to beat placebo,[109] leading to much talk of lacking "assay sensitivity." There were a total of 41 studies with active controls, which "for the most part," as Tom Laughren put it, "found no difference between the active drugs and, therefore, are very difficult to interpret."[110]

When the TCA imipramine trounced paroxetine in two of the studies, Leber commented, "In general, I think we are afraid of comparisons. They tend to be odious. I think the data on imipramine versus Paxil is an illustration of how dangerous it is to choose your source of data to illustrate a point which you believe in."[111]

In fact, paroxetine just sailed through the meeting of the advisory committee in October 1992. There were no tough questions, and the meeting adjourned by 12:25 P.M., virtually unheard of. Two months later, by December 1992, the FDA had approved paroxetine and it was on the market.

But the real world of psychopharm was slightly less ready than the FDA to trust in paroxetine's supposedly unrivaled efficacy, demonstrated on populations of the malcontent recruited through newspaper ads. The Danish University Antidepressant Group, less intimidated than SmithKline Beecham's trialists at the difficulties of studying hospital populations, compared paroxetine to the tricyclic antidepressant clomipramine in 102 hospitalized patients, and found clomipramine considerably more effective: At the end of 6 weeks, 56 percent of the patients with endogenous depression had a "complete response" to clomipramine, only 25 percent of the paroxetine patients. "The dominant finding in this study is the low rate of response with paroxetine which seems to outweigh the advantages in terms of fewer side effects and low toxicity."[112] This was among the first studies to demonstrate the superiority of the tricyclics to the SSRIs, an important point because the companies claimed that efficacy was equal but that the SSRIs had a superior side effects profile.

At the end of the saga of the SSRIs at the Food and Drug Administration—a saga that unleashed this rather ineffective drug class upon a public guileless in its belief in the ubiquity of "major depression"—one is left not so much with the feeling of a sellout as a failure of science. Of the operating rules that Leber seems to have borne into FDA at the beginning of the 1980s, several had become tattered by the time of his departure nearly 20 years later.

Of his commitment to speedy approval of NDAs: That certainly went out the window with Solvay's fluvoxamine (Luvox) and Lilly's fluoxetine (Prozac). Yet he seemed dead keen to get SmithKline Beecham's paroxetine (Paxil) and Pfizer's sertraline (Zoloft) through. This is scarcely evidence of a "sellout to industry," as his detractors, some of them animated by Scientology, have charged. But on the whole, this is a drug class that the FDA treated with kid gloves.

Of Leber's impatience with cant about neurotransmitters and nebulous neurocognitive concepts: This never wavered. He remained as skeptical about trendiness at the end of his tenure as at the beginning.

Of his commitment to comparing drugs only to placebo and not to other drugs: Leber never deviated. In 1996 he told Wyeth that even though you've shown that lorazepam beats diazepam in status epilepticus, you can't advertise it: ". . . the study cannot reliably speak to the comparative performance of Ativan [lorazepam] and Valium [diazepam] under conditions of actual use."[113] But setting difficult conditions for comparisons made it hard to discard inferior agents; it became a guarantee for diminishing the efficacy of the nation's stock of antidepressant medication. Effective tricyclics such as clomipramine became forgotten: The SSRIs were hyped as just as effective, and oh those nasty tricyclic side effects, never again will our patients have trouble with dry mouth.

Of his commitment to the primacy of data: With the doctrine of "unresponsive populations" and "failed trials," Leber did seem to be explaining away inconvenient findings, most manifest perhaps in the sertraline discussion at the advisory committee. A close analysis of the PDAC transcripts shows that, on occasion, he could be highly manipulative of the advisory committee, and often steered them toward the result he wanted.[114]

Of Leber's concept of the two depressions: In accepting the SSRIs as a universal remedy for depression of every sort, otherwise known as major depression, he really abandoned his own view. Early on in his tenure, in 1983, Leber said, "The risk we run . . . is what happens if you have a drug that is ineffective in a particularly dangerously ill segment of the population? If you put that drug on the market, you have what I would call dilution of the therapeutic armamentarium. You are displacing individuals from the opportunity of getting treated with an effective drug because you have an ineffective one on the market. So you want to look at those cases where the failure to treat depression is most dangerous."[115] This is precisely the point.

The dangerous illness in the mood area is melancholia. But by the time the SSRIs came along in the late 1980s, Leber had lost interest in melancholia and the notion of two depressions. At the sertraline PDAC hearing in 1990, Jeffrey Lieberman, then at Long Island Jewish Hospital, asked, do we know how many patients in these trials "may have been of the melancholic subtype"? Leber indicated that the question was beside the point; he doubted that there were any predictors of treatment response or outcome in "this great unwashed mass called depressed patients."

Lieberman replied, "There is significant evidence in terms of biologic measures [dexamethasone suppression test], as well as placebo response rates [very low], which are associated with melancholia as a subtype as opposed to the larger category of MDD [major depressive disorder]."

Leber: "I would like to see the meta-analysis on that."[116]

In waving the SSRIs through, Leber and colleagues at the FDA violated the basic principle of not diluting the armamentarium. They helped drive effective drugs for serious depression, such as the tricyclics and the MAOIs, off the market with a drug class that treated only nonmelancholia, if that. The consequences for American psychiatry, psychopharmacology, and patient treatment have been disastrous, as ineffective drugs are offered for an undifferentiated *DSM* diagnosis of depression that does not exist in nature.

What happened? Why was the FDA of old, something of a star chamber for subduing the pharmaceutical industry, replaced by this new FDA that seemed almost eager to approve even the most embarrassingly inadequate products? Because access to FDA archives comes to an end around 1982, this question is impossible to answer definitively at present.[117] Also, my own knowledge is largely confined to psychopharmaceuticals, whereas the question covers the entire FDA. Yet there are a couple of hints.

One new circumstance was biography. Bob Temple and Paul Leber evidently saw it as their mission, however compromised it sometimes was in reality, to accelerate drug approvals rather than lurk under the bridge as gnarled curmudgeons waiting to strike down popular drugs. Leber, perhaps in a moment of desperation during the sertraline fiasco, became quite explicit: "We are now beginning to get a class of second and third generation antidepressants which work. . . . There are no cardiovascular effects to speak of—relatively free of some of the things that have troubled us with some of the tricyclics in the males. Maybe the last three or four have been like that. . . . Anybody disagree with that assessment? I am not trying to make a commercial but. . . ."[118] This is not the begrudging, dyspeptic diction of the agency of yore.

Another new circumstance was sociological: the growing network of informal social ties between industry representatives and FDA officers. The correspondence in the archives in these years fairly bounces with reports of industry executives popping into FDA offices for chats. The arrival of Temple and Leber meant much more collaboration in the design of trials and the preparation of NDAs. Industry by this time was thoroughly cowed. Lou Lasagna noted in 1989 that, even in the face of "regulation by accretion," drugmakers do not normally speak up, fearing "the possibility for vindictiveness and retaliation by agency staff on the firm's other current or future filings."[119] In evaluating these complex NDAs, there was necessarily much to-ing and fro-ing at the agency's headquarters in the Parklawn Building, and regulatory scholar Paul Quirk writes, " . . . Having frequent contacts with industry representatives, getting to know and perhaps like them personally, and seeing their anxiousness to have drugs approved obviously will tend to create some sympathy for industry viewpoints and interests. Such contacts on a regular basis over a period of years may strongly shape the attitudes of FDA officials."[120] In the days of the cop-agency of the 1950s and '60s such contacts were, on the basis of my inspection of the archives, much less. And the whole sociology of a syncytium means that all members are on board for the same ends.

Finally, in the background were the continuous pressures from Congress and the Department of Health and Human Services to speed up drug approvals.[121] These pressures culminated in the Prescription Drug User Fee Act of 1992, in which the FDA collected fees from industry to accelerate the drug approval process. The pharmaceutical industry may well have been behind this push, but industry had virtually no direct leverage on the FDA. The fulcrum of power lay on Capitol Hill and at DHHS and certainly not in any direct influencing of the agency by industry: Respectful submissiveness was the only industry posture tolerated in the Parklawn Building.

Uptake

In the 1990s the SSRIs, together with their close cousins, the reuptake inhibitors of serotonin and norepinephrine (the SNRIs such as Wyeth's venlafaxine, launched in 1994 as Effexor), drove almost every other drug class in psychiatry, except the "atypical" or second-generation antipsychotics and the hyperactivity drugs, off the boards. How did they do this?

Partly by trashing the competition. The SSRIs, unlike their predecessors, were said to be free of "dependency." Yet drugmakers have always indicted the competition as addictive. Thomas Ban, professor of psychopharmacology at Vanderbilt University in Nashville, saw this badmouthing of the predecessors as an old story: "In my judgment the issue of dependence on meprobamate was used in replacing meprobamate with chlordiazepoxide [Librium] and diazepam [Valium], and the issue of dependence on benzodiazepines was used in trying to replace them with [SSRI] antidepressants. Now the issue of dependency is blown out of proportion with antidepressants. I am not trying to say that there is no dependency on these drugs but it is not those who need these drugs who become dependent on them."[122]

The SSRI makers unleashed a systematic campaign to demonstrate how addictive and dangerous the benzos, already tainted with this stigma since the 1960s, and the tricyclics were. David Sheehan, an Irish-trained psychiatrist at the University of South Florida who was heavily involved in consulting to industry, had a ringside seat: "It was a deliberate tactic. At major U.K. and international meetings, they would sponsor symposia on the dangers of benzodiazepines. . . . Hundreds and, in some cases, thousands of physicians would attend these well-orchestrated meetings, would listen to this stuff and get into a panic that maybe they were doing some kind of social harm and that their colleagues disapproved of this practice. The public and the media certainly began to disapprove." Sheehan said that a "feverish pitch was built up" so that when the first SSRIs arrived, physicians would switch their patients over. "Then everyone would live happily ever after and the benzodiazepines would go the way of the barbiturates or the bromides."[123]

The tactic worked. The uptake of the blockbuster SSRIs was breathtaking. Prozac hit the market in December 1987, and had sales of $125 million in 1988, $350 million in 1989, "more," said *Newsweek*, "than was spent on *all* antidepressants just two years earlier."[124] Driven heavily by Prozac, the world market for psychotropics rose from $2 billion in 1986 to $4.4 billion in 1991.[125] By March 1991 Prozac had been launched in 26 countries.[126] "No one doubts that downmood can be upmarket," said an editorial in the British medical weekly *Lancet*.[127]

Yet in 1991 the non-SSRI antidepressants were still holding their heads above water: At that point Prozac had only 28 percent of the U.S. market, whereas nortriptyline (Lilly's Aventyl) had 9 percent, amitriptyline (Merck's Elavil) 9 percent, and trazodone (Mead Johnson's Desyrel) 4 percent.[128]

Then the SSRI companies started piling on sales representatives. No quarter was to be given! By March 1993, SmithKline Beecham's Paxil, which had just been launched with the first-time use of that catchy acronym "SSRI," was being detailed by a U.S. sales force of 1,800, versus Lilly's dispatch of 1,600 reps for Prozac and Pfizer's 1,250 for Zoloft.[129] A year later, the big story was Zoloft, up 138 percent in sales in 1993 and taking off faster even than Prozac had. Even Paxil wasn't braking Zoloft's growth![130] Observers were stunned. No drug class in pharmaceuticals had ever witnessed this kind of growth before. In 2001, 3 of the top 10 drugs in the United States were SSRIs (Zoloft number 6, Paxil number 7, Prozac number 9).[131]

We fast-forward past all the stupendous numbers, to reach the most stupendous: According to the Agency for Healthcare Research and Quality, total expenditures on antidepressants in the United States increased from $5.1 billion in 1997 to $12.1 billion in 2004.[132] Depression, once understood as a serious illness that curled its victims into fetal crouches on their beds, was now up there with consumer electronics.

On a worldwide basis, the SSRIs had in fact hosed up much of the oxygen in the room. By 2001, SSRIs constituted 46.2 percent of all antidepressant sales; the drugs that affected both serotonin and norepinephrine (such as Effexor [venlafaxine]) constituted 18.5 percent; and other "second-generation antidepressants" 13.7 percent. Meanwhile, the classic (and truly effective) antidepressants had shrunk to a tiny fragment of all sales: tricyclics 1.2 percent, and monoamine oxidase inhibitors 0.8 percent.[133]

"The Emperor's New Drugs"

These stunning amounts of antidepressants were being prescribed for individuals who were defined as "depressed." In the United States, outpatients with the diagnosis of "depression" who received antidepressants rose from 37.3 percent in 1987 to 74.5 percent in 1997—and more than three-quarters of those antidepressants were SSRIs.[134] In 1997–98, according to the National Center for Health Statistics, 31.3 percent of all women who visited the doctor received an antidepressant.[135] Said one lifestyle journalist, "Doctors call them 'so what drugs' because when you're on them and something bad happens you just say, 'So what'?"[136]

Is there anything wrong with drugs that cause you to say "so what"? That's basically what alcohol does. Yet in the case of the SSRIs there were several serious problems that weren't at once apparent amidst the media hysteria about sales growth: They didn't work very well for depression (though were suitable for other indications); they were to be avoided in melancholia; and they were loaded with side effects.

The lacking effectiveness of the SSRIs was apparent, as we have seen, in the clinical trials. On the whole, the SSRIs failed about half of their trials. Tom Laughren at the FDA told the PDAC in September 2004, "First I want to turn to adult depression trials for drugs that we believe work. Looking at trials that on face should work, about half the time those trials fail."[137] Half the trials failing is not good for any drug.

The meeting at which this adult-trial information surfaced was specifically focused on the possible suicide potential of antidepressants prescribed to children and adolescents. The FDA asked, should a black box be placed on the antidepressant label as a pediatric suicide warning? But might that reduce their use, leaving genuinely suicidal patients untreated? Responding at a joint meeting the next day between the PDAC and the FDA's Pediatric Advisory Committee, Thomas Newman, professor of pediatric epidemiology at the University of California, San Francisco, said: "It would not be that bad if use of these drugs were diminished, I think, because we don't know whether they actually help most patients."[138] As Michael Thase at the University of Pittsburgh put it in 1999, "No currently approved [antidepressant] medication obtains intent-to-treat response rates of better than 60 percent—actually, intent-to-treat rates of 40–50 percent are commonplace—and 10 percent to 20 percent of antidepressant trials are ended prematurely because of adverse effects."[139] (Intent to treat means including in the analysis all patients present at the beginning of the trial.)

Drug and placebo response rates were in the same range. The Committee for Proprietary Medicinal Products of the European Community, according to the *Pink Sheet*, estimated in 1999, on the basis of recent antidepressant trials, "that between 25–55 percent of responders experience a placebo effect, with the investigational drug producing effects ranging 'between 40 percent and 65 percent in the same trials.'"[140] On the basis of statistics on over 100,000 patients randomized to either drug or placebo, gathered by the FDA for a hearing in December 2006 on antidepressants and suicide, there was a 50 percent response rate to the active agent and 40 percent to placebo. As David Healy calculates, "that means that for every 2.5 people treated with placebo, 1 responds. For every 2 treated with drug, there is 1 response. But 80 percent of these responses come from placebo and therefore it in fact takes 10 to be treated with an antidepressant to produce 1 specific drug response."[141] These statistics do not speak well for the efficacy of the SSRI antidepressants.

Moreover, the European Community data may have gauged the drug response too high for the real world, where patients always do less well than in trials (because so many real-world patients are removed from trial populations, such as the alcoholic and the suicidal). Insiders estimate that in actual clinical practice 1 patient in 3 responds to SSRI antidepressants. "We give them as a fringe benefit to make the companies richer," said one senior psychopharmacologist.[142] Irving Kirsch, a psychologist who subjected the SSRI trial data to a rigorous analysis, referred to them as "the emperor's new drugs."[143]

"Paul Leber predicted this day would come," said Karen Barth Menzies, a plaintiff's lawyer, of the pediatric suicide crisis, "when he said that the FDA would come under attack because they weren't as demanding as they ought to have been when they were looking at the efficacy of the antidepressant products."[144]

The SSRIs were particularly inappropriate in melancholic illness. This had become evident with the failure of almost all the trials in hospital depression.[145] "Fluoxetine may be less effective than tricyclic antidepressant drugs for the treatment of inpatients with severe melancholic depression," wrote Lars Gram of Odense University in Denmark in the *New England Journal of Medicine* in 1994, just as the Prozac rocket was screaming skyward. "It should not be the first choice of a drug for them."[146] In 1997 Jan Fawcett, at Rush Medical College in Chicago, found that the tricyclics reduced depressive symptoms among 51 percent of inpatients on a long-term basis, the SSRIs, 33 percent.[147] Said psychopharm insider Alan Schatzberg, head of psychiatry at Stanford University, in an interview about SSRIs in melancholia, "I know of almost no studies that show an SSRI is more effective, but they are tolerated, and I think that where people miss the point is, for the vast majority of patients who are more what Sherv Frazier [at McLean Hospital] used to call the walking worried, the walking wounded, the SSRI's are good drugs. . . . They help mild to moderate depression. But for the more severely ill depression, you see a lot more resistance to the SSRI's and a lot more combinations or whatever. I think the tricyclics, which were tougher to tolerate, were probably more effective agents."[148]

David Healy, director of the North Wales Department of Psychological Medicine, is less charitable than Schatzberg toward the SSRIs for any kind of depression: "It is highly likely that had the SSRIs been tested clinically in the 1950s they would never have been designated as antidepressants."[149] In truth, for such illnesses as obsessive-compulsive disorder, social anxiety, and other components of the marketbasket of nonmelancholic illness, the SSRIs do hold some promise. (When asked if they responded in *any* way to antidepressants, 50 percent of active treatment patients said yes, 30 percent of placebo patients said yes.)[150] But for "depression," in the undifferentiated sense of Bob Spitzer's "major depression," they have been a disaster of historic proportions.

The SSRIs were marketed as much safer than the tricyclics, which were said to abet suicides.[151] Yet safety is the last refuge of the scoundrel. If you can't beat the competition on efficacy, you can surely tease out some aspect of the side effects profile that beats them on "safety." Contrary to the original hype, the SSRIs have been accompanied by frequent and distressing side effects. One study of primary care in the United Kingdom found that two-thirds of SSRI patients had discontinued treatment by the end of the third month.[152] In 1998, Evelinda Trindade at the Canadian Coordinating Office for Health Technology Assessment in

Ottawa and her coworkers calculated "crude rates" of occurrence of 18 different kinds of adverse effects in 84 controlled trials with SSRIs and TCAs; they reported that statistically five of these adverse effects occurred significantly more often with TCAs than with SSRIs, whereas 7 adverse effects occurred significantly more often with SSRIs than with TCAs. There was no statistically significant difference between the two groups of drugs in patients who dropped out of these trials due to adverse effects.[153] The SSRI overall side effects advantage turned out to be an urban myth.

Of SSRI side effects, impotence has proven particularly troublesome. In 2002, in a study of all the new antidepressants, using a validated rating scale of impotence, Anita Clayton and collaborators found that "the prevalence of sexual dysfunction was similar among SSRIs . . . ranging from 36 percent to 43 percent." There were no statistically significant differences among the four SSRIs but the rates were far higher than for other new antidepressants such as bupropion (GlaxoSmith-Kline's Wellbutrin).[154] In fact, Wellbutrin sales had soared in the 1990s because of impotence fears associated with the SSRIs.[155] Insiders thought rates considerably higher than Clayton found. At a meeting of the FDA's PDAC in 1997, Carl Salzman of Harvard University was discussing the difficulty of getting companies to report side effects: "For me, the current classic example is the failure of Lilly to notice that Prozac produces sexual dysfunction until the drug was really out for years. The initial reporting was under one percent, then they grudgingly acknowledge two percent, they are currently grudgingly acknowledging 30 percent, but most clinicians find it's running 80 to 90 percent."[156]

In 1998 when David Healy and I interviewed Roland Kuhn, the Swiss psychiatrist who was first to discover the efficacy of the tricyclic antidepressants, he really had a good deal to say about impotence and Prozac: "They must have missed a digit," he said of Lilly's report of 3 percent impotence. "With my patients I find that almost every second one to whom the drug was given ends up with dysfunction in this area. Of course you have to take into account what age you are dealing with: if you give it to a 20-year-old, it does not crucially diminish his potency but if you give it to a 50-year-old . . . he will be much affected." Kuhn said that Prozac made the men impotent and the women inorgasmic.[157]

Impotence is not a disabling side effect. But neither is dry mouth, the kind of side effect characteristic of the tricyclic antidepressants. Dear Reader, which would you rather have: dry mouth or impotence?

Science as a Marketing Device

If the SSRIs had rested on a fundamental scientific mechanism in brain chemistry, a bit of marketing hype would have been excusable. The problem was that by the advent of the SSRI era of skyrocketing sales in the 1990s, the whole concept of serotonin deficiency as the basis of depressive illness had been exploded. Clinically, the use of drugs that interfered with serotonin reuptake did seem to have some efficacy. Yet the mechanism of the drugs' effectiveness, such as it was, surely lay elsewhere, and blocking serotonin reuptake was somehow beside the point. This was well known among neuroscientists, widely unknown among clinicians.

The nervousness among scientists about reuptake inhibition as the mechanism of drug action began in the 1980s, just as the companies' advertising copy screamed receptors and neurotransmitters. Trazodone "selectively inhibits serotonin uptake in the brain," proclaimed Mead Johnson in 1982 of what they had brand-named Desyrel.[158] (In fact, trazodone has only a weak effect on serotonin; it is not an SSRI.)

But behind the scenes, doubts were growing. A year after trazodone danced on stage in the United States, Barney Carroll, at a select conference in the Berlin suburb of Dahlem said, "The biogenic amine theory [serotonin, norepinephrine, dopamine] now more closely resembles a venerable flag that the field salutes than a tool we can work with effectively." Recent research, he said, pointed at the endocrine system. ". . . Twenty-five years after the tricyclic antidepressants were introduced, we do not know how they work nor on what disturbed systems."[159] Torgny Svensson, professor of pharmacology at the Karolinksa Institute in Stockholm who had come down to London in November 1985 for a conference at the Ciba Foundation on Portland Place, was skeptical of the whole business: "Perhaps looking at receptors isn't that important. . . . I think the receptor approach may not necessarily lead us to improved antidepressant therapies for the future. Perhaps we should ask totally different questions." He mentioned cerebral blood flow and how antidepressants might affect it. "So to some extent we may be studying artifacts, looking at footprints rather than at the actual animal we are hunting."[160]

Uneasiness grew that with the neurotransmitter-uptake approach, people were in fact looking at footprints while the animal lay shadowed in the forest. There were disorienting research findings, such as the discovery that the antidepressant drug tianeptine *increased* the neuronal reuptake of serotonin rather than inhibiting it, as SSRI theory insisted.[161] In the mid-1990s Fridolin Sulser's lab at Vanderbilt University demonstrated "that blockade of biogenic amine uptake is not a prerequisite for antidepressants to exert profound effects in brain."[162] So reuptake really didn't matter so much, after all.

Among insiders at exclusive little conferences far from the colorful drug ads, disquiet rose. In 1990 British psychopharmacologist Merton Sandler convoked a small group to talk about serotonin. John Evenden, an Astra research scientist, told the participants, "Pharmacologists often talk as if there is one neurone, with all these receptors on it, rather than many different types of neurones, many of which are 5-HT [serotonin] mediated and interconnected with all other types of neurones. The simplistic idea of 'the 5-HT neurone' does not bear any relation to reality." Stephen Peroutka, a Stanford neuroscientist, picked up on this: "The system is clearly extremely complex. The beta receptors on the heart provided a simple model system where one can truly measure drug-receptor interactions [notion of "beta-blockers"]. This may have led people to think that there would be neuronal systems for which we would find one function. That is not the case."[163]

Had these remarks reached the doctors, they would have served as early red flags. But they didn't. The ad copy ground on, celebrating the selective reuptake inhibition of serotonin. When in March 1997 the Wellcome Institute in London brought a group of pioneering figures in psychopharmacology together for a chat, George Beaumont, who as Geigy's chief advisor in England had once helped introduce the tricyclic imipramine—and later became a professor of psychopharmacology—said, "After all this thrust towards selectivity what is now happening is that we are almost back to square one. . . . So all this emphasis on separating neurotransmitter systems and identifying receptors seems really to have got us nowhere and we have gone back full circle to where we started in the 1950s. . . . Virtually all the clinical trials of agonists and antagonists of the various 5-HT receptors have produced results which are either equivocal or really of no great clinical significance. . . ."[164]

It remained for Arvid Carlsson, whose work had begun the whole interest in serotonin 40 years previously, to sound the death knell of the concept of serotonin deficiency as the cause of depression. He said in 2002, "[We must] abandon the simplistic hypotheses of there being either an abnormally high or abnormally low function of a given neurotransmitter."[165]

What had started out so bravely in the Brodie lab with the spectro-photofluorimeter and the rabbits, two with their eyes open, the others closed, had ended in hype. There is a science of neurotransmitters, but the science and clinical practice are completely divorced.[166] It turned out that serotonin did not offer the key to depression and that the true biochemistry of affective disorder lay yet unplumbed deep in the interior of the brain. This was a final bitter note in the SSRI story—that it rested on spin and not on truth.

Adieu

In 1975 Louis Lasagna, senior psychopharmacologist, said, "Unlike Gresham's law, good remedies seem, in general, to push out the bad."[167] Why didn't that happen with the SSRIs? Why were bad remedies permitted to drive out the good—and then to remain dominant for so long? There were really two reasons why the SSRIs overcame the wisdom of accumulated experience that has guided medicine over the years.

One reason was that pharmaceutical propaganda simply drowned out the informal corridor exchanges that generally determine a drug's success. The volume of sales rep noise in physicians' offices was turned up to unimaginable levels. Jamie Reedy worked in the early 1990s as a sales representative for Pfizer, flogging Zoloft among other drugs. The Pfizer reps used cases of Zoloft as a "Hail Mary": "To keep a sales call alive, it was worthwhile to resort to the Zoloft play," he said. He would tell the office staff, "You know, I also have Zoloft, Perhaps some of your coworkers—"

"Zoloft! We've never had samples before!" they cried.

"Excited, I asked how many samples they'd like."

"As many as you can give us!" said the receptionists and clerks.

Reidy writes, "I skipped across the parking lot to the Lumina, grabbed a large box containing 144 bottles of seven pills . . . and raced back inside, to find [the receptionist] laughing. Her smile grew upon seeing the case."[168]

In virtually all medical settings, not just the office, the volume was deafening. An insider describes the regular academic sessions at annual meetings of the American Psychiatric Association:

> The APA's printed statement that the [regular] presentations can
> have no [industry] sponsorship simply means no direct contracted

sponsorship; most of the presenters get a lot of their income from industry via speaking at drug dinners, consultancies, etc. and almost all of the posters [at poster sessions reporting new research] are reporting industry research. . . . I am under the impression that a lot of people's travel to the APA is industry paid, especially the people who are flown in from outside North America. So as I think about it, this may contribute to the relatively few nonphysician presentations and the overwhelming focus on drug treatments.[169]

Under these circumstances, when the SSRIs were introduced, the informal corridor exchanges and personal impressions of therapeutic results—the sum of which amount to the accumulated wisdom of experience—were drowned out. The volume simply overpowered the shoulder shrugs, raised eyebrows, and resigned hand movements that normally constitute the signaling of questionable therapeutic results. The shoulders were shrugged, but the medical pens continued to pump out Zoloft prescriptions.

The accumulated wisdom of experience may have failed with the SSRIs for a second reason as well: the overwhelming volume of patient demand. Patients knew about SSRIs from the media, from direct-to-consumer advertisements on television and in print media, and from their friends, and wanted them prescribed. Pharmaceutical companies paid television stars to mention drugs such as Zoloft on camera, not to influence physicians but to prompt patients to ask their doctor for the drug. For example, according to the *New York Times*, Pfizer hired actor Noah Wyle, then playing Dr. John Carter on the television drama *ER*, to kick off its campaign for Zoloft in posttraumatic stress disorder by appearing on the *Today* show to "raise awareness of the disorder." The interviewer "asked Mr. Wyle questions as if he were the doctor he plays on television."[170] This would be a powerful cue for patients to request the drug when they next visited the doctor in connection with stress. It's unusual for physicians to refuse a patient's request to prescribe a specific drug, because refusal would be pointless unless the request is grossly inappropriate, and it would break the therapeutic alliance between doctor and patient.

Thus, a source of medical wisdom that had guided the profession for much of its modern history—the accumulated store of experience inherited from the past to the present—became largely inoperative with the SSRIs. The informal operating rules that helped physicians sort out safety and efficacy with the barbiturates, the stimulants, the benzodi-azepines, the monoamine oxidase inhibitors, the tricyclic antidepressants, and other past effective drug classes were suspended as Prozac, Paxil, and Zoloft appeared. How exactly this occurred, and whether it will happen again, remain big questions that cannot be sorted out in depth in this book.

Let us step back a pace or two. What are the main lines of this story?

The triumph of the SSRIs rolled forward on at least three parallel sets of rails. One set was laid by the FDA, as it blackballed earlier generations of safe and effective drugs for reasons that had everything to do with empire building and little with public health. The playing field was left bare, and the SSRIs rushed on unopposed.

Another track was laid by Bob Spitzer, in the form of "major depression," a formless diagnosis in which virtually any set of psychoactive compounds, however weak, could clean up, because—and this is the third set of tracks, laid by Paul Leber—if you had only to show you could beat placebo and didn't have to demonstrate efficacy against the best players in the competition, the game would be yours. And it was. The SSRIs became for 2 decades the world's face of psychiatry. And now their patents have almost all expired. And no more are in development.

9
What Now?

This is the past. What do we learn from it?

On a psychopharmacology listserv, one participant, himself a psychiatrist, posted a message seeking help for his ailing wife. He thought, with a touch of professional rivalry, that her current psychiatrist was not serving her well, having prescribed two SSRIs.

"Does this make sense to anyone?" he asked the list. "Is there anything in the literature, or from people's experience, that supports the co-administration of two SSRIs?"

One member of the list responded,

> Who really knows what causes depression? And for that matter
> who really knows what neurotransmitters or pathways are
> involved? New agents in research do not even touch the
> serotonergic pathways. I take the path of "whatever works."
> Evidence-based medicine will never look at combinations and the
> like [which members of the list prescribe all the time] as it would
> not benefit the industry's bottom line. As clinicians we have to
> tinker with the tools we have and see what happens. Or have
> I missed something over these years? Our evidence usually is
> sitting in front of us and is known as the patient.[1]

These are words of wisdom: The evidence is in front of us and is how the patients respond to treatment.

We can find out all kinds of things by looking at the patients. An example: trazodone was a mildly effective antidepressant developed in Italy in the 1960s and marketed in the United States by Mead Johnson in 1982 as Desyrel; it had indifferent success. Today, trazodone is experiencing a big comeback, not as an antidepressant but as a hypnotic. In the world of everyday psychiatry, trazodone is loved for its gentle qualities and its affordable price, in contrast to the patent-protected sleep aids that cost the moon. Yet you will never see an ad in a medical journal for trazodone, nor will drug reps ever stop by your office with free samples in the hopes that your patients might start on it and stay with it.

Once you get away from the glossy ads in the journals, in psychiatry today it's the Wild West out there. Clinicians are experimenting constantly with different combinations of treatments, many of them from psychiatry's past, that promise new therapeutic effectiveness. They communicate their day-to-day experiences almost furtively on listservs such as this one, aware that they are pioneering the future of therapeutics in a way that industry will not countenance, because most of the older drugs are not patent protected; government agencies will not support this kind of clinical experimentation because the whole enterprise seems much too empirical for "science" and does not involve research in molecular genetics.

Academic psychiatry offers the image of a prescribing desert with just two tall cactuses, the SSRIs and the atypical antipsychotics. But in the real world it's a different story. Among community psychiatrists with a good knowledge of psychopharm, there's a thoughtful pioneering of combos of the most diverse and imaginative variety. This is not polypharmacy, the harmful proliferation of medications. It's combopharmacy of the kind that the Food and Drug Administration rejected in DESI, the realization that the brain offers multiple pathways to the remediation of illness.

So there's a big disconnect between what is happening in the trenches and in the world of official medicine. The young community psychiatrists combining remedies from the shelf like kitchen spices rarely publish, although communication among themselves in listservs is lively. Academics with honoraria from drug companies dominate the meetings with papers on patent-protected compounds for FDA-approved indications. But this kind of disconnect is not good for a field. It recalls the days when the bewigged courtiers of Louis XVI confronted the angry citizens of Paris over the barricades. Perhaps the conflict between the arid desert of academic psychiatry and the vitality of community practice will have a similar outcome.

Meanwhile at the commanding heights of psychiatry—the organizations, the government funders, the pharmaceutical industry—perspectives are much gloomier. We have invested billions of dollars in the neurosciences, psychiatry, and psychopharmacology in the hopes of promises of singing tomorrows. Yet the therapeutic payoff of these billions has been meager. Psychiatry's ability to make patients better is probably less today than at the time of the first drug set in the 1950s. For the pharmaceutical industry, the current pipeline of drug discovery and development is about empty, and will remain empty until the diseases become better defined. You can't develop drugs for diseases that don't exist—except perhaps in the pages of a consensus-generated diagnostic manual.

Bruce Charlton, a psychiatrist and medical editor in Newcastle upon Tyne and something of a gadfly on the haunches of Big Pharma, likens the mid-twentieth century—the era of the first drug set—to a "golden age of therapeutic progress." He said in 2005, "Future commentators will probably see the past few decades as something of a 'silver age' of scholasticism, rather like the late medieval period of highly professional logic-chopping and commentaries written on commentaries." A fallow period, much like our own time. A Renaissance of drug discovery, he ventures, lies yet in our future.[2]

Maybe. But there's much to be learned about nosology and drug discovery by looking at psychiatry's past. Canadian psychiatrist Julius Hoenig has written, "In the natural sciences old views and interpretations of observations are overtaken by new discoveries, and retain historical interest only; in the humanities this is never quite the case. Psychiatry has one foot in each of these disciplines and our heritage is not something we can simply leave to the historians."[3] These observations assume that psychiatry has in common with the other natural sciences that it, too, is capable of progressing to new concepts and discoveries. And of course it is. Yet in the areas of diagnosis and drug treatment this has not really happened. And absent progress, one must, with the historians, look to the past.

How about the first drug set of the 1950s? Do we turn our backs on the many effective compounds of those years on the grounds that there are no randomized controlled trials confirming their efficacy? No. That would be FDA-style thinking, not real-world thinking. Randomized controlled trials, done as the FDA likes them, are so expensive they can be conducted only by the government, such as by the National Institute of Mental Health, or by drug companies. No drug company will ever fund trials of its precious new agent head to head with Miltown, Marsilid, Librium, or Valium. Yet the evidence of the effectiveness of these drugs in the real world of medical practice is overwhelming: Generations of physicians prescribed them with benefit; millions of patients witnessed their own steady recoveries after receiving drugs now forgotten.

Unfair standards of evidence? Am I holding the recent SSRIs to a higher bar than the first drug set? Have millions of patients done well on the new antidepressants? Not as many as one might think. In 2003, the National Institute of Mental Health sponsored a large "naturalistic" trial, called STAR*D, of antidepressants as prescribed in the real world. The trial randomized patients who had failed the SSRI citalopram (Celexa) to one of three other currently popular antidepressants. Grateful patients finally to get something that really works? Not exactly. As measured by the Hamilton Depression Scale, remission rates were only 21 percent for bupropion (Wellbutrin), 18 percent for sertraline (Zoloft), and 25 percent for venlafaxine (Effexor).[4] The majority of patients in this large, government-sponsored trial failed to get better on any of the new drugs.

Many of the old psychopharmacologists liked to observe their patients carefully on the ward for the subtle contours of illness and response, different from patient to patient yet having certain commonalities. Current trials are nothing like this. They are conducted using newspaper ads to recruit large numbers of highly heterogeneous individuals whose disparate flutterings are then flattened into a few numbers with a standard rating scale. This may be a bad idea. The great Yale epidemiologist Alvan Feinstein called these large, double-blind trials that ignore "humanistic data . . . a dehumanized form of pseudoscience."[5] Trials of this nature are incapable of discerning a clinical response in a unitary biological disease entity.

Here is how Roland Kuhn, who discovered the effectiveness of imipramine, the first tricyclic antidepressant, went about his work: "My methods were entirely different from those which are nowadays applied in clinical research. I have never used 'controlled double-blind studies' with 'placebo,' 'standardized rating scales,' or the statistical treatment of records of large number of patients. Instead I examined each patient individually even every day, often on several occasions, and questioned him or her again and again."[6] The unitary disease entity whose drug responsiveness Kuhn confirmed was vital depression, a form of melancholia. Vital depression was not included in DSM-III. Today, Kuhn would be kicked out the door at the FDA. Have we lost something here?

In 1997, Merton Sandler, the dean of British psychopharmacology, asked, "Why did the three major breakthroughs in drug treatment all occur in the 1950s, and then nothing since then?"[7] (He was presumably talking about the MAOI iproniazid, in which he had a direct role, the antipsychotic chlorpromazine, and the TCA imipramine.) These breakthroughs occurred precisely because FDA-style trials using *DSM* diagnoses were not in force in the 1950s.

Here and there are little rivulets of curiosity about nuggets that may lie hidden undiscovered in the treasury book of psychopharmacology. "One resurrects the past," said Jon Cole in 1970, founder of the Psychopharmacologic Drug Service Center of the National Institute of Mental Health, the only nonindustry agency ever to sponsor large trials. "Sometimes there is gold in those distant hills," Cole continued. "The use of cocaine in depression is also an area which intrigues me. . . . To my knowledge, the use of cocaine in depression has not been reexamined since [the early 1930s]. It might be faster acting and more effective than existing antidepressants. Marijuana may also be worth looking into depression."[8] It is a sad commentary on subordinating the science of drug discovery to politics that almost 40 years later Cole's genial proposals have little prospect of follow-up.

As for the once despised amphetamines, they are making a comeback in the therapy of depression. "A new strategy for treating depression is to use the psychostimulants methylphenidate and dextroamphetamine," said psychiatrists Mario Roy and Jacques Bernier in 1999. In their view, the stimulants prompted the release of such neurotransmitters as norepinephrine into the synapse.[9]

At this writing, there has never been a more effective antidepressant drug than imipramine, launched in the American market as Tofranil in 1959. Fridolin Sulser, professor of psychopharmacology at Vanderbilt University, said in 2000, "Though new drugs were discovered, in my opinion, there is not a single one that is more efficacious and faster acting than the original antidepressants discovered almost 40 years ago by serendipity."[10]

And the MAOIs today? As one veteran psychopharmacologist told his colleagues in 2007, "These drugs should be in the armamentarium of every psychiatrist. . . . With a little medication and diet education . . . the older drugs work just fine. Parnate and Nardil (tranylcypromine and phenelzine) remain effective drugs, and not at $500 per month. This class of drugs contains the most effective antidepressant drugs. We need to overcome two generations of drug company misinformation about antidepressants."[11]

How helpful have the regulatory authorities been in this story? The Food and Drug Administration's continual interventions over the past 50 years really have been a testimonial to the maleficent nature of mixing medicine and politics: In an exercise like DESI, shrinking the nation's supply of useful drugs for the sake of bureaucratic empire building; in the SSRI era, waving through inferior agents on the grounds that comparing them to the best available drugs is just too darned difficult.

So contributions from the sterile heights of academic medicine and regulatory politics have ranged from nugatory to toxic.

What is the proper role of an agency such as the FDA? A busy meddlesomeness in the measurement of "efficacy" is probably a waste of taxpayer dollars and a hindrance to progress in drug discovery. Before 1962, the agency limited itself to the assessment of safety—this is a legitimate function, keeping the dangerous products off the market that, in the form of the "elixir of sulfanilamide" scandal, prompted the original safety legislation in 1938. (A poisonous solvent, diethylene glycol, added to the new sulfa drug killed 107 persons.)[12] Insisting on efficacy sounds good, but in fact doctors themselves are capable of judging whether the drugs are working or not; they don't need bureaucrats to tell them.

What's wrong with making sure drugs are effective? The problem is that effectiveness is assessed for a given indication, rather than just in general. So the FDA ends up determining the particular indication, then verifying the effectiveness of drugs for it. This invalidates the search for effective drugs if the indication chosen, such as "depression," doesn't really exist. In its quest for an ostensible public benefit—an effective drug supply—the FDA ends up degrading the development of pharmaceuticals and the practice of medicine by insisting upon indications that may be artifacts. A similar argument may be made for "schizophrenia," "attention deficit disorder," and other popular diagnostic categories whose scientific status is problematical. Why not let doctors themselves determine effectiveness using their own diagnostic acumen rather than let government bureaucrats distort the process in chasing a will-o'-the-wisp?

Also, insisting on vast trials for efficacy is a way of driving small companies out of the market and ensuring that only the big ones remain, because they are the only ones capable of financing efficacy trials that cost hundreds of millions of dollars.

Bottom line:

New drugs are needed with fewer side effects and more effectiveness than the industry standards today possess. New diagnoses are required that cut Nature closer to the joints and for which drugs of the future will have a powerful and highly specific effect. It is not necessarily wonderful that these old drugs remain among the most effective offerings in psychiatry, given that they have as many side effects as the newer drugs. But it is evidence of a crisis in psychiatry. Somehow, the field has lost its grip over diagnosis and therapeutics. Although other areas of medicine continue to make genuine advances in determining what is wrong with patients and treating them successfully, psychiatry is floundering in an ivory-tower-spun web of diagnoses that jumble different diseases together, in a mesh of patent-protected remedies that represent, if anything, a loss of knowledge rather than a gain. This is not progress.

Glossary

NB: Unless indicated otherwise, the date refers to the drug's introduction in the United States.

acetylcholine.   A neurotransmitter acting on the central nervous system and on the parasympathetic division of the autonomic nervous system; its effect was discovered in 1921 by Otto Loewi.

ADHD.   *See* attention deficit hyperactivity disorder.

Adrenalin.   A trademark for preparations of adrenaline.

adrenaline.   *See* epinephrine.

agranulocytosis.   A marked decrease in granulocytes, a type of white blood cell; it may occur as an iatrogenic effect of medication, including various psychopharmaceuticals.

Alertonic.   A combination product containing pipradrol, alcohol, thiamine, and a number of vitamins and minerals that the William Merrell company introduced in 1957 to "help lift mood promptly" and as an antifatigue agent.

allobarbital.   A barbiturate sedative patented in the United States in 1912 and marketed by Ciba as Dial.

alprazolam.   A benzodiazepine launched by Upjohn as Xanax in 1981, initially as an anxiolytic, later as an antipanic agent.

amitriptyline.   A tricyclic antidepressant that Merck brought out in 1961 as Elavil.

amobarbital.   A barbiturate sedative patented by Lilly in 1924 and marketed as Sodium Amytal.

amoxapine.   A tricyclic antidepressant with neuroleptic properties launched by Lederle as Asendin in 1980.

amphetamine.   (1) A drug class with a phenylethylamine structure that stimulates the sympathetic nervous system centrally and peripherally ("sympathomimetic"); (2) amphetamine sulfate is the generic name of Benzedrine in tablet form, marketed by Smith, Kline & French in 1935; the name *amphetamine* was conferred in 1938.

Amytal.   *See* amobarbital.

Anafranil.   *See* clomipramine.

anticholinergic.   A drug blocking the nerve impulse in the parasympathetic nervous system and opposing the stimulation of cholinergic neurons in the brain.

antineurotic.   Traditional term in materia medica revived by Carter-Wallace in 1965 in connection with tybamate (Solacen), formerly meaning drugs indicated for "nervous" illness.

antipsychotic.   Term coined by Canadian psychiatrist Heinz Lehmann in 1961 for a drug against psychosis, although many antipsychotics were also effective for anxiety and other indications. Chlorpromazine (1952) was the first real antipsychotic drug; *see also* neuroleptic. *See also* atypical antipsychotic.

anxiolytic.   An antianxiety medication.

aspartate salts.   A mixture of the potassium and magnesium salts of aspartic acid that Wyeth brought out in 1961 as the antifatigue agent Spartase.

Atarax.   *See* hydroxyzine.

Ativan.   *See* lorazepam.

atropine.   An alkaloid similar to belladonna derived from Solanaceae plants used as a muscle relaxant or antispasmodic, and as an antidepressant.

attention deficit hyperactivity disorder (ADHD).   The diagnosis was coined in the *Diagnostic and Statistical Manual, Third Edition (DSM-III)*, of the American Psychiatric Association in 1980 as attention deficit disorder (ADD). In the revised third edition (*DSM-III-R*) in 1987, it became attention deficit hyperactivity disorder.

atypical antipsychotics   are thought to have a mild side effects profile, especially with regard to extrapyramidal symptoms (abnormal movements); the first was clozapine (Clozaril), introduced in Germany in 1974, in the United States in 1990. Also known as second-generation antipsychotics to distinguish them from the first-generation antipsychotics (the "typicals") introduced in the 1950s, such as chlorpromazine.

atypical depression.   A diagnosis coined in 1959 for a subset of depressed patients differentially responsive to iproniazid; the diagnosis was revived in 1979 for depressions characterized by oversleeping, overeating, leaden fatigue, and a poor response to rejection.

azacyclonal.   A diphenylmethane derivative that is an isomer of the stimulant pipradrol; introduced by Merrell in 1955 as Frenquel for anxiety and psychosis.

barbital.   A hypnotic also known generically as diemal malonal barbitone, the first of the barbiturates, marketed in 1903 in Germany by Merck and Bayer as Veronal, by Schering as Medinal.

barbiturates.   A class of sedatives and anticonvulsants introduced in Germany in 1903 with barbital as first of the series. Often given as sodium salts, as in Sodium Amytal, although the "sodium" is frequently omitted.

benactyzine.   An anticholinergic agent of the diphenylmethane class with atropine-like effects that Merck brought out in 1957 as Suavitil as an antidepressant and "antiphobic" medication; in 1958 Wallace offered it as Deprol in combination with meprobamate.

Benadryl.   *See* diphenhydramine.

benzodiazepine.   A class of antidepressant, antianxiety, anticonvulsant, hypnotic, and muscle-relaxing drugs launched by Hoffmann-La Roche with Librium (chlordiazepoxide) in 1960 and Valium (diazepam) in 1963.

borderline personality disorder.   A psychoanalytically inspired diagnosis coined in 1938 that replaced "hysteria," and that entered the *DSM* series in 1980.

bupropion.   A PEA derivative that Burroughs-Wellcome introduced in 1986 as the antidepressant Wellbutrin. (GlaxoSmithKline bought Burroughs-Wellcome in 1995.)

butabarbital.   A barbiturate sedative patented by Lilly in 1932 and marketed by McNeil laboratories as Butisol Sodium.

captodiame (captodiamine).   An anxiolytic synthesized by Lundbeck in 1958 and marketed in Europe as Covatin, in the United States in 1958 by Ayerst as Suvren.

chloral hydrate.   A hypnosedative the clinical efficacy of which was discovered in 1869; it is still marketed, usually in the form of a syrup.

chlordiazepoxide. The first benzodiazepine, introduced as Librium for
    anxiety in 1960 by Hoffmann-La Roche.
chlorpheniramine. An antihistamine created by Schering Labs and
    marketed in 1949 as, among other formulations, Chlor-Trimeton;
    it became the basis of the first SSRI, zimeldine.
chlorpromazine. From the phenothiazine chemical class, the first of
    the antipsychotics/neuroleptics, synthesized by Rhône-Poulenc
    in 1950 and introduced in world markets in 1953 as Largactil,
    in the American market by Smith, Kline & French in 1954 as
    Thorazine.
citalopram. An SSRI patented by Lundbeck in 1977 and launched in
    Denmark in 1989 as Cipramil; by Forest Laboratories in the United
    States in 1998 as Celexa.
clomipramine. A tricyclic antidepressant that Geigy launched for
    obsessive-compulsive disorder as Anafranil, in France in 1967, in
    the United States in 1990.
clonazepam. A benzodiazepine introduced by Hoffmann-La Roche in
    France in 1973 as Rivotril, in the United States in 1975 as Clonopin
    (Klonopin); used also as an anticonvulsant.
Clonopin. *See* clonazepam.
clorazepate. Abbott's Tranxene, a benzodiazepine with a short half-life
    introduced as an anxiolytic in France in 1968, in the United States
    in 1972.
Dalmane. *See* flurazepam.
deanol was synthesized in 1904 but its acetamidobenzoate salt was
    prepared in 1957 by Riker Labs and marketed in 1958 as Deaner; it
    has been tried as a stimulant, an antihyperactivity and an
    antidementia agent.
delirium tremens. Delirium from alcohol withdrawal, often including a
    coarse tremor, vivid hallucinations, and agitated behavior.
Deprol. An antidepressant combination of benactyzine and
    meprobamate launched by Wallace in 1958.
deserpidine. A reserpine-type pentacyclic, isolated from the roots of
    Rauwolfia in 1955 and marketed by Abbott in 1957 as an
    antihypertensive and antipsychotic agent under the brand name of
    Harmonyl.
desipramine. A metabolite of imipramine that itself shows
    antidepressant efficacy, marketed by Geigy as Pertofrane in the
    United Kingdom in 1963 and in the United States in 1964.
Desyrel. *See* Trazodone.

Dexamyl.   A combination of Amytal and Dexedrine that Smith, Kline & French launched in 1950.

Dexedrine.   *See* dextroamphetamine.

dextroamphetamine.   In 1944 Smith, Kline & French brought out Dexedrine, an isomer of Benzedrine (racemic amphetamine), for "mild depression."

Diagnostic and Statistical Manual of Mental Disorders (DSM)   of the American Psychiatric Association, the standard classification of psychiatric illness, the first edition of which was published in 1952, the second (*DSM-II*) in 1968, the third (*DSM-III*) in 1980, the revised third (*DSM-III-R*) in 1987, the fourth (*DSM-IV*) in 1994, and the revised fourth (*DSM-IV-TR*, which stands for *Text Revision*), in 2000.

Dial.   *See* allobarbital.

diazepam.   A benzodiazepine of Hoffmann-La Roche, marketed as Valium in Italy in 1962, in the United States in 1963, for use as an antianxiety medication and as a muscle relaxant.

diphenhydramine.   An antihistamine marketed by Parke Davis in 1946 as Benadryl.

Doriden.   *See* glutethimide.

Dormison.   *See* methylparafynol.

dothiepin (dosulepin).   A tricyclic antidepressant developed in Czechoslovakia and launched in 1969 as Prothioden by Knoll in the United Kingdom; it was never licensed in the United States.

doxepin.   An antidepressant–antianxiety agent of the TCA class, introduced by Pfizer in the United States in 1969 as Sinequan.

DSM.   See *Diagnostic and Statistical Manual of Mental Disorders.*

ectylurea.   An aliphatic tranquilizer developed by Miles Laboratories and introduced by Ames in 1956 as Nostyn.

Effexor.   *See* venlafaxine.

Elavil.   *See* amitriptyline.

emylcamate.   An anxiolytic of the carbamate class, synthesized in 1912 and marketed in 1960 by Merck as Striatran.

endogenomorphic depression.   A term, coined in 1974 by Donald Klein, meaning any depression with the features of retardation, agitation, and dysphoria, regardless of whether precipitated or not.

endogenous depression.   A term coined in 1920 by German psychiatrist Kurt Schneider for a severe depression, thought to originate more or less spontaneously from within the brain and body and having many somatic symptoms, as opposed to a depression mainly of mood (reactive depression).

ephedrine. An alkaloid of the ephedra plant, isolated in 1887, used as a stimulant in traditional Chinese medicine and marketed as Ephedrine Sulphate by Lilly in 1926.

Epinephrine (adrenaline). A catecholamine hormone isolated from adrenal medulla in 1901, described as a "sympathomimetic amine" in 1910. (Catechol is a chemical structure.) Stimulates sympathetic division of the autonomic nervous system.

EPS. *See* extrapyramidal symptoms.

Equanil. *See* meprobamate.

Eskatrol Spansules. A combination of dextroamphetamine and prochlorperazine, introduced by Smith, Kline & French in 1959.

ethchlorvynol. Abbott brought out this short-acting aliphatic hypnosedative in 1955 as Placidyl.

ethinamate. A hypnosedative of the carbamate class that Lilly launched in 1955 as Valmid (later Valamin).

extrapyramidal symptoms (EPS). Muscle symptoms outside ("extra") the pyramidal tract: Nerve impulses that travel from the brain down the spinal cord outside the pyramidal tract—which is used for voluntary muscle movements—may cause involuntary muscle movements, a frequent side effect of antipsychotic medications.

5-hydroxytryptamine (5-HT). A synonym for serotonin.

fluoxetine. An SSRI patented by Lilly in 1975; it was trade named Prozac and marketed in Belgium in 1986, in the United States in 1988.

flurazepam. A short-half-life benzodiazepine that Hoffmann-La Roche launched in 1970 as Dalmane for insomnia.

fluvoxamine. An SSRI, patented in 1975 by Philips-Duphar (a subsidiary of Solvay), launched in Switzerland in 1983 as Floxyfral, in the United Kingdom in 1987 as Faverin, and in the United States in 1995 as Luvox, in this latter market specifically for use in obsessive-compulsive disorder.

Frenquel. *See* azacyclonal.

glutethimide. A hypnosedative of the piperidinedione class that Ciba launched in 1955 as Doriden.

Guillain-Barré syndrome. Described in 1916 by Georges Guillain and Alexandre J. Barré involving acute muscle weakness from demyelination.

Halcion. *See* triazolam.

Haldol. *See* haloperidol.

haloperidol.   First of the butyrophenone antipsychotics, launched by
    Janssen as Haldol in world markets in 1960 and in the United
    States in 1967.
hydrochlorothiazide.   A diuretic that Merck marketed in 1959 as
    HydroDiuril.
hydroxyphenamate.   A carbamate indicated for anxiety, launched by
    Armour in 1961 as Listica.
hydroxyzine.   An anxiolytic of the diphenylmethane class, synthesized
    by the Union Chimique Belge in 1956 and marketed that same year
    in the United States by Pfizer as Atarax.
hypnotic.   Sleeping medication.
imipramine.   First of the tricyclic antidepressants, marketed as Tofranil
    in Switzerland by Geigy in 1957, in 1959 in the United States.
indalpine.   An SSRI, patented in 1977 and launched in France by
    Fournier Frères-Pharmuka in 1983 as Upstène; never introduced in
    the United States.
Indonad.   A combination of barbital and cannabis indica, marketed in
    England in the 1930s and used as a hypnotic.
iproniazid.   One of the first inhibitors of monoamine oxidase (an
    MAOI), introduced by Hoffmann-La Roche as Marsilid for
    tuberculosis in 1951, for depression in 1957.
isocarboxazid.   An MAOI for depression that Hoffmann-La Roche
    launched in 1959 as Marplan.
Klonopin.   *See* clonazepam.
Largactil.   *See* chlorpromazine.
levomepromazine (later methotrimeprazine).   A phenothiazine
    synthesized in 1958 by Rhône-Poulenc, marketed in France in 1963
    as the neuroleptic Nozinan, in the United States in 1966 as
    Lederle's sedative/analgesic Levoprome; it acquired a reputation
    as an antimelancholic.
Librium.   *See* chlordiazepoxide.
Listica.   *See* hydroxyphenamate.
lithium.   An element, the antimanic efficacy of which was known in
    the nineteenth century, then reestablished in 1949; lithium also
    maintains depressed patients from relapse. Approved by the FDA
    in 1970, the drug was marketed in the United States variouslyby
    the Rowell Company, Smith, Kline & French, and Pfizer.
lorazepam.   A benzodiazepine that Wyeth brought out in Europe in
    1972 as Temesta among other trade names, in the United States in
    1977 as Ativan, for anxiety; efficacy in catatonia.

Luminal. *See* phenobarbital.

MAOIs. Monoamine oxidase inhibitors, a class of antidepressant drugs that blocks the breakdown of monoamines such as serotonin, dopamine, and norepinephrine in the brain by the enzyme monoamine oxidase. *See* iproniazid.

maprotiline. A tetracyclic antidepressant introduced by Ciba as Ludiomil in Germany in 1973, in the United States in 1981.

Marplan. *See* isocarboxazid.

Marsilid. *See* iproniazid.

melancholia. A well-defined recurrent and debilitating mood disorder characterized by high serum cortisol, slowing of mind and muscle, and pervasive apprehension and gloom, resulting in severe feelings of failure and low self-worth; it can deteriorate into psychosis. *Compare* nonmelancholia.

Mellaril. *See* thioridazine.

mepazine. A phenothiazine antipsychotic synthesized by Promonta in Germany in 1952 and introduced in the United States as Pacatal by Warner-Chilcott in 1957.

mephenesin. A propanediol member of the aromatic glycerol ethers, that Squibb brought out in 1954 as Tolserol; among the first of the "tranquilizers."

mephenoxalone. A heterocyclic tranquilizer of the oxazolidinone class introduced in Argentina in 1956 and in the United States in 1961 by Lederle as Trepidone.

meprobamate. An antineurotic drug of the dicarbamate class marketed as Miltown by Carter Products in 1955 and licensed to Wyeth as Equanil.

methamphetamine. A member of the amphetamine class, marketed by Abbott Laboratories in 1943 as Desoxyn.

methylparafynol (methylpentynol; meparfynol). An early tranquilizer and member of the carbinol drug class, launched by Schering in 1951 as Dormison for insomnia and anxiety; N-Oblivon, a carbamate congener, came out in 1955.

methylphenidate. A stimulant and antidepressant related in structure to amphetamine, launched as Ritalin in Switzerland in 1954, in the United States in 1956.

methyprylon. A hypnosedative of the piperidine class that Hoffmann-La Roche launched in 1955 as Noludar.

mianserin. A tetracyclic antidepressant developed by Organon and introduced in Germany in 1975 as Tolvin, in the United Kingdom in 1976 as Bolvidon (never licensed in the United States).

Miltown. *See* meprobamate.

monoamine neurotransmitters are molecules containing one amino (NH) group; biogenic monoamines include norepinephrine, serotonin, and dopamine.

monoamine oxidase inhibitors. *See* MAOIs.

Nardil. *See* phenelzine.

Navane. *See* thiothixine.

neuroleptic. A term of Greek origin meaning literally taking hold, a seizure; coined in 1955 to refer to the effects of phenothiazine medication, it became a synonym for antipsychotic. *See also* antipsychotic.

nialamide. An MAOI that Pfizer launched in 1959 as Niamid for depression.

Niamid. *See* nialamide.

nomifensine. A bicyclic antidepressant that Hoechst introduced in Germany in 1976 as Alival and in the United States in 1985 as Merital; it was withdrawn in 1986.

nonmelancholia. A heterogeneous and poorly circumscribed group of mood disorders with symptoms that may include dysphoria or mild depression, anxiety, tension, and general unhappiness; in terms of classification, a mixture of reactive depression, mixed anxiety-depression, dysthymia, and depressive character traits; collectively called *psychoneurosis* by nineteenth-century Austrian psychiatrist Richard von Krafft-Ebing. *Compare* melancholia.

noradrenaline. *See* norepinephrine.

norepinephrine. A neurotransmitter whose presence in the central nervous system was discovered in 1954.

nortriptyline. A tricyclic antidepressant that is an active metabolite of amitriptyline; developed by Merck and introduced by Lilly as Aventyl in the United Kingdom in 1963, in the United States in 1965.

olanzapine. A "second-generation," or "atypical," antipsychotic, marketed by Lilly in 1996 as Zyprexa.

oxanamide. A tranquilizer that Merrell synthesized in 1950 and introduced in 1958 as Quiactin.

oxazepam. A benzodiazepine that Wyeth brought out in 1965 as Serax for anxiety.

paraldehyde. A hypnosedative synthesized in 1872 and still marketed in the United States as Paral (by Forest Laboratories).

Parnate. *See* tranylcypromine.

paroxetine. An SSRI developed by Ferrosan in 1974 and introduced in the United States by SmithKline Beecham in 1993 as Paxil, and in the United Kingdom as Seroxat.

Paxil. *See* paroxetine.

PEA derivatives. Molecules having the basic phenylethylamine structure, of which amphetamine is a good example.

phenaglycodol. A propanediol-derivative tranquilizer that Lilly launched in 1957 as Ultran.

phenelzine. An MAOI that Warner-Chilcott brought out in 1959 as the antidepressant Nardil.

Phenergan. *See* phenothiazine.

pheniprazine. An MAOI introduced by Lakeside in 1959 as Catron for depression.

phenobarbital. A barbiturate sedative and anticonvulsant marketed in Germany by Bayer in 1911 as Luminal.

phenothiazine. A chemical class synthesized in 1883 linking two benzene rings with a nitrogen and a sulfur atom, creating the appearance of three rings; promethazine, synthesized in 1944 and marketed in the United States in 1951 as Phenergan, was the first of the phenothiazine antihistamines (later called antipsychotics) to be introduced in psychiatry, followed by chlorpromazine in 1952.

phenyltoloxamine. An antihistamine synthesized in 1949; the dihydrogen citrate form was brought out in 1952 by Bristol Labs as Bristamin, an over-the-counter antihistamine.

pimozide. An antipsychotic patented by Janssen in 1965, introduced as Orap in the United Kingdom in 1971, in the United States by McNeil in 1984; useful in Tourette's disease.

pipradrol. A stimulant marketed in 1955 by Merrell as Meratran.

Placidyl. *See* ethchlorvynol.

posttraumatic stress disorder (PTSD). A diagnosis that entered the *DSM* series with *DSM-III* in 1980, indicating mental symptoms that appear, often after a considerable interval, following trauma.

prazepam. A benzodiazepine that Warner-Lambert brought out in 1977 as Verstran, a muscle relaxant and anxiolytic.

prochlorperazine. A phenothiazine neuroleptic that Rhône-Poulenc developed; it was marketed in the United States by Smith, Kline & French in 1956 as Compazine.

promazine. A phenothiazine neuroleptic that Rhône-Poulenc patented in 1950, introduced by Wyeth Laboratories in 1956 as Sparine.

promethazine.   *See* phenothiazine.

propoxyphene.   Patented by Lilly in 1955; the dextro isomer was
     marketed in 1957 as the analgesic Darvon.

protriptyline.   A tricyclic antidepressant marketed by Merck in the
     United Kingdom in 1966 as Concordin, in the United States in 1967
     as Vivactil.

Prozac.   *See* fluoxetine.

PTSD.   *See* posttraumatic stress disorder.

pyrilamine.   The first antihistamine, synthesized by Rhône-Poulenc in
     1944 and marketed in the United States by Merck in 1948 as Neo-
     Antergan.

reactive depression.   A depression mainly of mood, unlike endogenous
     depression; term coined by German psychiatrist Kurt Schneider
     in 1920.

reserpine.   An antipsychotic derived from *Rauwolfia serpentina*,
     introduced for hypertension by Ciba in 1953 as Serpasil; Riker Labs
     brought out a mixture of alkaloids from the plant as Rauwidrine
     for "mood elevation" in 1954.

reuptake of a neurotransmitter.   The transport of the neurotransmitter
     from the synapse (the space between two neurons) back into the
     neuron that discharged it.

Ritalin.   *See* methylphenidate.

secobarbital sodium.   A short-acting barbiturate hypnotic synthesized in
     1934 and marketed by Lilly in 1936 as Seconal.

secondary amine.   *See* tertiary amine.

selective serotonin reuptake inhibitors.   *See* SSRIs.

Serax.   *See* oxazepam.

serotonin.   A neurotransmitter whose presence in the central nervous
     system was discovered in 1954.

Serpasil.   *See* reserpine.

sertraline.   An SSRI patented by Pfizer in 1981 and introduced in 1992
     as Zoloft.

Sodium Amytal.   *See* amobarbital.

spectrophotofluorimeter.   A device using fluorescence to assay the
     content of organic compounds, developed at the National Heart
     Institute in 1955.

SSRIs.   Selective serotonin reuptake inhibitors, a class of
     antidepressant and antianxiety agents that includes, among others,
     Lilly's Prozac (fluoxetine), GlaxoSmithKline's Paxil (paroxetine),
     Pfizer's Zoloft (sertraline), and Lundbeck/Forest's citalopram

(Celexa) and escitalopram (Lexapro). The acronym was coined by SmithKline Beecham (as the firm was then called) in 1993.

STAR*D.   The sequenced treatment alternatives to relieve depression, a drug trial commissioned by the National Institute of Mental Health and contracted to the University of Texas Southwestern Medical Center at Dallas; this large "naturalistic" study of responsiveness to current antidepressant agents in real-world settings began in 2003.

status epilepticus.   A continuous life-threatening series of generalized epileptic seizures.

Striatran.   See emylcamate.

Suavitil.   See benactyzine.

sulfonal (sulfonmethane).   A hypnosedative prepared by condensing ethyl mercaptan with acetone, it was synthesized by Bayer in 1885 and marketed as Sulfonalum Bayer.

sulfonethylmethane.   A hypnosedative prepared by condensing ethylmercaptan with methyl ethyl ketone, it was synthesized by Bayer in 1889 and marketed as Trional.

talbutal.   A barbiturate sedative synthesized in 1925 and marketed by Winthrop in 1955 as Lotusate.

tardive dyskinesia.   An extrapyramidal movement disorder caused by long-term administration of antipsychotic drugs, characterized by involuntary movements of the tongue, mouth, and extremities.

TCAs.   See tricyclic antidepressants.

tertiary amine,   such as amitriptyline, has two methyl groups (CH_3) attached to the nitrogen on the side chain; a "secondary" amine, such as desipramine, has one.

thalidomide.   A hypnosedative and immunomodulator synthesized by Chemie Grünenthal and patented in 1957, the agent was distributed on an investigational basis in the United States by Marion Merrell Dow as Kevadon; not licensed at the time owing to its teratogenic effects (later available for multiple myeloma and leprosy under a special program).

thioridazine.   A phenothiazine antipsychotic that Sandoz synthesized in 1958 and introduced in the United States in 1959 as Mellaril.

thiothixine.   An antipsychotic of the thioxanthene series, introduced by Pfizer in 1967 as Navane.

Thorazine.   See chlorpromazine.

thymoleptic.   An early synonym for tricyclic antidepressant.

tianeptine.   A tricyclic antidepressant that increases serotonin reuptake, synthesized in 1970; Servier marketed it in France in 1983 as Stablon; not registered in the United States.

Tofranil.   See imipramine.

Tolserol.   See mephenesin.

tranquilizer.   A popular name in the 1950s for drugs whose main action was deemed to be tranquility, including chlorpromazine (Thorazine/Largactil), reserpine (Serpasil), and meprobamate (Miltown/Equanil).

tranylcypromine.   An MAO inhibitor introduced for depression by Smith, Kline & French as Parnate in the United Kingdom in 1960, in the United States in 1961.

trazodone.   A bicyclic antidepressant/hypnotic developed by Angelini in Italy and marketed there in 1972 as Trittico, in the United States by Mead Johnson in 1982 as Desyrel.

triazolam.   A benzodiazepine hypnotic with a short half-life that Upjohn launched as Halcion in the United Kingdom in 1979, in the United States in 1982.

tricyclic antidepressants (TCAs).   A group of antidepressant drugs that has the appearance of containing three fused rings; Geigy launched the first TCA, imipramine (Tofranil), in 1957 in Switzerland, 1959 in the United States.

Trional.   See sulfonethylmethane.

tryptophan.   An amino acid that is a precursor of serotonin, isolated in 1902.

tybamate.   A meprobamate-type minor tranquilizer introduced by Carter-Wallace as Solacen in 1965 as an "antineurotic."

uptake of a neurotransmitter.   See reuptake.

Valium.   See diazepam.

Valmid.   See ethinamate.

venlafaxine.   An antidepressant with a selective effect on the reuptake of both serotonin and norepinephrine (SNRI), patented by Wyeth in 1984 and marketed in 1994 in the United States as Effexor.

Verstran.   See prazepam.

Wellbutrin.   See bupropion.

Xanax.   See alprazolam.

Zelmid.   See zimelidine.

zimelidine (zimeldine).   The first SSRI antidepressant, synthesized by Astra-Hässle in 1969 and launched in Europe in 1981 as Zelmid.

ziprasidone.   An "atypical" (less EPS) antipsychotic that Pfizer marketed in 2001 as Geodon.

Zoloft.   See sertraline.

Zyprexa.   See olanzapine.

NOTES

NOTES TO CHAPTER 1

1. William M. Wardell and Louis Lasagna, *Regulation and Drug Development* (Washington, DC: American Enterprise Institute for Public Policy, 1975), 30.

2. Louis Lasagna, discussion, in Joseph D. Cooper, ed., *The Efficacy of Self-Medication*, Philosophy and Technology of Drug Assessment 4 (Washington, DC: Smithsonian Institution, 1973), 168, 156. The conference took place in 1972.

3. United States Food and Drug Administration, FDA Oral History Program, "Interview with William W. Goodrich, Office of the General Counsel, 1939–1971 (Part 2)," Oct. 15, 1986, www.fda.gov/oc/history/oralhistories/goodrich/part2.html (accessed July 4, 2002).

NOTES TO CHAPTER 2

1. Shakespeare, *Cymbeline*, act III, scene 2.

2. Casebook of Frederick Parkes-Weber, 1913–, 77, Contemporary Medical Archives Center, Wellcome Library, London.

3. Société Suisse de Psychiatrie, "Comptes-rendus des séances, 21–22 juin 1930 à Neuchâtel et à Perreux," *Schweizer Archiv für Neurologie und Psychiatrie* 27(1931): 174–183. Hans Walther gave the lecture on "Pharmacologie und Psychiatrie," summary, 175, but many other contributions touched on this theme; the title of the meeting, "Pharmakologie et Psychiatrie," appeared in the announcement in *Annales Médico-psychologiques*, 12th ser., 88 (1930): 186.

4. James M. Adair, *Medical Cautions for the Consideration of Invalids* (Bath: Cruttwell, 1786), 13.

5. Charles F. Mullett, ed., *The Letters of Doctor George Cheyne to Samuel Richardson (1733–1743)* (Columbia: University of Missouri, 1943), 47, letter of Feb. 3, 1738.

6. L[ouis] Mayer, "Menstruation im Zusammenhange mit psychischen Störungen," *Beiträge zur Geburtshilfe und Gynäkologie* 1 (1872): 111–134, quote 127.

7. On the impact of the isolation of hyoscyamine, see Henry Wetherill, "The Modern Hypnotics," *American Journal of Insanity* 46 (1889): 28–47, esp. 29.

8. Ian Tait, discussion, in *Wellcome Witnesses to Twentieth Century Medicine*, ed. E. M. Tansey (London: Wellcome Institute for the History of Medicine, 1998), 2: 169. The green medicine also contained a barbiturate.

9. Luigi Belloni, introduction, to S[ilvio] Garattini et al., eds., *Psychotropic Drugs* (Amsterdam: Elsevier, 1957), v–ix.

10. Conrad Arnold Elvehjem et al., "The Isolation and Identification of the Anti-Black Tongue Factor," *Journal of Biological Chemistry* 123 (1938): 137–149.

11. John H. Stokes et al., "The Action of Penicillin in Late Syphilis Including Neurosyphilis," *JAMA* 126 (Sept. 9, 1944): 74–79.

12. H[ugh] E[dward] De Wardener et al., "Cerebral Beriberi (Wernicke's Encephalopathy): Review of 52 Cases in a Singapore Prisoner-of-War Hospital," *Lancet* 1 (Jan. 4, 1947); see, on this, Edward Shorter, *Historical Dictionary of Psychiatry* (New York: Oxford University Press, 2005), 303–304.

13. A[dolphus] E. Bridger, *Depression: What It Is and How to Cure It* (London: Hogg, 1892), 51–52.

14. Arvid Carlsson, "Rise of Neuropsychopharmacology," interview, in *The Psychopharmacologists*, ed. David Healy, 1: 51–80 (London: Chapman and Hall, 1996), quote 77.

15. On the pharmacology of opium, see Louis S. Goodman and Alfred Gilman, *The Pharmacological Basis of Therapeutics*, 2nd ed. (New York: Macmillan, 1955), 216–217. All editions of this classic textbook contain a discussion of opium, yet this edition provides probably the most extensive.

16. On the history of opium in psychiatry, see Matthias M. Weber, "Die 'Opiumkur' in der Psychiatrie: Ein Beitrag zur Geschichte der Psychopharmakologie," *Sudhoffs Archiv* 71 (1987): 31–61.

17. See Hermann E. E. Engelken, "Familie Engelken, 1742–1919," in *Deutsche Irrenärzte*, ed. Theodor Kirchhoff, 1: 223–227 (Berlin: Springer, 1921).

18. See Geert Benning, *Das Opium in der deutschen Psychiatrie des 19. Jahrhunderts* (Göttingen doctoral diss., Wurm, 1936), 13–14. The author was a family member.

19. R[ichard] von Krafft-Ebing, *Lehrbuch der Psychiatrie* (Stuttgart: Enke, 1879), 1: 255.

20. Ludwig J. Pongratz, ed., Günter Elsässer [autobiographical account], *Psychiatrie in Selbstdarstellungen* (Berne: Huber, 1977), 54–81, quote 62.

21. Post to psycho-pharm@psycom.net, Mar. 13, 2007. The members of this listserv did not necessarily realize they were posting for attribution, and I am preserving their anonymity.

22. See Bela Issekutz, *Die Geschichte der Arzneimittelforschung* (Budapest: Kiado, 1971), 68.

23. Trevor Turner, *A Diagnostic Analysis of the Casebooks of Ticehurst House Asylum, 1845–1890*, Psychological Medicine Monograph Supplement 21 (Cambridge: Cambridge University Press, 1992), 59, table 12.

24. Heinrich Böttger, "Bericht über die Heil- und Pflegeanstalt für Gemüths- und Nervenkranke Asyl Carlsfeld bei Halle a. S.," *Deutsche Klinik* (Feb. 25, 1865): 79–80, quote 80.

25. Max Cloetta, discussion comment following A. Ulrich, "Ueber die psychischen Wirkungen des Broms und über die Brombehandlung von melancholischen Verstimmungen," *Correspondenz-Blatt für Schweizer Aerzte* 46 (1916): 504, comment 505.

26. N. Mutch, "Proprietary Remedies, with Special Reference to Hypnotics," *BMJ* 1 (Feb. 24, 1934): 319–322, see 322, table 5.

27. See *Rote Liste 1939, Preisverzeichnis deutscher pharmazeutischer Spezialpräparate*, 3rd ed. (Berlin: Fachgruppe Pharmazeutische Erzeugnisse, 1939), 330.

28. See Peter Gay, *Freud: A Life for Our Time* (New York: Norton, 1988), 43–44.

29. David F. Musto, *The American Disease: Origins of Narcotics Control* (New Haven: Yale University Press, 1973), 7.

30. Leo Alexander testimony, "Before the Secretary, Department of Health, Education and Welfare, Food and Drug Administration. In the Matter of: Depressant and Stimulant Drugs," Docket No. FDA-DAC-1, Aug. 5, 1966: 2742 ("Meprobamate Hearings"). Obtained from FDA through the Freedom of Information Act.

31. Norbert Matussek, "The Neurotransmittter Era in Neuropsychopharmacology: Reflections of a Neuropsychopharmacologist," in *The Neurotransmitter Era in Neuropsychopharmacology*, ed. Thomas A. Ban and Ronaldo Ucha Udabe, 193–200 (Buenos Aires: Polemos, 2006), quotes 195.

32. Vincenzo Cervello, "Sull'azione fisiologica della paraldeide," *Archivio per le Scienze Mediche* 6 (1882): 177–214.

33. Henry McIlwain considers urethane (1885) among the first "attempt[s] to design a therapeutic agent." Yet urethane was quickly displaced by the less toxic barbiturates. Henry McIlwain, *Chemotherapy and the Central Nervous System* (Boston: Little, Brown, 1957), 24–25.

34. Emil Fischer and J[osef] von Mering, "Ueber eine neue Klasse von Schlafmitteln," *Therapie der Gegenwart* 44 (1903): 97–101. For details, see Edward Shorter, *History of Psychiatry* (New York: Wiley, 1997), 37, 202–207.

35. Alex A. Cardoni, "Fifty Years of Psychopharmacology: An Interview with Benjamin Wiesel," *Connecticut Medicine* 55 (1991): 409–411, quote 409.

36. Louis Lasagna, discussion, in Joseph D. Cooper, ed., *The Philosophy of Evidence*, Philosophy and Technology of Drug Assessment 3 (Washington, DC: Interdisciplinary Communication Associates, 1972), 78.

37. For details see Shorter, *Historical Dictionary of Psychiatry*, 37.

38. See *The People of the State of New York, Respondent v. William Esposito and Anthony Esposito, Appellants*, Court of Appeals of New York, 287 N.Y. 389; 39 N.E.2d 925; 1942 N.Y. LEXIS 1100; 142 A.L.R. 956, decided Jan. 22, 1942, 4.

39. Frank J. Curran, "Current Views on Neuropsychiatric Effects of Barbiturates and Bromides," *Journal of Nervous and Mental Disease* 100 (1944): 142–169, see 143.

40. Lord Horder, "Use of Narcotics in the Treatment of Nervous and Mental Patients," *BMJ* 2 (Oct. 6, 1934): 619–621, quote 621.

41. See Virginia Woolf to Vita Sackville-West, Feb. 4, 1929, in Nigel Nicolson et al., eds., *The Letters of Virginia Woolf*, vol. 4, 1929–1931 (New York: Harvest/ HBJ, 1978), 13.

42. W[illiam] J. Bleckwenn, "Sodium Amytal in Certain Nervous and Mental Conditions," *Wisconsin Medical Journal* 20 (1930): 693–696, quotes 694.

43. Erich Lindemann, "The Psychopathological Effect of Sodium Amytal," *Journal of the Society for Experimental Study of Biology and Medicine* 28 (1931): 864–866, quote 865.

44. Erich Lindemann, "Psychological Changes in Normal and Abnormal Individuals Under the Influence of Sodium Amytal," *AJP* 88 (1932): 1083–1091.

45. Erich Lindemann, "Symptomatology and Management of Acute Grief," *AJP* 101 (1944): 141–148.

46. Joel Fort, "The Problem of Barbiturates in the United States of America," *Bulletin on Narcotics* 16 (Jan.–Mar. 1964): 17–35, quote 18.

47. Eskaphen B Elixir advertisement, *New York State Journal of Medicine* 50 (1950): 1897.

48. Joan-Ramon Laporte et al., "Patterns of Use of Psychotropic Drugs in Spain in an International Perspective," in *Clinical Pharmacology in Psychiatry: Bridging the Experimental-Therapeutic Gap*, ed. Lars F. Gram et al., 18–31 (London: Macmillan, 1983), quote 24.

49. Marcel Proust to Natalie Barney, undated letter, in Natalie Clifford Barney, *Aventures de l'esprit* (Paris: Editions Émile-Paul Frères, 1929), 66.

50. Matthias M. Weber, *Die Entwicklung der Psychopharmakologie im Zeitalter der naturwissenschaftlichen Medizin* (Munich: Urban, 1999), 110.

51. R[onald] D[ick] Gillespie, discussion, "Hypnotic Drugs: Uses and Dangers," *BMJ* 2 (Dec. 30, 1933): 1213–1214, quote 1214.

52. L. I. M. Castleden, "Hypnotic Drugs," *The Practitioner* 137 (1936): 358–368, see 364–367.

53. W. E. Hambourger, "A Study of the Promiscuous Use of the Barbiturates: Their Use in Suicides," *JAMA* 112 (Apr. 8, 1939): 1340–1343.

54. Annakatri Ohberg et al., "Alcohol and Drugs in Suicides," *BJP* 169 (1996): 75–80; in defined daily doses (DDD) per 1,000 population in 1987, the barbiturates had a relative suicide risk of 105.3, the benzodiazepines 0.3.

55. Louis Lasagna, "The Newer Hypnotics," *Medical Clinics of North America* 41 (1957): 359–368, quote 365.

56. Harold Simmons, discussion, "[BMA] Section of Neurology, Psychological Medicine and Mental Diseases," *BMJ* 2 (Aug. 4, 1934): 223.

57. Goldberg had prepared the table at the request of Gerhard Zbinden, Hoffmann-La Roche's vice president for research. See *Drug Abuse Control Amendments of 1965. Hearings Before the Committee on Interstate and Foreign Commerce, House of Representatives, 89th Congress, 1st Session, on H.R. 2. Jan. 27–Feb. 10, 1965* (Washington, DC: U.S. Government Printing Office, 1965), table at 293.

58. Edward G. Egan (Gane's Chemical Works) to Hearing Clerk, Department of Health, Education and Welfare, Feb. 14, 1966, National Archives and Records Administration, College Park, MD (NARA), RG 88 (Records of the Food and Drug Administration), 88–74–2, (hearing material, 1965–1966), box. 50.

59. WHO Expert Committee on Addiction-Producing Drugs, *13th Report*, WHO Technical Report Series 273 (Geneva: World Health Organization, 1964), 9.

60. "Schedule II Controls for Barbiturates," *F-D-C Reports/Pink Sheet*, Nov. 20, 1972: T&G-8.

61. Worldwide, large amounts of barbiturate continue to be manufactured. For the International Narcotics Control Board's Schedule III barbiturates (amobarbital, butabarbital, cyclobarbital, and pentobarbital), see INCB, *Psychotropic Substances, Statistics for 2002* (New York: United Nations, 2004), 33–36; for the Schedule IV barbiturates (a list of seven including barbital and phenobarbital), see 48–50. These data are unreliable guides to national levels of consumption as so much product is exported.

62. Max Fink, interview with Edward Shorter and David Healy, Oct. 25, 2002, Nissequogue, New York.

63. Jules Angst, "Myths of Psychopharmacology," interview, in *The Psychopharmacologists*, ed. David Healy, 1: 287–307 (London: Chapman and Hall, 1996), quote 296.

64. L[azar] Edeleano, "Ueber einige Derivate der Phenylmethacrylsäure und der Phenylisobuttersäure," *Berichte der Deutschen Chemischen Gesellschaft*, 20 (1887): 616–622. In retrospect, it is not exactly clear what compound Edeleano synthesized, and this was agonized over long in court. See *Smith, Kline & French Laboratories v. Clark & Clark et al.*, No. 9048. United States Circuit Court of Appeals, Third Circuit. 157 F.2d 725; U.S. App. LEXIS 3910; 70 U.S.P.Q. (BNA) 382, Aug. 6, 1946 decided, 2.

65. See Kinnosuke Miura, "Aus der chirurgisch-ophthalmologischen Universitätsklinik in Tokio (Japan): Vorläufige Mittheilung über Ephedrin, ein neues Mydriaticum," *Berliner Klinische Wochenschrift*, 24 (Sept. 19, 1887): 707, reporting the work of "Prof. Dr. Nagai." In 1885 G. Yamanashi had isolated an impure form of the alkaloid.

66. See K. K. Chen and Carl F. Schmidt, "Action and Clinical Use of Ephedrine," *JAMA* 87 (Sept. 11, 1926): 836–842. See also Carl F. Schmidt, "Pharmacology in a Changing World," *Annual Review of Physiology* 23 (1961): 1–14, esp. 5. Walter Sneader, *Drug Discovery: The Evolution of Modern Medicines* (Chichester: Wiley, 1985), 100.

67. Jokichi Takamine, "The Blood-Pressure-Raising Principle of the Suprarenal Glands—A Preliminary Report," *Therapeutic Gazette* 25 (1901): 221–224.

68. G[eorge] Barger and H[enry] H. Dale, "Chemical Structure and Sympathomimetic Action of Amines," *Journal of Physiology* 41 (1910): 19–59.

69. C[arl] Mannich and W. Jacobsohn, "Ueber Oxyphenyl-alkylamine und Dioxyphenyl-alkylamine," *Berichte der Deutschen Chemischen Gesellschaft* 43 (1910): 189–197.

70. For a guide to PEA derivatives, see Lundbeck Institute, *Psychotropics 2002/03* (Copenhagen: Lundbeck Institute, 2003), 385–400.

71. P. Burnat et al., "L'Ecstasy: Psychostimulant, hallucinogène et toxique," *Presse Médicale* 25 (Sept. 14, 1996): 1208–1212.

72. For a helpful summary of both drugs, and of almost all other drugs discussed in this book, the reader is referred to Frank Ayd, Jr., *Lexicon of Psychiatry, Neurology and the Neurosciences*, 2nd ed. (Philadelphia: Lippincott, 2000), 595–598.

73. S. J. Peroutka, discussion, in Merton Sandler et al., eds., *5-Hydroxytryptamine in Psychiatry: A Spectrum of Ideas* (Oxford: Oxford University Press, 1991), 20.

74. Desoxyn advertisement, in *New York State Journal of Medicine* 47 (1947): 1473. On 1943 as the launch year of methamphetamine, see Eric Colman, "Anorectics on Trial: A Half Century of Federal Regulation of Prescription Appetite Suppressants," *Annals of Internal Medicine* 143 (2005): 380–385.

75. Ernst Späth, "Ueber die *Anhalonium*–Alkaloide: I. Anhalin und Mezcalin," *Monatshefte für Chemie* 40 (1919): 129–154.

76. S. Weir Mitchell, "Remarks on the Effects of Anhelonium Lewinii (the Mescal Button)," *BMJ* 2 (Dec. 5, 1896): 1625–1629. On its isolation, see A. Heffter, "Ueber Cacteenalkaloide," *Berichte der Deutschen Chemischen Gesellschaft* 29 (1896): 216–227.

77. Havelock Ellis, "Mescal: A New Artificial Paradise," *Contemporary Review* 73 (1898): 130–141, quote 141.

78. George Piness, Hyman Miller, and Gordon A. Alles, "Clinical Observations on Phenylaminoethanol Sulphate," *JAMA* 94 (Mar. 15, 1930): 790–791.

79. *Smith, Kline & French v. Clark & Clark*, 8.

80. The details in this section are based on Nicolas Rasmussen, "Making the First Anti-Depressant: Amphetamine in American Medicine, 1929–1950," *Journal of the History of Medicine and Allied Sciences* 61 (2006): 288–314. Rasmussen had access to the Alles papers; further details are also in *Smith, Kline & French v. Clark & Clark*. On 1932 as the marketing date for the first amphetamines, see Sherwin Gardner to the secretary, July 12, 1979, National Archives and Records Administration, RG 88, General Subject Files, 88-85-49, box 33.

81. Council on Pharmacy and Chemistry, "Reports of the Council," *JAMA* 111 (July 2, 1938): 27. See also *Smith, Kline & French Laboratories v. Clark & Clark et al.*, No. C-2311; United States District Court for the District of New Jersey, 62 F. Supp. 971; 1945 U.S. Dist. LEXIS 1899; 66 U.S.P.Q. (BNA) 440, Sept. 1, 1945, 2.

82. Myron Prinzmetal and Wilfred Bloomberg, "The Use of Benzedrine for the Treatment of Narcolepsy," *JAMA* 105 (Dec. 21, 1935): 2051–2054.

83. A. S. Peoples and E[ric] Guttmann, "Hypertension Produced with Benzedrine: Its Psychological Accompaniments," *Lancet* 1 (May 16, 1936): 1107–1109, quotes 1108–1109.

84. Erich Guttmann and William Sargant, "Observations on Benzedrine," *BMJ* 1 (May 15, 1937): 1013–1015, quote 1014.

85. Abraham Myerson, "Effect of Benzedrine Sulfate on Mood and Fatigue in Normal and in Neurotic Persons," *AMA Archives of Neurology and Psychiatry* 36 (1936): 816–822, quote 817.

86. M[orrris] H. Nathanson, "The Central Action of Beta-aminopropylbenzene (Benzedrine)," *JAMA* 108 (Feb. 13, 1937): 528–531, quote 531.

87. Dwight L. Wilbur et al., "Clinical Observations on the Effect of Benzedrine Sulfate: A Study of Patients with States of Chronic Exhaustion, Depression and Psychoneurosis," *JAMA* 109 (Aug. 21, 1937): 549–554.

88. Torald Sollmann, *A Manual of Pharmacology*, 7th ed. (Philadelphia: Saunders, 1948), 385.

89. United States Patent Office, Patent 2,276,508, issued Mar. 17, 1942.

90. Compare the numbers of Benzedrine and Dexedrine advertisements in the *New York State Journal of Medicine* in 1946: 267 (Benzedrine), 1883 (Dexedrine).

91. Benzedrine advertisement, *New York State Journal of Medicine* 41 (Jan. 15, 1941): 185.

92. Advertisement for Benzedrine, see *New York State Journal of Medicine* 47 (1947): 2082; advertisement for Dexedrine, see *New York State Journal of Medicine* 48 (1948): 2193.

93. Among the historians to pick up on the amphetamines as the "first generation" of antidepressants are Shorter, *Historical Dictionary of Psychiatry* (2005), 20–21; and Nicolas Rasmussen, "First Anti-Depressant Amphetamine" (2006).

94. Desoxyn advertisement, *New York State Journal of Medicine* 47 (1947): 1473. The factual basis of the claim was probably Eugene Davidoff, "A Comparison of the Stimulating Effect of Amphetamine, Dextroamphetamine and Dextro-N-Methyl Amphetamine (Dextro-Desoxyephedrine)," *Medical Record* 156 (1943): 422–424. Davidoff had conducted several trials of amphetamines.

95. Advertisement for Methedrine, *New York State Journal of Medicine* 50 (1950): 2750.

96. Jean Delay, "Pharmacological Explorations of the Personality: Narco-Analysis and Methedrine Shock," *Proceedings of the Royal Society of Medicine* 42 (1949): 491–496, quote 491–492.

97. G[erald] de M[ontjoie] Rudolf, "Treatment of Depression with Sympathomimetic Preparations," *The Practitioner* 174 (1955): 180–183.

98. Editorial "Drugs in the Treatment of Depression," *Lancet* 1 (May 21, 1955): 1065.

99. John L. Simon and Harry Taube, "A Preliminary Study on the Use of Methedrine in Psychiatric Diagnosis," *Journal of Nervous and Mental Disease* 104 (1946): 593–596.

100. T. M. Ling and L. S. Davies, "The Use of Methedrine in the Diagnosis and Treatment of the Psychoneuroses," *AJP* 109 (1952): 38–39. See also John T. Hutchinson, "The Value of Drugs in the Treatment of Neuroses," *British Journal of Clinical Practice* 10 (1956): 541–544, esp. 543.

101. Sheila McNulty, "Needles and Haystacks," *Financial Times Weekend*, Aug. 20, 2005, W1.

102. Benjamin Cohen and Abraham Myerson, "The Effective Use of Phenobarbital and Benzedrine Sulfate (Amphetamine Sulfate) in the Treatment of Epilepsy," *AJP* 95 (1938): 371–393, quote 387.

103. Edward C. Reifenstein and Eugene Davidoff, "Benzedrine Sulfate Therapy," *New York State Journal of Medicine* 39 (1939): 42–57, quote 52.

104. Abraham Myerson, "The Reciprocal Pharmacologic Effects of Amphetamine (Benzedrine) Sulfate and the Barbiturates," *NEJM* 221 (Oct. 12, 1939): 561–564, quotes 562. The article referred to in the quote was Myerson et al., "The Effect of Amphetamine (Benzedrine) Sulfate and Paredrine Hydrobromide on Sodium Amytal Narcosis," *NEJM* 221 (Dec. 28, 1939): 1015–1019. Paredrine is hydroxyamphetamine.

105. Jacques S. Gottlieb and Frank E. Coburn, "Psychopharmacologic Study of Schizophrenia and Depressions: Intravenous Administration of Sodium Amytal and Amphetamine Sulfate Separately and in Various Combinations," *AMA Archives of Neurology and Psychiatry* 51 (1944): 260–263.

106. Jacques S. Gottlieb, "The Use of Sodium Amytal and Benzedrine Sulfate in the Symptomatic Treatment of Depressions," *Diseases of the Nervous System* 10 (1949): 50–52, quotes 50–51.

107. D. Legge and Hannah Steinberg, "Actions of a Mixture of Amphetamine and a Barbiturate in Man," *British Journal of Pharmacology* 18 (1962): 490–500, quote 499.

108. Benzebar advertisement, *New York State Journal of Medicine* 48 (1950): 1897.

109. The first Dexamyl advertisement, *New York State Journal of Medicine* 50 (1950): 511.

110. See J. M. Gowdy (at DMR) to Louis Lasher (at Bureau of Field Administration), Feb. 28, 1963: "In the past we have taken the position that it would be difficult to show medically that 'Dexamyl' or similar drugs lend themselves readily to addicting or non-medical use/abuse." NARA, RG 88, General Subject Files, 1964/65, box 3754.

Notes to Chapter 3

1. Harry H. Pennes, "The Nature of Drugs with Mental Actions and Their Relation to Cerebral Function," *Bulletin of the New York Academy of Medicine* 33 (1957): 81–88, quote 81.

2. The term "first drug set" was coined by Thomas Ban in the 1960s, then revived in his "Selective Drugs Versus Heterogeneous Diagnoses: Towards a New Methodology in Psychopharmacologic Research," *Psiquiatria Biol.* 7 (1999): 177–189.

3. "Wyeth's Spartase Came from 'Entirely New Development in Therapy,'" *F-D-C Reports/Pink Sheet*, Jan. 15, 1962, 20.

4. Robert S. Roe (director, BPS) to commissioner, Oct. 28, 1958, NARA, RG 88, General Subject Files, box 2534.

5. Joseph Sadusk (head of Bureau of Medicine) to George Larrick (commissioner), Mar. 17, 1965, NARA, RG 88, General Subject Files, box 4248.

6. Frank Fish, discussion, in E. Beresford Davies, ed., *Depression: Proceedings of the Symposium Held at Cambridge 22 to 26 September 1959* (Cambridge: Cambridge University Press, 1964), 349.

7. Paul Hoch and Joseph Zubin, eds., *Anxiety: The Proceedings of the 39th Annual Meeting of the American Psycho-Pathological Association, Held in New York City, June, 1949* (New York: Grune & Stratton, 1950).

8. F[rank] M. Berger and W. Bradley, "The Pharmacological Properties of Dihydroxy (2-Methylphenoxy)-Propane (Myanesin)," *British Journal of Pharmacology* 1 (1946): 265–272. Myanesin is a brand name for the generic mephenesin. For the synthesis of mephenesin see Petar Zivkovic, "Ueber eine neue Bildungsart von Äethern des Glyzerins mit Phenolen," *Monatshefte für Chemie* 29 (1908): 951–958; for the history of the glycerol ethers see Louis

Goodman and Alfred Gilman, eds., *The Pharmacological Basis of Therapeutics*, 2nd ed. (New York: Macmillan, 1955), 206–207.

9. Frank Berger interview, by Edward Shorter, Aug. 10, 2006, in New York.

10. F[rank] M. Berger and W. Bradley, "Muscle-Relaxing Action of Myanesin," *Lancet* 252 (Jan. 18, 1947): 97.

11. Berger interview.

12. On mephenesin in anxiety, see Louis S. Schlan and Klaus R. Unna, "Some Effects of Myanesin in Psychiatric Patients," *JAMA* 140 (June 25, 1949): 672–673.

13. Tolserol advertisement, *Diseases of the Nervous System* 12 (1951): 2.

14. Berger interview.

15. Berger interview.

16. The FDA considered mephenesin to be a tranquilizer. See "Tranquilizer Classifications," *F-D-C Reports/Pink Sheet*, April 1, 1957, 7–8. In one of the many miscarriages of the Drug Efficacy Study Implementation (DESI, which is discussed in greater detail in Chapter 6 of this book), in 1972 the FDA withdrew mephenesin as lacking in efficacy. See Compliance Evaluation Branch to All Regional Food and Drug Directors, May 1, 1972, mandating the withdrawal of the drug from its many manufacturers. NARA, RG 88, General Subject Files, box 4647, 505.52.

17. Benjamin Rush, *Medical Inquiries and Observations upon the Diseases of the Mind*, 3rd ed. (1812; repr., Philadelphia: Grigg, 1827), 179.

18. See Hugo J. Bein, "Biological Research in the Pharmaceutical Industry with Reserpine," in *Discoveries in Biological Psychiatry*, ed. Frank J. Ayd, Jr. and Barry Blackwell, 142–154 (Baltimore: Ayd Medical Communications, 1984), quote 143. Some writers attribute the coining of "tranquilizer" to Frank Berger, yet the evidence for this is poor. To be sure, in his 1946 article on the pharmacology of mephenesin, Berger says, "Administration of small quantities of these substances to mice, rats, or guinea pigs caused tranquillization, muscular relaxation, and a sleep-like condition from which the animals could be roused." F[rank] M. Berger and W. Bradley, "The Pharmacological Properties of Dihydroxy (2-Methylphenoxy)-Propane (Myanesin)," *British Journal of Pharmacology* 1 (1946): 265–272, quote 265. Yet the reference is a glancing one and the authors do not again return to the concept in that article or in subsequent work. Paul Janssen attributes coinage of the term to Nathan Kline, who in a restaurant conversation is supposed to have urged Berger to call Berger's new drug meprobamate a "tranquillizer." "What the world really needs is a 'tranquillizer,'" Kline is supposed to have said. "The world needs tranquility." See Paul Janssen, "From Haloperidol to Risperidone," interview, in *The Psychopharmacologists*, ed. David Healy, 2: 39–70 (London: Chapman and Hall, 1998), quote 59. The story may or may not be apocryphal; the first advertisement for Miltown, Wallace Laboratories' brand of meprobamate, called it "an entirely new type of tranquilizer." *New York State Journal of Medicine* 56 (1956): 5.

19. Serpasil advertisement, *New York State Journal of Medicine* 53 (1953): 3076.

20. Rauwiloid advertisement, *New York State Journal of Medicine* 53 (1953): 1628–1629.

21. Robert W. Wilkins, "Clinical Usage of Rauwolfia Alkaloids, Including Reserpine (Serpasil)," *Annals of the New York Academy of Sciences* 59 (1954): 36–44, quote 43.

22. Rauwidrine advertisement, *New York State Journal of Medicine* 54 (1954): 915.

23. "FDA Seizes 'Tranquil,'" *F-D-C Reports/Pink Sheet*, Mar. 4, 1957, 11–12.

24. "Tranquilizer Classifications," *F-D-C Reports/Pink Sheet*, Apr. 1, 1957, 7–8.

25. For the first Dormison advertisement, see *New York State Journal of Medicine* 51 (1951): 2213; Alexandre Blondeau, *Histoire des laboratoires pharmaceutiques en France et de leurs médicaments* (Paris: Cherche Midi, 1994), 2: 167–168. On sorting out methylparfynol (meparfynol) and its congeners, see *The Merck Index*, 9th ed. (Rahway, NJ: Merck, 1976), 5666, nos. 5671, 5672.

26. On scientific use of the term *antineurotic*, see, for example, Karl Rickels, chair of session on "Antineurotic Agents," in Daniel E. Efron, ed., *Psychopharmacology: A Review of Progress, 1957–1967*, Public Health Service Pub. No. 1836 (Washington, DC: GPO, 1968), 137.

27. Renate Weber, "Die Ritalin-Story," *Deutsche Apotheker Zeitung* 141 (2001): 1091–1093. See also Leandro Panizzon, "La Preparazione di Piridil-e Piperidil-arilacetonitrili," *Helvetica Chimica Acta* 27 (1944): 1748–1756; R. Meier et al., "Ritalin, eine neuartige synthetische Verbindung mit spezifischer zentralerregender Wirkungskomponente," *Klinische Wochenschrift* 32 (May 15, 1954): 445–450.

28. Ritalin advertisement, *Diseases of the Nervous System* 17 (1956): 68.

29. Ritalin advertisement, *JAMA*, 163 (Apr. 13, 1957): 4–5.

30. J. Cole and P. Glees, "Ritalin as an Antagonist to Reserpine in Monkeys," *Lancet* 270 (Mar. 24, 1956): 338.

31. A. Drassdo et al., "Untersuchungen über ein neuartiges, zentrales Stimulans (Ritalin)," *Medizinische Klinik* 49 (May 28, 1954): 892–893.

32. "Other Interesting Figures Disclosed by the Import Tabulation," *F-D-C Reports/Pink Sheet*, July 30, 1956, 6.

33. John T. Ferguson, "Treatment of Reserpine-Induced Depression with a New Analeptic: Phenidylate [*sic*]," *Annals of the New York Academy of Sciences* 61 (1955): 101–107.

34. Adolph L. Natenshon, "Clinical Evaluation of Ritalin," *Diseases of the Nervous System* 17 (1956): 392–396, quote 395. The 39 fatigued, depressed patients were a subset of the 89 in this open trial. See also A. B. Kerenyi et al., "Depressive States and Drugs—III. Use of Methylphenidate (Ritalin) in Open Psychiatric Settings and in Office Practice," *Canadian Medical Association Journal* 83 (Dec. 10, 1960): 1249–1254.

35. Peter E. Siegler et al., "A Comparative Study of the Effects of Methylphenidate and a New Piperidine Compound (SCH 5472)," *Current Therapeutic Research* 2 (1960): 543–553, see 550, table 5.

36. Karl Rickels et al., "Pemoline and Methylphenidate in Mildly Depressed Outpatients," *Clinical Pharmacology and Therapeutics* 11 (1970): 698–710, quote 709.

37. Council on Drugs, American Medical Association, "New and Nonofficial Drugs," *JAMA* 163 (Apr. 20, 1957): 1479–1480.

38. A placebo-controlled trial finding Ritalin ineffective in hospital depression was A. A. Robin and S. Wiseberg, "A Controlled Trial of Methylphenidate

(Ritalin) in the Treatment of Depressive States," *Journal of Neurology, Neurosurgery and Psychiatry* 21 (1958): 55–57.

39. Paul De Haen, "Diseases and Their Remedies—Quarterly Review of Drugs," *New York State Journal of Medicine* 73 (1973): 2168–2173, quote 2169. In fairness, some did argue that methylphendiate and the stimulants ended up making depression worse, after an initial uplift. The argument was that in depression, as Charles Shagass had shown, the stimulation threshold was already quite high (Shagass, "The Sedation Threshold: A Method for Estimating Tension in Psychiatric Patients," *Electroencephalography and Clinical Neurophysiology* 6 [1954]: 221–233). Giving stimulants thus was thought to make the condition worse. This viewpoint is quite theoretical, though, and the practical evidence of methylphenidate's benefit in nonmelancholic depression is considerable.

40. B[ernard] J. Ludwig and E. C. Piech, "Some Anticonvulsant Agents Derived from 1,3 Propanediols," *Journal of the American Chemical Society* 73 (Dec. 1951): 5779–5781.

41. See Henry Hoyt's testimony, *Hearings Before the Subcommittee on Antitrust and Monopoly of the Committee on the Judiciary, United States Senate, 86th Congress, 2nd Session, Pursuant to S. Res. 57, Part 16: Administered Prices in the Drug Industry (Tranquilizers), Jan. 21–29, 1960* (Washington, DC: GPO, 1960), 9146–9150. Hereafter cited as *Kefauver Hearings (Tranquilizers)*.

42. These details from Berger interview. On Berger's compensation and commercial arrangements for meprobamate, see also "Administered Prices: Drugs," *Report of the Committee on the Judiciary, United States Senate, Made by Its Subcommittee on Antitrust and Monopoly, Pursuant to S. Res. 52, 87th Congress, First Session June 27, 1961* (Washington, DC: GPO, 1961), 140–144. Hereafter cited as *Kefauver Hearings Report*.

43. Miltown advertisement, *New York State Journal of Medicine* 56 (1956): 5.

44. For hostility to Deprol, see the testimony of Heinz Lehmann and Fritz Freyhan at the Senate's *Kefauver Hearings Report*, 178–179, and *AMA Drug Evaluations, Evaluated by the AMA Council on Drugs* (Chicago: AMA, 1971), 229.

45. For example, William Karliner, interview by Edward Shorter and Max Fink, Apr. 6, 2004, New York.

46. Frank Ayd, Jr., interview by David Healy, Dec. 13, 1998: 10–11, American College of Neuropsychopharmacology (ACNP), Oral History Project; I am grateful to Thomas Ban for making the transcript available.

47. Lowell S. Selling, "Clinical Study of a New Tranquilizing Drug: Use of Miltown," *JAMA* 157 (Apr. 30, 1955): 1594–1596.

48. Leo E. Hollister et al., "Meprobamate in Chronic Psychiatric Patients," *Annals of the New York Academy of Sciences* 67 (1957): 789–798, quote 798. The paper was given at a symposium in 1956 organized by Frank Berger. In the large number of clinical trials of meprobamate for nervous, anxious, and nonmelancholic conditions, most were positive. Yet the citation of this literature often proved highly selective. Weatherall, in a hostile article, strove to put the worst possible face on the "tranquillizers." Weatherall, "Tranquillizers," *BMJ* 1 (May 5, 1962): 1219–1224; as evidence of the uselessness of meprobamate he cited two underpowered trials: M. J. Raymond et al., "A Trial of Five

Tranquilizing Drugs in Psychoneurosis," *BMJ* 2 (July 13, 1957): 63–66; Herbert Koteen, "Use of a 'Double-Blind' Study Investigating the Clinical Merits of a New Tranquilizing Agent," *Annals of Internal Medicine* 47 (1957): 978–989. Weatherall cited Tucker (1957) to demonstrate the inadequacy of meprobamate in chronic schizophrenics. Kenneth Tucker and Harold Wilensky, "A Clinical Evaluation of Meprobamate Therapy in a Chronic Schizophrenic Population," *AJP* 113 (1957): 698–703. For a positive early trial beating placebo, see E. D. West et al., "Controlled Trial of Meprobamate," *BMJ* 2 (Nov. 24, 1956): 1206–1209. An interesting exercise in toting up these underpowered and relatively meaningless trials is David J. Greenblatt and Richard I. Shader, "Meprobamate: A Study of Irrational Drug Use," *AJP* 127 (1971): 1297–1303, who concluded the benzodiazepines were superior. This is possible, but does not necessarily mean that meprobamate was a bad drug.

49. FDA, "In the Matter of Depressant and Stimulant Drugs," docket no. FDA-DAC-1, session of Aug. 18, 1966: 3519–3521, U.S. Food and Drug Administration, Division of Dockets Management, Rockland, MD; obtained through the Freedom of Information Act (FOIA). Hereafter cited as "Meprobamate Hearings."

50. Joseph C. Borrus, "Meprobamate in Psychiatric Disorders," *Medical Clinics of North America* 41 (1957): 327–337, quote 334.

51. These statistics were entered as evidence in congressional hearings; *Drug Abuse Control Amendments of 1965. Hearings Before the Committee on Interstate and Foreign Commerce, House of Representatives, 89th Congress, First Session, on H.R. 2, Feb. 9, 1965, Serial no. 89-1* (Washington, DC: GPO, 1965), 293.

52. Berger interview.

53. Frank J. Ayd, Jr., "The Early History of Psychopharmacology," *Neuropsychopharmacology*, 5 (1991): 71–84, quote 73–74.

54. Information Carter-Wallace supplied for *Carter-Wallace, Inc.* v. *Wolins Pharmacal Corp.*, No. 70 C 45; United States District Court for the Eastern District of New York, 326 F. Supp. 1299; 1971 U.S. Dist. LEXIS 14734; 168 U.S.P.Q. (BNA) 566; 1971 Trade Cas. (CCH) P73,488. Filed Feb. 5, 1971, p. 1. Carter became Carter-Wallace in 1965.

55. "AM Psychiatric Assn's Kline Hits Unfavorable Tranquilizer Publicity at Senate Hearing," *F-D-C Reports/Pink Sheet*, June 10, 1957, 10.

56. Estes Kefauver, in *Kefauver Hearings (Tranquilizers)*, 9145.

57. See, for example, "New Tranquilizer Market Strategy," *F-D-C Reports/Pink Sheet*, Nov. 5, 1956, 11–12.

58. Frank Ayd testimony, Meprobamate Hearings, July 29, 1966: 2084–2085.

59. Jean Delay, "Introduction au colloque international," in Delay, ed., *Colloque international sur la chlorpromazine, Paris, 20–22 octobre 1955* (Paris: Doin, 1956), 3–6.

60. Pierre Deniker, discussion, in Nathan S. Kline, ed., *Psychopharmacology Frontiers: Proceedings of the Psychopharmacology Symposium, Second International Congress of Psychiatry, Zurich, 1957* (Boston: Little, Brown, 1958), 424; Deniker meant signs of Parkinsonism.

61. World Health Organization, *Ataractic and Hallucinogenic Drugs in Psychiatry Report of a Study Group*, Technical Report Series, no. 152 (Geneva:

WHO, 1958), 22–23. In the United States this distinction was reflected in Jonathan O. Cole and C. Jelleff Carr, "A Synoptic Review of Psychoactive Drugs," in Seymour Fisher, ed., *Child Research in Psychopharmacology* (Springfield, IL: Thomas, 1959), 3–20. They said, "The main drug groups to be considered are: *the major tranquilizers*, those with apparent efficacy in the treatment of hyperactivity and disturbed behavior in psychotic patients; the *minor tranquilizers* [for] . . . neurotic and psychosomatic reactions." They added as further groups the *"nonbarbiturate sedatives"* and the *"antidepressive agents,"* 4. Italics in original. The symposium was held in 1958.

62. Heinz Lehmann, "New Drugs in Psychiatric Therapy," *Canadian Medical Association Journal* 85 (Nov. 18, 1961): 1145–1151. The term "antipsychotic" was certainly in use before Lehmann "coined" it. See, for example, the Senate testimony of A. Dale Console, *Administered Prices: Hearings Before the Subcommittee on Antitrust and Monopoly of the Committee on the Judiciary, United States Senate, 86th Congress, 2nd Session, Pursuant to S. Res. 238, Part 18, Apr. 13, 1960* (Washington, DC: GPO, 1960), 10391. "Drugs like chlorpromazine and reserpine should really be called antipsychotic drugs. They play a definite role in patients with psychoses. They were given the unfortunate term 'tranquilizer.'" Console was a former medical director of Squibb. This European concept of "neurolepsis" became a license for American psychiatrists to run up the doses of drugs such as chlorpromazine to astonishingly high levels.

63. See Tofranil advertisement, *JAMA* 174 (Sept. 10, 1960): 303.

64. The term *antianxiety* had been used in previous advertisements for other agents without suggesting it was a separate therapeutic class. Merck launched Elavil (amitriptyline) in 1961 as "a potent antidepressant with effective anti-anxiety properties," *Diseases of the Nervous System* 22 (1961): 361. The Librium advertisement is in *JAMA* 190 (Dec. 28, 1964): 64–65. Academic psychopharmacology tended at first not to accept Hoffmann-La Roche's argument that Librium was not a tranquilizer. See Jonathan O. Cole et al., "Drug Therapy," in *Progress in Neurology and Psychiatry*, 15 (1960): 540–576, esp. 543.

65. Paul Charpentier, "Sur la constitution d'une diméthylamino-propyl-N-phénothiazine," *Comptes Rendus Hebdomadaires des Séances de l'Académie des Sciences* 225 (July–Dec. 1947): 306–308.

66. See, for example, Jean Thuillier, *Ten Years That Changed the Face of Mental Illness*, trans. Gordon Hickish (1981; repr. London: Dunitz, 1999), 32.

67. Thomas Ban, personal communication, Apr. 9, 2007.

68. For an authoritative account, see David Healy, *The Creation of Psychopharmacology* (Cambridge: Harvard University Press, 2002).

69. Thorazine advertisement, *Diseases of the Nervous System* 16 (1955): 227.

70. Thomas Ban, personal communication, Oct. 8, 2007.

71. See for example M[aurice] Lacomme, H[enri] Laborit et al., "Note sur un essai d'analgésie obstétricale potentialisée par association de dolosal et de 45–50 R. P. en perfusion intra-veineuse. Étude de 175 cas," *Bulletin de la Fédération des Sociétés de Gynécologie et d'Obstétrique de Langue Française*, 4 (1952): 558–562.

72. J[ean] Delay et al., "Etude de 300 dossiers de malades psychotiques traités par la chlorpromazine en service fermé depuis 1952," in Delay, ed., *Colloque international sur la chlorpromazine, Paris, 20–22 octobre 1955* (Paris: Doin, 1956), 228–235.

73. See Edward Shorter and David Healy, *Shock Therapy: The History of Electroconvulsive Treatment in Mental Illness* (New Brunswick, NJ: Rutgers University Press, 2007).

74. J[ean] Sigwald and D[aniel] Bouttier, "L'utilisation des propriétés neuroplégiques du chlorhydrate de chloro-3(diméthylamino-3'-propyl)-phénothiazine en thérapeutique neuro-psychiatrique," *Presse médicale* 61 (Apr. 25, 1953): 607–609, quote 608.

75. J[ean] Sigwald et al., "'Ambulatory' Treatment with Chlorpromazine," *Journal of Clinical and Experimental Psychopathology and Quarterly Review of Psychiatry and Neurology* 17 (1956): 57–69, quote 68.

76. John T. Hutchinson, "The Value of Drugs in the Treatment of Neuroses," *British Journal of Clinical Practice* 10 (1956): 541–544, quote 541.

77. P[aul] Kielholz, "Über die Largactilwirkung bei depressiven Zuständen und Manien sowie bei der Entziehung von Morphin- und Barbitursüchtigen," *Schweizer Archiv für Neurologie und Psychiatrie*, 73 (1954): 291–309.

78. Heinz Lehmann, "Psychopharmacotherapy," interview, in *The Psychopharmacologists*, ed. David Healy, 1: 159–186 (London: Chapman and Hall, 1996), quote 160.

79. Douglas Goldman, "The Effect of Chlorpromazine on Severe Mental and Emotional Disturbances," in *Chlorpromazine and Mental Health: Proceedings of the Symposium Held . . . June 6, 1955, Warwick Hotel, Philadelphia, Pennsylvania*, ed. Smith, Kline & French Laboratories, 19–40 (Philadelphia: Lea & Febiger, 1955), quote 32–33.

80. Max Fink and Donald F. Klein, "Behavioral Reaction Patterns with Phenothiazines," *Archives of General Psychiatry* 7 (1962): 449–459, quotes 454. A simultaneous analysis of the patients randomized to imipramine showed that the relationship did not run the other way: The depressed patients responded well, the schizophrenic significantly less so. Klein and Fink, "Psychiatric Reaction Patterns to Imipramine," *AJP* 119 (1962): 432–438.

81. A word of caution: Precisely as a result of a large, early RCT sponsored by the Psychopharmacology Research Branch of the National Institute for Mental Health, imipramine was found in general superior to chlorpromazine as an antidepressant. Allen Raskin et al., "Differential Response to Chlorpromazine, Imipramine, and Placebo," *Archives of General Psychiatry* 23 (1970): 164–173.

82. Pierre Deniker and T[herèse] Lempérière, "Drug Treatment of Depression," in *Depression: Proceedings of the Symposium Held at Cambridge 22 to 26 September 1959*, ed. E. Beresford Davies, 214–215 (Cambridge; Cambridge University Press, 1964), quote 215.

83. Deniker must have misspoken. There is no levopromazine. On levomepromazine (methotrimeprazine, Nozinan) as an antimelancholic, see T[homas] Ban and L. Schwarz, "Systematic Studies with Levomepromazine," *Journal of Neuropsychiatry* 5 (1963): 112–117; H[enri] Baruk, "Principes et direction pratique de la thérapeutique des états dépressifs," *Annales Moreau de Tours* 2 (1965): 71–73.

84. The drug company Pfizer has officially been Pfizer-Roerig since 1953; Roerig is now a division of Pfizer. The company no longer uses "Roerig" in its drug advertising and shall be referred throughout the text simply as Pfizer.

85. Nathan Kline, discussion, in *Biogenic Amines and Affective Disorders: Proceedings of a Symposium held in London 18–21 January 1979*, ed. T[orgny] Svensson and A[rvid] Carlsson (Copenhagen: Munksgaard, 1980), 131.

86. Navane (thiothixene) advertisement, *Diseases of the Nervous System* 28 (1967), unpaginated.

87. Max Fink, "Hy Denber: An Appreciation," *Neuropsychopharmacology* 23 (2000): 474–475.

88. Even today, Pfizer is unable to resist the temptation—doubtless quite legitimate—to market its antipsychotics as antidepressants. See Lisa L. Stockbridge (FDA regulatory reviewer) to Rita Wittich (Pfizer VP, worldwide regulatory strategy), Sept. 13, 2002, reproaching Pfizer for permitting its sales representatives at the APA meeting in Philadelphia in May 2002 to "misrepresent Geodon [ziprasidone] as having antidepressant effects similar to the selective serotonin reuptake inhibitors (SSRIs)," www.fda.gov/cder/warn/2002/10790.pdf (accessed Dec. 3, 2003).

89. John E. Overall, Leo E. Hollister, Merlin Johnson, and Veronica Pennington, "Nosology of Depression and Differential Response to Drugs," *JAMA* 195 (Mar. 14, 1966): 946–948. On Pennington, see Edward Shorter, *Historical Dictionary of Psychiatry* (New York: Oxford University Press, 2005), 310.

90. For an overview see Mary M. Robertson and M[ichael] R. Trimble, "Major Tranquillisers Used as Antidepressants," *Journal of Affective Disorders* 4 (1982): 173–193; Gordon Parker and Gin Malhi, "Are Atypical Antipsychotic Drugs Also Atypical Antidepressants?" *Australian and New Zealand Journal of Psychiatry* 35 (2001): 631–638.

91. Saul H. Rosenthal and Charles L. Bowden, "A Double-Blind Comparison of Thioridazine (Mellaril) Versus Diazepam (Valium) in Patients with Chronic Mixed Anxiety and Depressive Symptoms," *Current Therapeutic Research* 15 (1973): 261–267, quote 261.

92. Marsilid advertisement, *New York State Journal of Medicine* 57 (1957): 2036–2037.

93. J[ohn] H. Gaddum and H. Kwiatkowski, "The Action of Ephedrine," *Journal of Physiology* 94 (1938): 87–100.

94. Thomas Ban calls the evidence on behalf of the hypothesis "tenuous." "Pharmacotherapy of Depression: A Historical Analysis," *Journal of Neural Transmission* 108 (2001): 707–716, see 709.

95. Merton Sandler, "Monoamine Oxidase Inhibitors in Depression: History and Mythology," *Journal of Psychopharmacology* 4 (1990): 136–139.

96. Irving J. Selikoff et al., "Toxicity of Hydrazine Derivatives of Isonicotinic Acid in the Chemotherapy of Human Tuberculosis," *Quarterly Bulletin of Sea View Hospital* 13 (1952): 17–26.

97. Irving J. Selikoff et al., "Treatment of Pulmonary Tuberculosis with Hydrazine Derivatives of Isonicotinic Acid," *JAMA* 150 (Nov. 8, 1952): 973–980, quote 977.

98. For a more discouraging view of the psychiatric side effects of iproniazid, see Robert G. Bloch et al., "The Clinical Effect of Isoniazid and Iproniazid in the Treatment of Pulmonary Tuberculosis," *Annals of Internal Medicine* 40 (1954): 881–900.

99. E. A[lbert] Zeller et al., "Influence of Isonicotinic Acid Hydrazide (INH) and 1-Isonicotinyl-2-isopropyl Hydrazide (IIH) on Bacterial and Mammalian Enzymes," *Experientia* 8 (Sept. 15, 1952): 349–350.

100. Gordon R. Kamman et al., "The Effect of 1-Isonicotynl 2-Isopropyl Hydrazide (IIH) on the Behavior of Long-Term Mental Patients," *Journal of Nervous and Mental Diseases* 118 (1953): 391–407. For another early negative report, see Jackson A. Smith, "The Use of the Isopropyl Derivative of Isonicotinylhydrazine (Marsilid) in the Treatment of Mental Disease," *American Practitioner Digest of Treatment* 4 (1953): 519–520.

101. George E. Crane, "The Psychiatric Side-Effects of Iproniazid," *AJP* 112 (1956): 494–501, quote 499.

102. John C. Saunders, discussion, in E. A. Zeller, ed., "Amine Oxidase Inhibitors," *Annals of the New York Academy of Sciences* 80 (1959): 551–1038, quote 719. The conference was in 1958.

103. Frank Ayd said, "Nate persuaded Saunders to leave Ciba and join him at Rockland State." Ayd, "The Discovery of Antidepressants," in Healy, *Psychopharmacologists* 1: 81–110, quote 93.

104. At the 1958 conference (720), Saunders gave "p. 152" of the proceedings of the 1955 conference as the source for his contribution. The 1955 reference: Jacques S. Gotttlieb, ed., *Pharmacologic Products Recently Introduced in the Treatment of Psychiatric Disorders*, American Psychiatric Association, Psychiatric Research Reports 1 (Washington, DC: APA, 1955). Neither that page, nor any other in the 1955 volume, bears Saunders' name.

105. Alfred Pletscher, "Iproniazide: Prototype of Antidepressant MAO-Inhibitors," in *Reflections on Twentieth-Century Psychopharmacology*, ed. Thomas A. Ban et al., 174–177 (Budapest: Animula, 2004), see 175. This version is confirmed by Arvid Carlsson, who was a fellow in Brodie's lab between circa July 1955 and January 1956; Carlsson remembers that Kline visited the Brodie lab on numerous occasions and was "inspired" when Pletscher told him about iproniazid. Arvid Carlsson interview by David Healy and Edward Shorter, Feb. 27, 2007, in Gothenburg, Sweden, 6. Some accounts have Kline discovering the drug during a visit to Warner Laboratories, for example, Sandler, "Monoamine Oxidase Inhibitors," 137.

106. Harry P. Loomer, John C. Saunders, and Nathan S. Kline, "A Clinical and Psychodynamic Evaluation of Iproniazid as a Psychic Energizer," in *Research in Affects*, American Psychiatric Association, Psychiatric Research Reports 8, ed. Marc H. Hollender (Washington, DC: APA, 1957), quote 138.

107. George Simpson, "Clinical Psychopharmacology," interview, in Healy, *Psychopharmacologists* 2: 285–305, see 292.

108. Frank J. Ayd, Jr., "A Preliminary Report on Marsilid," *AJP* 114 (1957): 459. See also R. L. de Verteuil and H[einz] E. Lehmann, "Therapeutic Trial of Iproniazid (Marsilid) in Depressed and Apathetic Patients," *Canadian Medical Association Journal* 78 (Jan. 15, 1958): 131–133. About a third of patients

with a mixed set of diagnoses improved, yet the trialists discontinued their study when they had a death from liver failure and a high incidence of complications.

109. Ayd interview, "The Discovery of Antidepressants," in Healy, *Psychopharmacologists* 1: 81–110, 95.

110. See Sandler, "Monoamine Oxidase Inhibitors," 138; John C. Saunders, "Lasker Award: Priority Claim," *JAMA* 191 (Mar. 8, 1965): 161; John Clarke Saunders, obituary, *New York Times*, Mar. 29, 2001: A25.

111. Sandler, "Monoamine Oxidase Inhibitors," 137. See also Nathan Kline testimony, *False and Misleading Advertising (Prescription Tranquilizing Drugs). Hearings Before a Subcommittee of the Committee on Government Operations, 85th Congress, 2nd session, Feb. 11–26, 1958* (Washington, DC: GPO, 1958), 15. For Kline's account of the group's discovery of the antidepressant efficacy of the MAOIs, see his Lasker Award lecture, "The Practical Management of Depression," *JAMA* 190 (Nov. 23, 1964): 732–740.

112. C. M. B. Pare and M[erton] Sandler, "A Clinical and Biochemical Study of a Trial of Iproniazid in the Treatment of Depression," *Journal of Neurology, Neurosurgery and Psychiatry* 22 (1959): 247–251, quote 251.

113. Alexander P. Dukay, discussion, in Zeller, "Amine Oxidase Inhibitors," 668, who made fun of an enthusiastic investigator who discovered the smile also on placebo patients in a trial. The conference was held at the New York Academy of Sciences in November 1958.

114. Carl Breitner, discussion, in Zeller, "Amine Oxidase Inhibitors," 742–744; Breitner, "Marsilid in Catatonic Schizophrenia," *AJP* 114 (1958): 941.

115. David C. English, discussion, in Zeller, "Amine Oxidase Inhibitors," 807. On the drug treatment of psychotic depression see Conrad M. Swartz and Edward Shorter, *Psychotic Depression* (New York: Cambridge University Press, 2007).

116. Zale A. Yanof, discussion, in Zeller, "Amine Oxidase Inhibitors," 752.

117. Nathan S. Kline, "Clinical Experience with Iproniazid (Marsilid)," *Journal of Clinical and Experimental Psychopathology and Quarterly Review of Psychiatry and Neurology* 19, no. 1 (1958): 72–79, see 73.

118. Samuel W. Joel, "Twenty Month Study of Iproniazid Therapy," *Diseases of the Nervous System* 20 (1959): 521–524, quote 524. Joel's article appeared a year before the contribution that is thought to have initiated the modern era of OCD treatment: J. Guyotat et al., "L'imipramine en dehors des états dépressifs," *Journal de Médecine de Lyon* 41 (1960): 367–375.

119. Nathan S. Kline, "Clinical Experience with Iproniazid (Marsilid)," *Journal of Clinical and Experimental Psychopathology and Quarterly Review of Psychiatry and Neurology* 19, no. 1 (1958): 72–79, quote 76.

120. Nathan Kline, discussion, in *Psychopharmacology Frontiers*, ed. Nathan Kline (Boston: Little, Brown, 1957), 433.

121. Samuel Joel, personal communication, Aug. 6, 1997.

122. Theodore R. Robie, "Iproniazid Chemotherapy in Melancholia," *AJP* 115 (1958): 402–409.

123. E. D. West and P. J. Dally, "Effects of Iproniazid in Depressive Syndromes," *BMJ* 1 (June 13, 1959): 1491–1494, quote 1491–1492.

124. "Roche's Marsilid Pick–Up Program," *F-D-C Reports/Pink Sheet*, Apr. 21, 1958, 19–20.

125. See George Larrick (commissioner, FDA) to Louis Gershenfeld (Philadelphia College of Pharmacy and Science), July 27, 1959, NARA, RG 88, General Subject Files, box 2698.

126. "Hoffmann-La Roche Marsilid," *F-D-C Reports/Pink Sheet*, Apr. 14, 1958, 2.

127. On these events, see *Interagency Coordination in Drug Research and Regulation. Hearings Before the Subcommittee on Reorganization and International Organizations of the Committee on Government Operations, United States Senate, 87th Congress, 2nd Session. Agency Coordination Study, Aug 1 and 9, 1962, Part 1* (Washington, DC: GPO, 1963), 518–521.

128. Guy Walters to B. S. Mansueto, Sept. 24, 1965, NARA, RG 88, General Subject Files, 1964/65, box 3755.

129. "M-A-O-I New Drug Era," *F-D-C Reports/Pink Sheet*, June 8, 1959, 18.

130. "Lakeside's Catron," *F-D-C Reports/Pink Sheet*, Nov. 30, 1959, 18.

131. Leo Alexander and Austin W. Berkeley, "The Inert Psychasthenic Reaction (Anhedonia) as Differentiated from Classic Depression and Its Response to Iproniazid," *Annals of the New York Academy of Sciences* 80 (1959): 669–679.

132. Martin Roth, "The Phobic Anxiety-Depersonalization Syndrome," *Proceedings of the Royal Society of Medicine* 52 (1959): 587–596, quote 594.

133. Thomas Ban, personal communication, Aug. 20, 2002.

134. Alfred Pletscher, "The Discovery of Antidepressants: A Winding Path," *Experientia* 47 (1991): 4–8, quote p. 6.

135. "New Drug Developments," *F-D-C Reports/Pink Sheet*, June 15, 1959, 16.

136. August Bernthsen, "Zur Kenntnis des Methylenblau und verwandter Farbstoffe," *Chemische Berichte (Berichte der Deutschen Chemischen Gesellschaft)* 16 (1883): 2896–2904.

137. Alan Broadhurst, discussion, in *Wellcome Witnesses to Twentieth Century Medicine*, ed. E. M. Tansey et al., 2: 138–139 (London: Wellcome Trust, 1998).

138. The following account is based on "The Imipramine Dossier," in *From Psychopharmacology to Neuropsychopharmacology in the 1980s*, ed. Thomas A. Ban et al., 282–352 (Budapest: Animula, 2002).

139. Roland Kuhn [autobiographical essay], in *Psychiatrie in Selbstdarstellungen*, ed. Ludwig J. Pongratz, 219–257 (Berne: Huber, 1977), quote 236.

140. Ban, "Imipramine Dossier," 311–312, 325.

141. Ibid., 301.

142. Ibid., 318. For details on Schneider and vital depression, see Shorter, *Historical Dictionary of Psychiatry*, 83.

143. Ban, "Imipramine Dossier," 337.

144. R[oland] Kuhn "Über die Behandlung depressiver Zustände mit einem Iminodibenzylderivat (G 22355)," *Schweizerische Medizinische Wochenschrift* 87 (Aug. 31, 1957): 1135–1140, quote 1136

145. The usage "Thymoleptikum" stemmed from a Geigy employee named Oeschger with a background in philology. See Kuhn to Jules Angst, July 5, 1999; I am grateful to David Healy for sharing with me a copy of this letter; see also Matthias M. Weber, *Die Entwicklung der Psychopharmakologie im Zeitalter der naturwissenschaftlichen Medizin* (Munich: Urban, 1999), 166. On "timolepsia"

in Spanish psychiatry see Antonio Mestre, "Consideraciones con Motivo de Algunos Terminos Tecnicos," *Revista Cubana: Periodico Mensual de Ciencias, Filosofia, Literatura Y Bellas Artes* (Havana), 6 (1887), 97–108, esp. 107-108.

146. See Kuhn interview in Healy, *Psychopharmacologists* 2: 102–103. Kuhn places the conversation with Boehringer at the 1958 Congress in Rome. See Kuhn, "Corrections of Statements in the Publication by David Healy on the History of the Discovery of Modern Antidepressants," in Ban, *From Psychopharmacology to Neuropsychopharmacology*, 301–308, esp. 304.

147. R[aymond] Coirault et al., "Mode d'action du G 22 355–Chlordydrate de N-(y-diméthyl-amino-propyl-)iminodibenzyle—où Tofranil en pathologie mentale," in *Neuropsychopharmacology: Proceedings of the First International Congress of Neuro-Pharmacology (Rome, September 1958)*, ed. P[hilip] Bradley et al., 520–526 (Amsterdam: Elsevier, 1959), quote 523.

148. Jean Thuillier, "Ten Years That Changed Psychiatry," interview, in *The Psychopharmacologists*, ed. David Healy, 3: 543–559 (London: Arnold, 2000), see 549–550.

149. Roland Kuhn, "From Imipramine to Levoprotiline: The Discovery of Antidepressants," in Healy, *Psychopharmacologists* 2: 93–118, see 107–108.

150. H[einz] E. Lehmann et al., "The Treatment of Depressive Conditions with Imipramine (G 22355)," *Canadian Psychiatric Association Journal* 3 (1958): 155–164, quote 161.

151. Alan Broadhurst, "Before and After Imipramine," interview, in Healy, *Psychopharmacologists* 1: 111–134, quote 119. Hilda C. Abraham et al., "A Controlled Clinical Trial of Imipramine (Tofranil) with Out-patients," *British Journal of Psychiatry* 109 (1963): 286–293.

152. Healy, *Psychopharmacologists* 3: 117, 119.

153. Donald F. Klein, "Commentary by a Clinical Scientist in Psychopharmacological Research," *Journal of Child and Adolescent Psychopharmacology* 17 (2007): 284–287, quote 284.

154. J[ean] Delay and P[ierre] Deniker, "Efficacy of Tofranil in the Treatment of Various Types of Depression: A Comparison with Other Antidepressant Drugs," in *McGill University Conference on Depression and Allied States, Montreal, Mar. 19–21, 1959, Canadian Psychiatric Association Journal* 4, special suppl. (1959): S100–S112, quote S109; see also S103, table 2. Some of these patients were also treated with neuroleptic drugs and the results, as Delay and Deniker admitted, did not have "statistical purity." They controlled their trials with 45 patients on Marsilid, and the two drugs came out about even, though the subcategories contain so few patients as to make the comparison statistically meaningless.

155. Gerald L. Klerman and Jonathan O. Cole, "Clinical Pharmacology of Imipramine and Related Antidepressant Compounds," *Pharmacological Reviews* 17 (1965): 101–141, quote 118.

156. Thomas Ban, personal communication, Mar. 28, 2007.

157. Fritz Freyhan, "Clinical Effectiveness of Tofranil in the Treatment of Depressive Psychoses," *McGill University Conference* (1959): S86–S89.

158. Frank Ayd, discussion, ibid., S135.

159. Interview with Walter Brown, by Edward Shorter and Max Fink, Feb. 16, 2006, in Tiverton, Rhode Island, 26.

160. See Conrad M. Swartz and Edward Shorter, *Psychotic Depression* (New York: Cambridge University Press, 2007).

161. For a balanced view of the risks and benefits of the tricyclic antidepressants, see Thomas Ban, *Psychopharmacology* (Baltimore: Williams & Wilkins, 1969), 270–289.

162. Alfred Pletscher, "The Discovery of Antidepressants," 7.

163. Alexander Glassman, interview, Dec. 10, 2003, 11, American College of Neuropsychopharmacology (ACNP), Oral History Project. I am grateful to Thomas Ban for a copy of this transcript. Whether the tricyclics are really associated with a higher suicide rate than other drug classes has never really been clarified. A powerful British database of over 172,000 patients taking antidepressants found that fluoxetine (Prozac) and mianserin (Bolvidon, among other brands in the United Kingdom) had exceptionally high suicide rate per 10,000 person years on the drug (19.0 per 10,000 person years, and 16.1 respectively), the tricyclics all below "average" (taking dothiepin's rates of 8.7 per 10,000 person years as the average). Susan S. Jick et al., "Antidepressants and Suicide," *BMJ* 310 (Jan. 28, 1995): 215–218, see table 3, 216. See also J. G. Edwards' editorial in the same issue, 205–206. It is often difficult, however, to know which drug was the actual cause of death in suicide victims taking several different agents.

164. S. Weir Mitchell, "On the Use of Bromide of Lithium," *American Journal of the Medical Sciences* 60 (1870): 443–445. See also for early lithium use, William A. Hammond, *A Treatise on Diseases of the Nervous System* (New York: Appleton, 1871), 381. Lithium-rich springs ("crazy water") in the United States had offered what was essentially lithium treatment for decades.

165. Accounts may be found in F. Neil Johnson, *The History of Lithium Therapy* (London: Macmillan, 1984); Edward Shorter, *History of Psychiatry* (New York: Wiley, 1997), 255–257; see also "Fifty Years of Treatments for Bipolar Disorder: A Celebration of John Cade's Discovery," *Australian and New Zealand Journal of Psychiatry* 33, suppl. (1999).

166. John F. J. Cade, "Lithium Salts in the Treatment of Psychotic Excitement," *Medical Journal of Australia* 2 (Sept. 3, 1949): 349–352.

167. See, for example, A[ndré] Plichet, "Le traitement des états maniaques par les sels de lithium," *Presse Médicale* 62 (June 5, 1954): 869–870; see also the comments of Paris psychiatrist S. Follin, discussion, who prescribes lithium for its "action remarquable sur les états d'excitation maniaque," 744. The comment follows H[ans] Steck, "Le syndrome extrapyramidal et diencéphalique au cours des traitements au largactil et au serpasil," *Annales Médico-Psychologiques* 112 (1954): 737–743.

168. See Shorter, *Historical Dictionary*, 162.

169. Mogens Schou, "Lithium: Personal Reminiscences," *Psychiatric Journal of the University of Ottawa* 14 (1989): 260–262, see 261.

170. M[ogens] Schou et al., "The Treatment of Manic Psychoses by the Administration of Lithium Salts," *Journal of Neurology, Neurosurgery and Psychiatry* 17 (1954): 250–260, quote 255.

171. Felix Post [interview], in *Talking About Psychiatry*, ed. Greg Wilkinson, 157–177 (London: Gaskell, 1993), see 167.

172. Anne E. Caldwell makes this point. "History of Psychopharmacology," in *Principles of Psychopharmacology*, 2nd ed., ed. William G. Clark et al., 9–40 (New York: Academic, 1978), see 30.

173. See Shepherd interview in Healy, *Psychopharmacologists* 2: 249. The passage in the initial interview was even more explicit than the published version. See also Healy interview with Schou, "Lithium," 267.

174. M[ichael] Shepherd, "Evaluation of Psychotropic Drugs (2): Depression, Part II—1969," in *Principles and Practice of Clinical Trials*, ed. E. L. Harris, et al., 208–216 (Edinburgh: Livingstone, 1970), esp. 214–216.

175. Alec Coppen, "Biological Psychiatry in Britain," interview, in Healy, *Psychopharmacologists* 1: 265–286, quote 274.

176. Reyss Brion, discussion, in Jean-M. Sutter, ed., "Psychopharmacologie," *L'Encéphale* 62, suppl. (1973): 68. "Les lithinés du docteur Gustin."

177. Samuel Gershon and Arthur Yuwiler, "Lithium Ion: A Specific Pharmacological Approach to the Treatment of Mania," *Journal of Neuropsychiatry* 1 (1960): 229–241; Eddie [sic] Kingstone, "The Lithium Treatment of Hypomanic and Manic States," *Comprehensive Psychiatry* 1 (1960): 317–320. The paper had been rejected by the *American Journal of Psychiatry*.

178. Ronald R. Fieve, "Lithium: From Introduction to Public Awareness," in *The Triumph of Psychopharmacology and the Story of CINP*, ed. Thomas Ban et al., 258–260 (Budapest: Animula, 2000), quote 259.

179. Ralph N. Wharton and Ronald R. Fieve, "The Use of Lithium in the Affective Psychoses," *AJP* 123 (1966): 706–712.

180. Ronald R. Fieve et al., "The Use of Lithium in Affective Disorders: I. Acute Endogenous Depression," *AJP* 125 (1968): 487–491.

181. Jonathan Cole, telephone interview, July 17, 2002. See also "FDA to Approve Lithium," *F-D-C Reports/Pink Sheet*, Feb. 23, 1970, T&G 1.

182. Discussion comment of Robert Prien at NIMH, in FDA, Psychopharmacological Drugs Advisory Committee, 31st Meeting, vol. 1, Sept. 21, 1989, on NDA 18–276, Xanax (alprazolam): 195; obtained through the FOIA.

183. A[lec] Coppen et al., "Prophylactic Lithium in Affective Disorders: A Controlled Trial," *Lancet* 2 (Aug. 7, 1971): 275–283. Some NIMH research is seen as establishing the view that lithium is ineffective in the treatment of unipolar depression. Yet the study had only 12 unipolar patients, of whom 8 failed to improve (as opposed to 40 bipolar patients, of whom 8 failed to improve). Such a slender finding should never have been regarded as definitive. Frederick K. Goodwin et al., "Lithium Response in Unipolar Versus Bipolar Depression," *AJP* 129 (1972): 44–47.

184. See Tom G. Bolwig and Edward Shorter, eds., "Melancholia: Beyond DSM, Beyond Neurotransmitters," *Acta Psychiatrica Scandinavica* 115, no. 433 (February 2007): 136–183.

185. Jair C. Soares and Samuel Gershon, "The Psychopharmacologic Specificity of the Lithium Ion: Origins and Trajectory," *Journal of Clinical Psychiatry* 61, no. 9 (2000): 16–22, quotes 17–18.

186. The number of children hospitalized for "bipolar disorder" increased fivefold between 1996 and 2004; the increase for adolescents was fourfold. See

Joan Arehart-Treichel, "Kids' Hospitalizations Have Researchers Puzzled," *Psychiatric News*, June 15, 2007, 8.

187. Dennis Charney, discussion, in FDA, Psychopharmacologic Drugs Advisory Committee, Meeting No. 44, Feb. 6, 1995 [valproate in mania]: 135; obtained through FOIA.

188. Robert L. Bowman et al., "Spectrophotofluorometric Assay in the Visible and Ultraviolet," *Science* 122 (July 1, 1955): 32–33.

189. Marthe Vogt, "The Concentration of Sympathin in Different Parts of the Central Nervous System Under Normal Conditions and After the Administration of Drugs," *Journal of Physiology* 123 (1954): 451–481.

190. A. H. Amin, T. B. B. Crawford, and J[ohn] H[enry] Gaddum, "The Distribution of Substance P and 5–Hydroxytryptamine in the Central Nervous System of the Dog," *Journal of Physiology* 126 (1954): 596–618. On Gaddum and serotonin keeping us sane, see Gaddum, "Drugs Antagonistic to 5–Hydroxytryptamine," in *Ciba Foundation Symposium on Hypertension,* ed. G. E. W. Wolstenholme et al., 75–77 (London: Churchill, 1954), quote 77; on Gaddum's own LSD experiment, see Dick Barlow, "Receptors and the Chemist," interview, in Healy, *Psychopharmacologists* 3: 157–173, esp. 162.

191. D. W[ayne] Woolley and E. Shaw, "A Biochemical and Pharmacological Suggestion About Certain Mental Disorders," *Proceedings, National Academy of Sciences* 40 (1954): 228–231, quote 230.

192. See Robert Kanigel, *Apprentice to Genius: The Making of a Scientific Dynasty* (New York: Macmillan, 1986).

193. Alfred Pletscher, Parkhurst A. Shore, and Bernard B. Brodie, "Serotonin Release as a Possible Mechanism of Reserpine Action," *Science* 122 (Aug. 26, 1955): 374–375. According to Arvid Carlsson, it was Park Shore who had this idea first, but all three have now passed on and it will probably never be possible to sort out the exact credit for this epochal discovery. Carlsson interview by Healy and Shorter, Feb. 27, 2007, 8.

194. Fridolin Sulser, "The Noradrenergic Second Messenger Cascade: Switch from Presynaptic to Postsynaptic Receptor-Mediated Events," in *The Neurotransmitter Era in Neuropsychopharmacology*, ed. Thomas A. Ban et al., 56–64 (Buenos Aires: Polemos, 2006), quote 53.

195. Bernard B. Brodie and Parkhurst A. Shore, "A Concept for a Role of Serotonin and Norepinephrine as Chemical Mediators in the Brain," *Annals of the New York Academy of Sciences* 66 (1957): 631–642, photo 635.

196. Julius Axelrod, "The Fate of Adrenaline and Noradrenaline," in *Ciba Foundation Symposium . . . On Adrenergic Mechanisms*, ed. R. Vane et al., 28–39 (Boston: Little, Brown, 1960), quote 37.

197. Julius Axelrod et al., "Effect of Psychotropic Drugs on the Uptake of H³-Norepinephrine by Tissues," *Science* 133 (Feb. 10, 1961): 383–384.

198. Arvid Carlsson and Margit Lindqvist, "Effect of Chlorpromazine or Haloperidol on Formation of 3-Methoxytryptamine and Normetanephrine in Mouse Brain," *Acta Pharmacologica et Toxicologica* 20 (1963): 140–144.

199. Jacques Glowinski and Julius Axelrod, "Inhibition of Uptake of Tritiated-Noradrenaline in the Intact Rat Brain by Imipramine and Structurally Related Compounds," *Nature* 204 (Dec. 26, 1964): 1318–1319.

200. Brian E. Leonard, "Fifty Years of Psychopharmacology," in Ban and Udabe, *The Neurotransmitter Era*, 21–23, quote 21.

201. Ibid., 22.

202. All authorities agree that this bon mot is Warren Gerard's. But I have been unable to source it in his writings.

203. G. S. Duboff of the University of Michigan asking a question of Amedeo S. Marrazzi, discussion, D. V. Siva Sankar, ed., conference on "Some Biological Aspects of Schizophrenic Behavior," in *Annals of the New York Academy of Science* 96 (1962): 226; conference April 6–8, 1961.

NOTES TO CHAPTER 4

1. Surprisingly, there is no comprehensive history of the Food and Drug Administration. This paragraph is based on Donna Hamilton, "A Brief History of the Center for Drug Evaluation and Research," www.fda.gov/cder/about/history/Histext.htm, accessed July 13, 2002; and John P. Swann, "Food and Drug Administration," in *A Historical Guide to the U.S. Government*, ed. George Thomas Kurian, 248–254 (New York: Oxford University Press, 1998).

2. On the chronology of this reopening of the addiction discussion, see "What Is a Habit-Forming Drug?" *F-D-C Reports/Pink Sheet* Apr. 12, 1956, 6–8.

3. A key early document, cited repeatedly in the coming years, was Frederick Lemere, "Habit-Forming Properties of Meprobamate," *AMA Archives of Neurology and Psychiatry* 76 (1956): 205–206. In 13 of the 600 patients for whom he had prescribed meprobamate, there had been "excessive self-medication"; 10 of these were former alcoholics. An additional 9 patients after this original 600 "took increasing amounts of meprobamate to achieve the same effects." This slender report formed the Magna Carta of the antimeprobamate efforts.

4. "Tranquilizer 'Addicting,'" *F-D-C Reports/Pink Sheet*, Nov. 12, 1956, 18.

5. "Tranquilizer Addiction," *F-D-C Reports/Pink Sheet*, May 27, 1957, 12–14. Nathan Eddy also wrote an influential WHO report in 1965 suggesting the concept of "drug dependence" instead of "drug addiction" or "drug habituation." Nathan B. Eddy, II. Halbach, Harris Isbell, and Maurice H. Seevers, "Drug Dependence: Its Significance and Characteristics," *WHO Bulletin* 32 (1965): 721–733. Interestingly, Seevers, professor of pharmacology at the University of Michigan, was also a member of the scientific advisory board of the pro-industry lobby, Tobacco Industry Research Committee. This alliance of civil servants and pro-tobacco industry scientific advisors was clearly keen to spin the robust traditional concept of "addiction" into directions that would be hard to operationalize, and easy to politicize.

6. Carl F. Essig and John D. Ainslie, "Addiction to Meprobamate (Equanil, Miltown)," *JAMA* 164 (July 20, 1957): 1382.

7. "Miltown-Equanil Habituation," *F-D-C Reports/Pink Sheet*, Aug. 26, 1957, 16.

8. "Tranquilizers Useful, Not Proved Addictive," *F-D-C Reports/Pink Sheet*, Feb. 25, 1957, 7.

9. *Hearings Before the Subcommittee on Antitrust and Monopoly of the Committee on the Judiciary, United States Senate, 86th Congress, 2nd Session, Part 16:*

Administered Prices in the Drug Industry (Tranquilizers) (Washington, DC: GPO, 1960), 9028. Hereafter cited as *Kefauver Hearings (Tranquilizers)*.

10. "Kline Defends Miltown Against Addiction Allegations," *F-D-C Reports/ Pink Sheet*, June 10, 1957, 10.

11. Ibid., 10–11.

12. Robert H. Felix testimony to Blatnik House subcommittee investigating tranquilizers, quoted in *F-D-C Reports/Pink Sheet*, Mar. 3, 1958, 19.

13. *Kefauver Hearings (Tranquilizers)*, 9145.

14. Ibid., 9119.

15. "Supplementary Statement by Senator Hubert H. Humphrey," *Hearings Before the Subcommittee on Reorganization and International Organizations of the Committee on Government Operations, United States Senate, 88th Congress, 1st session, Agency Coordination Study, Part 5, June 19, 1963* (Washington, DC: GPO, 1964), 2812–2832, quotes 2821–2822.

16. "Fraternization-With-Industry and Other Charges v. FDA Splattered All Over Kefauver Hearing Room by Disgruntled Dr. Babs Moulton," *F-D-C Reports/Pink Sheet*, June 2, 1960, 11.

17. "Tranquilizer 'Addicting,'" 8–10.

18. See Kenneth D. Campbell (Acting Director, Drug and Device Branch) to Ralph G. Smith (acting medical director), July 25, 1960, NARA RG 88, General Subject Files, box 2887, 511.09. The FDA did, however, begin a crackdown on street sales of amphetamine. See *F-D-C Reports/Pink Sheet*, Nov. 2, 1959: 22–23.

19. C. E. Beisel (Advisory Opinions Branch, Division of Industry Advice) to Louis M. Moore, Feb. 28, 1964, NARA, RG 88, UD-WW, E35, General Subject Files, 1964.

20. See Peter Barton Hutt, "Balanced Government Regulation of Consumer Products," *Symposium on "Who Regulates the Regulator . . ." Institute of Food Technologists, Anaheim, CA, June 7, 1976*, Pub. Series PS-7601: 5 (Rochester, NY: Center for the Study of Drug Development, Departments of Pharmacology and Toxicology and of Medicine, University of Rochester Medical Center, Fall 1976). Hutt was chief counsel for FDA, 1971–75.

21. [Food and Drug Administration], *Report of Second Citizens Advisory Committee on the Food and Drug Administration to the Secretary of Health, Education, and Welfare, October, 1962* (Washington, DC: U.S. DHEW/FDA, 1962), 32.These statistics also include some personnel in the Bureau of Biological and Physical Sciences responsible for drug approvals.

22. "No Bromide and Acetanilid-Bromide 'Crusade' for FDA," *F-D-C Reports/ Pink Sheet*, Sept. 16, 1957, 6.

23. "Fraternization-With-Industry," 6–9.

24. George S. Leong, in discussion, in Joseph D. Cooper, ed., *The Philosophy of Evidence* (Washington, DC: Interdisciplinary Communication Associates, 1972), 93, the proceedings of a 1971 conference.

25. Louis Lasagna in discussion, Craig D. Burrell, ed., *Drug Assessment in Ferment: Multinational Comparisons* (Washington, DC: Interdisciplinary Communication Associates, 1976), 149, the proceedings of a 1973 conference.

26. "Fraternization-With-Industry," 10–11.

27. J. Kenneth Kinney (supervisory inspector) to Director, Seattle District, Nov. 29, 1961, NARA, RG 88, General Subject Files, box 3054, 515.04.

28. Monte O. Rentz to Ted M. Hopes (Inspector, San Francisco District), Oct. 13, 1960, NARA RG 88, General Subject Files, box 2893, 515.

29. Edward M. Grundlach to Winton B. Rankin (assistant commissioner FDA), Nov. 19, 1963, NARA RG 88, General Subject Files, box 3568, 505.5.

30. Arthur Ruskin to Office of the Commissioner, Jan. 31, 1963, NARA RG 88, General Subject Files, box 3578, 515.04

31. Rufus King, *The Drug Hang-Up: America's Fifty-Year Folly* (New York: Norton, 1972), see ch. 22: 229–239.

32. See the testimony at the meprobamate hearings of Samuel Kaim, chief of research at the Veterans Administration, Meprobamate Hearings, Aug. 3, 1966, 2437. For a full citation, see below. He had, however, heard of Roger Egeberg, then medical director of the Los Angeles County Department of Charities, who had been a member of the White House Ad Hoc Panel on Drug Abuse in 1962 (Egeberg counted as a liberal and later, as Assistant Secretary for Health and Scientific Affairs, de-emphasized the supposed dangers of marijuana).

33. *The President's Advisory Commission on Narcotic and Drug Abuse, Final Report* (Washington, DC: GPO, Nov. 1963); for list of addicting and nonaddicting drugs ("Exhibit I"), see 10. The members were Judge E. Barrett Prettyman, chair; James P. Dixon, MD; James S. Dumpson; Roger O. Egeberg, MD; Harry M. Kimball; Austin H. MacCormick; Rafael Sanchez-Ubeda, MD.

34. Amedeo Marrazzi, in discussion, in D. V. Siva Sankar, ed., "Some Biological Aspects of Schizophrenic Behavior," *Annals of the New York Academy of Sciences* 96 (1962): 335, proceedings of a conference held in April 1961.

35. George P. Larrick, testimony, *Drug Control Amendments of 1965. Hearings Before the Committee on Interstate and Foreign Commerce, House of Representatives, 89th Congress, First Session, on H.R. 2, Jan 27, 28; Feb 2, 9, and 10, 1965* (Washington, DC: GPO, 1965), 24. Larrick added, "My testimony today isn't exclusively my testimony. I am speaking for the Department" (89).

36. Ibid., 250

37. Ibid., 87.

38. Ibid., 346–347.

39. Ibid., 362.

40. "Depressant and Stimulant Drugs: Proposed Listing of Additional Drugs Subject to Control," FDA 21 CFR Part 166, *Federal Register* 31 (Jan. 18, 1966): 565; this is also in NARA, RG 88–74–2 (Hearing Files), box 42, together with administrative correspondence.

41. The 39-volume transcript of the hearings, amounting to 4683 manuscript pages, is at FDA: "In the Matter of Depressant and Stimulant Drugs," docket no. FDA-DAC-1, June 27–Sept. 16, 1966, U.S. Food and Drug Administration, Division of Dockets Management, Rockland, MD; obtained through the Freedom of Information Act. On the background, see Meprobamate Hearings, June 27, 1966: 2–5. The prehearing began June 14 and is part of the record.

42. "FDA Rebuttal to Industry Drug Bill Testimony Before House Interstate," *F-D-C Reports/Pink Sheet*, Sept. 3, 1962, S-2–S-8, quote S-4.

43. It is unclear when this committee was actually struck. On the basis of other evidence, it was already in existence in 1965. Yet its second meeting took place on April 25–26, 1966; FDA, Advisory Committee on Abuse of Depressant and Stimulant Drugs, Summary of Proceedings, Second Meeting. NARA, RG 88, UD-WW, E9, Acc. 88–79–49.

44. On this committee, see Meprobamate Hearings, Henry Brill testimony, June 29, 1966, 335. See also FDA, Advisory Committee on Abuse of Depressant and Stimulant Drugs, Summary of Proceedings, Third Meeting, June 29–30, 1966, 4, NARA, RG 88, UD-WW, E9, 88–79–49. The committee included two warhorses in the federal battle against the tranquilizers: New York State asylum chief Henry Brill, who would testify against meprobamate at the FDA hearings, and Harris Isbell, director of the Addiction Research Center of the National Institute for Mental Health in Lexington, Kentucky, and adviser to the World Health Organization about "drugs liable to production addiction." Brill became a reliable addiction watchdog within the FDA as chair in the 1970s of the Controlled Substances Advisory Committee.

45. FDA, Advisory Committee on Abuse of Depressant and Stimulant Drugs, Summary of Proceedings, Second Meeting, April 25–26, 1966: 6, NARA, RG 88, UD-WW, E9, 88–79–49. "Appendix B," which listed the minor tranquilizers the committee had decided to spare, was not preserved in the archival copy of the meeting minutes. A version evidently doctored by the FDA was given to a federal court on July 10, 1972. The FDA had refused to produce this report for the petitioner at the time of the 1966 hearing. In an astonishing about-face in the record, as discussed in detail in Chapter 5, the memorandum summarizing the Advisory Committee's deliberations that the FDA finally produced for the court showed the committee as recommending that the minor tranquilizers *be placed under control*. (This memorandum did not contain the committee's original "Appendix B.") See *Hoffmann-La Roche, Inc., Petitioner v. Richard G. Kleindienst, Attorney General of the United States*. No. 71–1299. United States Court of Appeals for the Third Circuit, 478 F.2d I; 1973 U.S. App. LEXIS 10840, decided Mar. 28, 1973, 14, 20; http://web.lexis-nexis.com (accessed Sept. 24, 2005).

46. Paul A. Palmisano (acting director, Bureau of Medicine), memorandum, to Advisory Committee on the Abuse of Stimulant and Depressant Drugs, June 13, 1966. Attached to FDA, Advisory Committee on Abuse of Depressant and Stimulant Drugs, Summary of Proceedings, Third Meeting, June 29–30, 1966, NARA, RG 88, UD-WW, E9, 88–79–49.

47. William L. Hanaway to Hearing Clerk, DHEW, Jan. 10, 1966, NARA, RG 88–74–2, box 50.

48. Frederick M. Garfield (FDA Bureau of Regulatory Compliance) to J. K. Kirk (assistant commissioner for operations), May 13, 1966, NARA, RG 88, box 3891, 515.

49. When in 1964 an Indianapolis physician noted that Librium and meprobamate were much less harmful than the public feared, the FDA agreed with him: "This is admittedly a difficult public relations area . . . ." James L. Trawick, Director (FDA Division of Consumer Education) to Nelson N. Kaufman, Feb. 11, 1964, NARA, RG 88, General Subject Files, 1964, UD-WW, E-35.

50. Kenneth Lennington to Directors of Districts, May 17, 1966, NARA, RG 88, General Subject Files, box 3891, 515.

51. Bennie Moxness to file, memorandum of telephone conversation, May 19, 1966, NARA, RG 88, General Subject Files, box 3891, 515.

52. Ibid.

53. Ibid.

54. Ibid.

55. John Merandino, memorandum of conference, May 23, 1966; NARA, RG 88, box 3891, 515.

56. Margaret Milliken to Dennis McGrath, memorandum, May 23, 1966; NARA, RG 88, box 3891, 515.

57. This evidence came out in Murphy's testimony at the Librium-Valium Hearings: Before the Secretary, Department of Health, Education and Welfare, Food and Drug Administration, "In the Matter of: Depressant and Stimulant Drugs," docket no. FDA-DAC-2, Washington, DC, Oct. 6, 1966: 3812–3814, NARA, RG 88–74–2 (Hearing material), box 49: 3777–3778.

58. On Lasagna's apparent role as informal advisor to the hearing examiner, see Frank Berger interview, Aug. 10, 2006, 1.

59. John Finlator (director of Bureau of Drug Abuse Control), memorandum, to Commissioner James L. Goddard, June 15, 1966, NARA, RG 88, General Subject Files, box 3891, 515.

60. Meprobamate Hearings, June 14, 1966, 14.

61. Melvin Sabshin testimony, Meprobamate Hearings, Aug. 1, 1966, 2170–2196.

62. Frank Ayd testimony, Meprobamate Hearings, July 29, 1966, 2017–2021. In fairness, there were experts, though not at this hearing, who felt that meprobamate increased suicidality. See the testimony of James A. Knight, professor of psychiatry at Tulane University, who at the Librium-Valium Hearings argued that meprobamate increased depression "and with increased depression then his [patient's] risk of suicide would increase." He therefore said he would not use meprobamate with "agitated depression." Librium and Valium, he said, were superior drugs. Librium-Valium Hearings, Oct. 12, 1966, 4368.

63. Herman Denber testimony, Meprobamate Hearings, Aug. 11, 1966, 3102–3107.

64. Leo Alexander testimony, Meprobamate Hearings, Aug. 5, 1966, 2750.

65. Edward Annis testimony, Meprobamate Hearings, July 29, 1966, 1978–1979.

66. Joseph Bordenave testimony, Meprobamate Hearings, Aug. 1, 1966, 2280.

67. Minutes, Controlled Substances Advisory Committee, July 24, 1974, 2, NARA, RG88, UD-WW, E1, 88–80–3. Again at the meeting of Nov. 20–21, 1974, members expressed concern about listing leading to underutilization of controlled drugs and to overutilization of noncontrolled drugs, particularly analgesics.

68. Meprobamate Hearings, Aug. 12, 1966, 3325; Aug. 30, 4112.

69. N. N. Alberstadt, memorandum of telephone conversation with Carl Essig, May 23, 1966, NARA, RG 88, General Subject Files, box 3891, 515. The basis of Essig's expertise was a one-page research note cowritten with John D. Ainslie, "Addiction to Meprobamate," *JAMA* 164 (July 20, 1957): 1382, on the reactions of three patients taking very large doses following

sudden withdrawal, in addition to the dog research. A fuller version of this Essig-Ainslie report circulated within the FDA, prompting discussion of an addictiveness warning. Yet the FDA pulled back from this, evidently on grounds of not wanting to give meprobamate a competitive disadvantage. See *F-D-C Reports/Pink Sheet*, Jan. 6, 1958, 17. Ten years later Essig published further results of dog-addiction research, "Addiction to Nonbarbiturate Sedative and Tranquilizing Drugs," *Clinical Pharmacology and Therapeutics* 5 (1964): 334–343. In 1974, FDA's own Controlled Substances Advisory Committee cast doubt on such animal tests as a means of determining the "dependence potential" of a drug. See CSAC Minutes, July 24–25, 1974, 7, NARA RG 88, UD-WW, E1, 88–80–3.

70. "Test Dogs Killed by Tranquilizer," *New York Times* July 6, 1966, 27.

71. Carl Essig testimony, Meprobamate Hearings, July 5, 1966, 605; he showed the movie at 602–604.

72. Carl Essig testimony, Meprobamate Hearings, July 5, 1966, 637.

73. John Ewing testimony, Meprobamate Hearings, June 27, 1966, 647.

74. Jefferson Davis Bulla testimony, Meprobamate Hearings, Aug. 10, 1966, 3072.

75. John Ewing, re-testimony, Meprobamate Hearings, Aug. 22, 1966, 3719.

76. "DSD" (Dorothy S. Dobbs), telephone memo, to Office of the General Counsel, May 24, 1966, NARA, RG 88–74–2, box 46.

77. Jerome Jaffe testimony, Meprobamate Hearings, July 1, 1966, see, for example, 467.

78. Jerome Jaffe re-testimony, Meprobamate Hearings, Sept. 16, 1966, 4722–4767.

79. Meprobamate Hearings, Sept. 15, 1966, 4588.

80. Meprobamate Hearings, Aug. 26, 1966, 4024–4025.

81. Meprobamate Hearings, Sept. 14, 1966, 4344.

82. Proposed Rule Making, Department of Health, Education and Welfare, Food and Drug Administration. "Meprobamate: Proposed Findings of Fact and Conclusions and Tentative Order Regarding Listing Drug as Subject to Control," *Federal Register* 32 (Apr. 13, 1967): 5933–5938.

83. Alexander testimony, Meprobamate Hearings, Aug. 5, 1966, 2745–2746.

84. An editorial in *JAMA*, apropos of the Essig note and similarly based on anecdotes and worst-case scenarios, spoke of "intoxication . . . from deliberate ingestion of very large amounts of the drug." The point of the editorial was not to single out meprobamate but to observe that it had side effects, as did all drugs, and that it "should be administered with the same discretion as other therapeutic agents." See *JAMA*, 164 (July 20, 1957): 1332–1333.

85. Frederic Riederer appeared before the hearing three times, on July 6, Aug. 26, and Sept. 14. Frank Berger had obtained from U.S. DHEW, Office of Vital Statistics, data on the pharmaceutical agents used in suicides, 1954–1963. Although the exact construction of his categories was subject to give-and-take during the examination and cross-examinations of the hearing, it is apparent that by far the commonest agents in suicides were barbiturates, and that meprobamate was buried in a minority role among the "tranquilizers." Berger's paper "The Drugs Used to Commit Suicide" may be found at

NARA RG 88–74–2, box 46. The data in table 3, "Suicide from Poisoning by Drugs in 1963," were published in Frank Berger, "Social Implications of Psychotropic Drugs," in Silvio Garattini et al., eds., *Advances in Pharmacology and Chemotherapy* (New York: Academic, 1972), 105–118.

86. In 1958, for example, a pharmacist in Milledgeville, GA, wrote the FDA to find out how much Benzedrine he could dispense without a prescription. Answer: none. See Cilver Kidd to FDA, June 25, 1958, NARA RG 88, General Subject Files, box 2535, 511.09.10.

87. "Tranquilizer D-H Case," *F-D-C Reports/Pink Sheet*, July 1, 1957, 15; "Tranquilizer D-H Violations," *F-D-C Reports/Pink Sheet*, Aug. 26, 1957, 15. According to FDA historian John Swann, FDA enforcement of prescription requirements in general began with a Supreme Court decision in 1948. Swann, "FDA's Encounter with Goof Balls, Bennies Before DEA," *News Along the Pike* [FDA CDER newsletter] 3, no. 4 (Apr. 1997): 5.

88. Frank Berger interview, Aug. 10, 2006, 4.

89. See Walter Sullivan, "Drugs Approved Before '62 Face Rescreening," *New York Times*, Mar. 19, 1966, 1.

90. FDA Oral History Program, "Interview with William W. Goodrich, Office of the General Counsel, 1939–1971," p. 8 of 12 in printout, http://www.fda. gov/oc/history/oralhistories/goodrich (accessed July 4, 2002).

91. The manufacturer, Smith, Kline & French, had requested hearings on tranylcypromine (Parnate). But in a sudden reversal under its new medical director Joseph Sadusk, the FDA returned Parnate to market before the hearings began. See editorial "Tranylcypromine Sulfate," *JAMA* 189 (Sept. 7, 1964): 766–767.

92. *Carter-Wallace, Inc., Petitioner, v. John W. Gardner, Secretary of Health, Education, and Welfare, and James L. Goddard, Commissioner of Food and Drugs, Respondents*, No. 12200, United States Court of Appeals for the Fourth Circuit, 417 F.2d 1086; 1969 U.S. App. LEXIS 10181. Decided Nov. 4, 1969.

93. "Meprobamate 'Abuse' Control by BNDD Begins July 6," *F-D-C Reports/Pink Sheet*, June 8, 1970, 18.

94. "Meprobamate Sales by AMHO & Carter, 1961–76," *F D C Reports/Pink Sheet*, Nov. 5, 1962, 7.

95. Dorothy S. Dobbs to Paul A. Bryan (special assistant for DESI), Nov. 26, 1969, FDA, DESI files, #9698, box 8, no. 1730; obtained through the Freedom of Information Act (FOIA).

96. John Jennings (acting director, Bureau of Medicine) to Charles C. Edwards (FDA commissioner), Feb. 2, 1970, DESI files, #9698.

97. William W. Goodrich to John Jennings, Feb. 24, 1970. DESI files, #9698.

98. Barrett Scoville to deputy director, Bureau of Drugs, Jan. 10, 1974, NARA RG 88, General Subject Files, box 5035, 515. See Lino Covi et al., "Length of Treatment with Anxiolytic Sedatives and Response to Their Sudden Withdrawal," *Acta Psychiatrica Scandinavica* 49 (1973): 51–64.

99. Edward Kennedy and eight other congresspersons to Dockets Management Branch, FDA, Sept. 13, 2002, http://www.fda.gov/ohrms/ dockets/dailys/102/Sep02/091802/80027f41.pdf (accessed Aug. 2005).

100. Thomas Ban, interview, Aug. 20, 2002.

1. Tybamate advertisement: "When only an antineurotic can help your patient," *JAMA*, 193 (Sept. 6, 1965): 252.

2. Before the Secretary, Department of Health, Education and Welfare, Food and Drug Administration, "In the Matter of: Depressant and Stimulant Drugs," docket no. FDA-DAC-2, Washington, DC, Oct. 6, 1966, 3812–3814, NARA, RG 88–74–2 (Hearing materials), box 49. Hereafter cited as Librium-Valium Hearings.

3. Neil Kessel, "Psychiatric Morbidity in General Practice," in "The Medical Use of Psychotropic Drugs: A Report of a Symposium Sponsored by the Department of Health and Social Security . . . 1–2 July 1972," *Journal of the Royal College of General Practitioners* 23, suppl. 2 (1973): 11–15, quote 12.

4. Andy J. Rose, "Controversies in Practice," in *Benzodiazepines Divided: A Multidisciplinary Review*, ed. Michael Trimble, 61–64 (Chichester: Wiley, 1983), quote 61.

5. See the various contributions in the symposium Hoffmann-La Roche organized for Librium's launch. Titus Harris, ed., "Symposium on Newer Antidepressant and Other Psychotherapeutic Drugs . . . Nov. 13–14, 1959," *Diseases of the Nervous System* 21, suppl. (March 1960), "farmer's frau," 21. On gin and Librium, see M. Marinker, "The Doctor's Role in Prescribing," in *Journal of the Royal College of General Practitioners* 23, suppl. no. 2 (1973): 26–30, quote 27. The symposium at which this paper was given rang with snooty talk about the barrenness of life on English housing estates. Historian Susan L. Speaker challenges the stereotype of a tranquilizer-addicted society passively consuming large quantities of psychoactive drugs. "From 'Happiness Pills' to 'National Nightmare': Changing Cultural Assessment of Minor Tranquilizers in America, 1955–1980," *Journal of the History of Medicine* 52 (1997): 338–376.

6. Joseph M. Tobin and Nolan D. C. Lewis, "New Psychotherapeutic Agent, Chlordiazepoxide: Use in Treatment of Anxiety States and Related Symptoms," *JAMA* 174 (Nov. 5, 1960): 1242–49, quote 1247.

7. Alec Jenner, discussion, in E. M. Tansey et al., eds., *Wellcome Witnesses to Twentieth Century Medicine* (London: Wellcome Trust, 1998), 2: 152–153. For his original report, see F. A. Jenner et al., "A Controlled Trial of Methaminodiazepoxide (Chlordiazepoxide, 'Librium') in the Treatment of Anxiety in Neurotic Patients," *Journal of Mental Science* 107 (1961): 575–582.

8. R[alph] W. Gerard, "Drugs for the Soul: The Rise of Psychopharmacology," *Science* 125 (1957): 201–203, quote 201.

9. Librium advertisement, *Diseases of the Nervous System* 21 (March, 1960): 122–123.

10. "How's Business?" *F-D-C Reports/Pink Sheet*, Oct. 17, 1960, 19.

11. Edgar A. Buttle, Hearing Examiner, "Report Including Recommended Findings and Conclusions Re Potential for Abuse of the Drugs Librium and Valium," Apr. 7, 1967, 44–45, FDA, docket no. FDA-DAC-2, NARA, RG 88–74–2, box 51.

12. U.S. Department of Health, Education, and Welfare, Task Force on Prescription Drugs, *Background Papers, The Drug Users* (Washington, DC: Office of the Secretary, Dec. 1968), App. A: 38.

13. Mrs. Mae M. to William Dworkin, FDA, Sept. 28, 1973, NARA, RG 88, box 4866. She said she took Librium and Valium alike.

14. Carl Salzman, in discussion, special issue on "Innovative Treatment Strategies," *Journal of Clinical Psychiatry* 51, suppl. (Oct. 1990): 31.

15. National Prescription Audit, Therapeutic Category Report, Ten-Year Trend, 1963–72, NARA, RG 88, uncataloged.

16. American Medical Association, *AMA Drug Evaluations* (Chicago: AMA, 1971), 227.

17. International sales of meprobamate have remained robust to this day. In 2001, 252,000 kg (277 U.S. tons) of meprobamate were manufactured worldwide. International Narcotics Control Board (INCB), *Psychotropic Substances, Statistics for 2002* (New York: United Nations, 2004), Schedule IV, D2, 174.

18. National Prescription Audit.

19. Lawrence K. Altman, "Valium, Most Prescribed Drug, Is Center of a Medical Dispute," *New York Times*, May 19, 1974, 1.

20. For a list, see Lundbeck Institute, *Psychotropics 2002/2003* (Skodsborg, Denmark: Lundbeck, 2003), 9–11.

21. Valium advertisement, *JAMA*, 208 (Apr. 28, 1969): 644–645.

22. See *Use and Misuse of Benzodiazepines. Hearing Before the Subcommittee on Health and Scientific Research of the Committee on Labor and Human Resources, United States Senate, 96th Congress, First Session, Sept. 10, 1979* (Washington, DC: GPO, 1980), 241–242.

23. For a listing, see Donald F. Klein and John M. Davis, *Diagnosis and Drug Treatment of Psychiatric Disorders* (Baltimore: Williams & Wilkins, 1969), 380, table 33A.

24. "Hoffmann-La Roche's Worldwide Drug Volume . . ." *F-D-C Reports/Pink Sheet*, July 26, 1971, 3–5.

25. Serax advertisement, *JAMA*, 193 (Sept. 6, 1965): 64–65.

26. Leo Sternbach, the Roche chemist who synthesized the first benzos, dilated upon this point in an interview. See "Leo H. Sternbach, interview by Tonja Koeppel, 12 March 1986" (Philadelphia: Chemical Heritage Foundation, Oral History Transcript #0043), 31.

27. John F. Tallman et al., "Receptors for the Age of Anxiety: Pharmacology of the Benzodiazepines," *Science* 207 (Jan. 18, 1980): 274–281.

28. "Top 20 Branded Products of 1988," *Scrip*, Jan. 19, 1990, 24.

29. Lundbeck Institute, *Psychotropics*, 18–19.

30. Frank J. Ayd, Jr., "The Early History of Modern Psychopharmacology," *Neuropsychopharmacology* 5 (1991): 71–84, see 81.

31. INCB, *Psychotropic Substances*, 174.

32. Librium-Valium Hearings, Oct. 5, 1966, 3678–3679.

33. Librium advertisement, *JAMA* 174, no. 10 (Nov. 5, 1960): 253–254.

34. See, for example, Jules Angst et al., "Co-morbidity of Anxiety and Depression in the Zurich Cohort Study of Young Adults, " in *Comorbidity of*

Mood and Anxiety Disorders, ed. Jack D. Maser et al., 123–127 (Washington, DC: American Psychiatric Press, 1990), see 134–135, tables 10, 11. On mixed anxiety-depression as the commonest form of depression, see Paula J. Clayton, "Depression Subtyping: Treatment Implications," *Journal of Clinical Psychiatry* 59, suppl. 16 (1998): 5–12, see 8, fig. 2.

35. D[onald] A. W. Johnson in discussion, in Michael Trimble, ed., *Benzodiazepines Divided* (Chichester: Wiley, 1983), 65.

36. T. B. Üstün et al., "Primary Mental Health Services: Access and Provision of Care," in *Mental Illness in General Health Care: An International Study,* ed. Ustün and N. Sartorius (Chichester: Wiley, 1995), 358, table 6.

37. H. Angus Bowes, "The Role of Librium in an Out-Patient Psychiatric Setting," *Diseases of the Nervous System* 21, suppl. (Mar. 1960): 20–22, quote 20–21.

38. Bernard Carroll, discussion, FDA, Psychopharmacologic Drugs Advisory Committee, Transcript [dothiepin/antidepressant labeling], vol. 2, Dec. 4, 1981, II-98–99; obtained from FDA through the Freedom of Information Act.

39. Joseph M. Tobin and Nolan D. C. Lewis, "New Psychotherapeutic Agent, Chlordiazepoxide: Use in Treatment of Anxiety States and Related Symptoms," *JAMA* 174 (Nov. 5, 1960): 1242–1249, quote 1247.

40. Alan F. Schatzberg and Jonathan O. Cole, "Benzodiazepines in Depressive Disorders," *Archives of General Psychiatry* 35 (1978): 1359–1365, quote 1364.

41. T. K. Birkenhäger et al., "Benzodiazepines for Depression? A Review of the Literature," *International Clinical Psychopharmacology* 10 (1995):181–195.

42. Dr. Rathbone in discussion, "Symposium on Chlordiazepoxide: A Scientific Meeting . . . January 14, 1961," *Diseases of the Nervous System* 22, suppl. (1961): 34–35.

43. T. A. Furukawa et al., "Antidepressant and Benzodiazepine for Major Depression (Cochrane Review)," *Cochrane Library* 3 (Oxford: Update Software, 2002), quote at 8 of 18. [Oct. 22, 2002].

44. Thomas Ban, personal communication, Mar. 3, 2007.

45. "Depressant and Stimulant Drugs," 21 CFR Part 166, *Federal Register,* 31 (Jan 18, 1966): 565.

46. The existence of these two communications was later revealed in court: *Hoffmann-La Roche, Inc., Petitioner* v. *Richard G. Kleindienst, Attorney General of the United States.* No. 71–1299. United States Court of Appeals for the Third Circuit, 478 F.2d I; 1973 U.S. App. LEXIS 10840, decided Mar. 28, 1973, 15; http://www.web.lexis-nexis.com (accessed Sept. 24, 2005). If Hoffmann-La Roche had known of their existence earlier, its lawsuit, as well as the 1966 hearings that prompted it, might have had a different outcome.

47. Memorandum of telephone conversation between Dr. Lee Gordon (Roche) and Dr. M[atthew] J. Ellenhorn, July 31, 1963, NARA, RG 88, General Subject Files, box 3568, 505.5.

48. Memorandum of interview, Aug. 22, 1963, between Dr. Lee Gordon (Roche) and Matthew J. Ellenhorn, Arthur Egelman, John H. Moling, and J. Hauser (all FDA), NARA, RG 88, box 3568, 505.5.

49. Valium advertisement, *JAMA* 186 (Dec. 21, 1963): 60.

50. Memorandum of meeting, Apr. 13, 1964; present were numerous Roche executives, representatives of Roche's advertising agency, and FDA staffers. NARA, RG 88, General Subject Files, UD-WW, E35, 505.51.

51. Ed C. to Joseph Sadusk (FDA), Jan. 18, 1966, NARA, RG 88, General Subject Files, box 3891, 515.

52. H. J. Bulgerin to FDA, Feb. 5, 1966, NARA, RG 88–74–2 (Hearing Materials), box 50.

53. John J. Jennings (New Drug Surveillance Branch) to Matthew J. Ellenhorn (Chief, New Drug Surveillance Branch), Oct. 27, 1964, NARA, RG 88, General Subject Files, box 4248, 505.53.

54. Memorandum of telephone conversation between A. H. Pate (Case Review Branch) and Charles Llewellen (Duke University), July 14, 1966; NARA, RG 88, General Subject Files, box 3885, 505.5

55. William Goodrich (FDA assistant general counsel) to Henry L. Verhulst, July 29, 1966, NARA RG 88, General Subject Files, box 3891, 515.

56. John Finlator to James L. Goddard, July 29, 1966; NARA, RG 88, box 3891, 515.

57. Ibid.

58. Librium-Valium Hearings, Oct. 12, 1966, 4340.

59. Buttle, "Report" (1967), 111–114, NARA, RG 88–74–2 (hearing material), box 51.

60. Librium-Valium Hearings, Feb. 28, 1967, 5102.

61. A later comprehensive review found little evidence of addiction to the benzos, either in patients or nonpatients: "Nonmedical use of benzodiazepines in the general population is rare and of little or no consequence." Furthermore, "There is virtually no recreational or other inappropriate use of benzodiazepines among patients for whom these drugs are prescribed." The author pooh-poohed "psychological dependence," and said that physical dependence arose only in prolonged use. "Withdrawal symptoms may be uncomfortable but are rarely severe." James H. Woods et al., "Use and Abuse of Benzodiazepines," *JAMA* 260 (Dec. 16, 1988): 3476–3480, quote 3479.

62. Thomas D. Finney, Jr., was the lead Hoffmann-La Roche lawyer. Librium-Valium Hearings, Feb. 28, 1967, 5139–5140. T. Gordon Reilly led the government's case.

63. Librium-Valium Hearings, Oct. 4, 1966, 3607–3608.

64. Edward Senay, an associate professor of psychiatry at the University of Chicago, said at a 1976 roundtable, "We asked 216 patients coming into the Illinois Drug Abuse program what they had used in the past 48 hours. Twenty-eight of the 216 said they had used Valium. Almost all of that use was in combination with other drugs, with heroin by far the most common. . . . Street people frequently do not know what drug they are taking." See Senay in discussion, in Leo E. Hollister, ed., "Valium: A Discussion of Current Issues," *Psychosomatics* 18 (1977): 44–58, quote 56. The roundtable discussion was held May 20, 1976.

65. Hoffmann-La Roche to Hearing Clerk, DHEW, Feb. 17, 1966, "Comment," 30, table 3, NARA, RG 88–27–2 (Hearing Materials), box 48.

66. Librium-Valium Hearings, Oct. 123, 1966: 4235–4306.

67. Librium-Valium Hearings, Feb. 28, 1967: 5125–5126.

68. Annakatri Ohberg et al., "Alcohol and Drugs in Suicides," *BJP* 169 (1996): 75–80, see 77, table 3.

69. Librium-Valium Hearings, Oct. 21, 1966: 4463.

70. Buttle, "Report," 106, 111–112.

71. "Librium/Valium Drug Abuse Listing Decision," *F-D-C Reports/Pink Sheet* June 24, 1968: T&G-9. In January 1968 Goddard let FDA's relevant advisory committee know that he had as yet made no decision "as to whether he will uphold the hearing examiner's recommendation to control these two drugs [Librium and Valium]." Food and Drug Administration, "Abuse of Depressant and Stimulant Drugs Advisory Committee, Minutes of the Ninth Committee Meeting," Jan. 23, 1968: 8; NARA, RG 88, UD-WW, E9, 88–79–49.

72. "Finch & Mitchell Disagree . . ." *F-D-C Reports/Pink Sheet* June 9, 1969: 34–36.

73. "Librium, Valium & Meprobamate Deleted from BNDD's Proposed Bill," *F-D-C Reports/Pink Sheet*, May 5, 1969: 4–5

74. "Proposed Rule Making. Department of Justice, Bureau of Narcotics and Dangerous Drugs, Depressant and Stimulant Drugs," 21 CFR Part 320, *Federal Register* 34 (May 21, 1969): 7968–7974, quotes 7973–74.

75. FDA, Advisory Committee on Abuse of Depressant and Stimulant Drugs, Summary of Proceedings, Second Meeting, April 25–26, 1966: 6, NARA, RG 88, UD-WW, E9, 88–79–49.

76. This letter, an internal FDA communication, was mentioned in Lexis/Nexis Mar. 28, 1973, 15. See next note.

77. See *Hoffmann-La Roche, Inc., Petitioner* v. *Richard G. Kleindienst, Attorney General of the United States*. No. 71–1299. United States Court of Appeals for the Third Circuit, 478 F.2d I; 1973 U.S. App. LEXIS 10840, decided Mar. 28, 1973, see 14, 20; http://www.web.lexis-nexis.com (accessed Sept. 24, 2005). The advisory committee's actual "report" was not present in the files. We have only the minutes of what the committee decided in session. What purported to be the one-page report was reprinted in the court's opinion, 20 of 21. This report listed the drugs claimed to be in the committee's "Appendix B," but it did not include a copy of Appendix B.

78. Ibid., 18.

79. "Two Tranquilizers, Librium and Valium, Face Strict Control," *New York Times*, June 2, 1975, 27.

80. Ibid.

81. FDA Controlled Substances Advisory Committee, Minutes, Nov. 20, 1974: 2, NARA, RG 88, UD-WW, E1, 88–00–03.

82. Alec Jenner, discussion, in E. M. Tansey et al., eds., *Wellcome Witnesses to Twentieth Century Medicine* (London: Wellcome Trust, 1998), 2: 152–153.

83. Buried in the long "proposed rule making" was the sentence, "Librium and Valium have been taken in excessive amounts for extended periods of time by individuals to the point that they have become physically dependent on the drug." Two of the three authorities for the sentence were the animal pharmacologists Nathan Eddy and Harris Isbell in Lexington, Kentucky. *Federal Register* 34 (May 21, 1969): 7971.

84. J[onathan] L. Katz et al., "Abuse Liability of Benzodiazepines," in *Benzodiazepines: Current Concepts*, ed. I. Hindmarch et al., 181–198 (Chichester: Wiley, 1990), quote 194.

85. S[idney] Brandon, "Clinical Use of Benzodiazepines in Anxiety and Panic Disorders," in Hindmarch, *Benzodiazepines*, 111–139, quote 112.

86. Leo H. Hollister et al., "Withdrawal Reactions from Chlordiazepoxide ('Librium')," *Psychopharmacologia* 2 (1961): 63–68, quote 67.

87. Hollister apparently regretted the government's misconstruction of his real views. In court hearings on Librium and Valium in 1971, as a member of BNDD's advisory board, Hollister submitted a memo on behalf of Hoffmann-La Roche's appeal, expressing the belief, in the words of the *Pink Sheet* reporter, "that virtually all CNS stimulants and depressants 'or any other neuro-psychopharmacologic agents can be the subject of abuse,' but he argued that Librium and Valium are not abused significantly and lack 'substantial potential for abuse.' 'Interim control of these drugs,' Hollister said, 'would be disruptive and unwise from the standpoint of both the patients . . . and the prescribing physician.'" "Librium-Valium Abuse Listing Would Cut Sales . . .," *F-D-C Reports/Pink Sheet*, Apr. 12, 1971, 8.

88. Lino Covi et al., "Factors Affecting Withdrawal Response to Certain Minor Tranquilizers," in *Drug Abuse: Social and Psychopharmacological Aspects*, ed. Jon O. Cole et al., 93–108 (Springfield: Thomas, 1969).

89. L[ino] Covi et al., "Length of Treatment with Anxiolytic Sedatives and Response to Their Sudden Withdrawal," *Acta Psychiatrica Scandinavica* 49 (1973): 51–64.

90. Herman X to "Director," Oct. 15, 1979, NARA, RG 88, General Subject Files, 88–85–49, box 33, 515.231; attached to Robert Wetherell (assoc. commissioner, Legislative Affairs) to Sen. Richard S. Schweiker, Nov. 6, 1979.

91. M[alcolm] Lader, "Benzodiazepines—The Opium of the Masses," *Neuroscience* 3 (1978): 159–165, quote 163.

92. Peter Tyrer et al., "Benzodiazepine Withdrawal Symptoms and Propanolol," *Lancet* 1 (Mar. 7, 1981): 520–522.

93. H. Petursson and M. H. Lader, "Withdrawal from Long-term Benzodiazepine Treatment," *BMJ* 283 (Sept. 5, 1981): 643–645, quote 643.

94. Heather Ashton, "Benzodiazepine Withdrawal: An Unfinished Story," *BMJ* 288 (Apr. 14, 1984): 1135–1140.

95. H. C. Sh. to Henry E. Simmons (FDA Bureau of Drugs), Dec. 23, 1972, NARA, RG 88, General Subject Files, box 4867.

96. Barbara Gordon, *I'm Dancing As Fast As I Can* (New York: Harper & Row, 1979).

97. *James Scott Brady . . . Plaintiffs* v. *John J. Hopper, Jr., M.D.*, Civil Action No. 83-JM-451. United States District Court for the District of Colorado. 570 F. Supp. 1333; 1983 U.S. Dist. LEXIS 13755, Sept. 14, 1983. LexisNexis Academic, quote 2 of 5 (accessed July 29, 2005).

98. *Ricky Jones, Plaintiff,* v. *Nurse Ehlert . . . defendants*, Case No. 88-C-103. United States District Court for the Eastern District of Wisconsin. 704 F. Supp. 885; 1989 U.S. Dist. LEXIS 1093, Jan. 31, 1989, Decided. LexisNexis Academic, (accessed July 29, 2005).

99. "Librium-Valium Controls," *F-D-C Reports/Pink Sheet*, Oct. 12, 1970, 23–24. On Dodd's hostility to the "tranquilizers," see Rufus King, *The Drug Hang-Up: America's Fifty-Year Folly* (New York: Norton, 1972), 275.

100. "Sen. Dodd Describes Librium and Valium As 'Killer' Drugs," *F-D-C Reports/Pink Sheet*, Oct. 19, 1970.

101. "Agnew Joins Hue & Cry," *F-D-C Reports/Pink Sheet* June 29, 1970, T&G-2.

102. *Hearing Before the Subcommittee on Health and Scientific Research of the Committee on Labor and Human Resources, United States Senate, 96th Congress, 1st Session, On Examination on the Use and Misuse of Valium, Librium, and Other Minor Tranquilizers, Sept. 10, 1979* (Washington, DC: GPO, 1980), 1. For the articles, see 348–416.

103. "'Traceable' Prescriptions for Controlled Drugs," *F-D-C Reports/Pink Sheet*, Aug. 13, 1990, 8.

104. See H. Westley Clark, "Policy and Medical-Legal Issues in the Prescribing of Controlled Substances," *Journal of Psychoactive Drugs* 23 (1991): 321–328. The sun figure of speech is not Dr. Clark's.

105. "Federal Agency Lists Most Widely Abused Drugs," *JAMA* 236 (Aug. 2, 1976): 432.

106. William T. Robinson (supervisory inspector, FDA) to Director, N.Y. District, Mar. 28, 1963; NARA, RG 88, General Subject Files, box 3578, 515.

107. See Hollister, discussion, in Leo E. Hollister, ed., "Valium: A Discussion of Current Issues," *Psychosomatics* 18 (1977): 44–58, quotes 56.

108. "Drug Abuse Warning Network, Phase IV Report, May 1975–April 1976" (BNDD Contract No. 72–47. Submitted by IMS America, Ltd): 8; copy at Brown University, Providence, R.I., SuDocs J 24.2: D84/13/975–976.

109. FDA, Bureau of Drugs, Minutes, Drug Abuse Advisory Committee, Meeting No. 6, Feb. 5, 1980: 15–17, NARA, RG 88, UD-WW, E-29, 86–00–86.

110. As Gene R. Haislip, deputy assistant administrator, Office of Diversion Control, Drug Enforcement Administration, wrote in 1991, "Approximately one out of every three [DAWN] mentions (33.5 percent) in 1990 was for a licitly manufactured substance. The dominant group for licit drugs continues to be the benzodiazepines," accounting for 8 of the top 14 mentions of licensed ("licit") drugs. Haislip slaked the efforts of industry and medical practitioners to resist even tougher controls: "Certainly we have ample evidence that some practitioners fear the creation of data systems which will expose the nature of their prescribing activity." If patients suffered because their providers were loathe to find themselves on a DEA register, Haislip concluded it was just too bad: "Controls are intended to protect the entire public, of which patients are a smaller but critically important subset." Gene R. Haislip, "Drug Diversion Control Systems, Medical Practice, and Patient Care," in *Impact of Prescription Drug Diversion Control Systems on Medical Practice and Patient Care*, NIDA Research Monograph Series, no. 131, ed. National Institute on Drug Abuse, 120–131 (Rockville, MD: NIDA, 1993), quotes 120, 127, 128. The conference at which the paper was presented took place in 1991.

111. National Institute on Drug Abuse, *Annual Data, 1985: Data from the Drug Abuse Warning Network* (Rockville, MD: Department of Health and Human

Services, Public Health Service, Alcohol, Drug Abuse, and Mental Health Administration; series 1, no. 5), 24, table 2.06a.

112. Ibid., 148, table 6.10.

113. Ibid., 164, table 6.18.

114. Ibid., 134, table 6.03.

115. "French BDZ Guidelines Out Soon?" *Scrip*, Dec. 12, 1990: 8.

116. Jean-Pierre Dupuy et al., *L'invasion pharmaceutique*, 2nd ed. (Paris: Seuil, 1974), 201.

117. INCB, *Psychotropic Substances*, 40–41.

118. Hannes Petursson and Malcolm Lader, "Benzodiazepine Withdrawal Syndrome," in *New Psychiatric Syndromes: DSM-III and Beyond*, ed. Salman Akhtar, 177–190 (New York: Aronson, 1983), quote 177.

119. Malcolm Lader, discussion, in Ruth Chinnery et al., eds., *Pharmacodynamic, Pharmacokinetic and Clinical Aspects on Oxazepam and Related Benzodiazepines: Oxazepam Symposium, Stockholm, Nov. 14–15, 1977* (Copenhagen: Munksgaard, 1978), 122–123.

120. Lader, "Benzodiazepines," quotes 163, 164.

121. The monograph appeared in 1978. The quote is from the following source: John Marks, "The Benzodiazepines—Use and Abuse," in Hans Georg Classen, et al., eds., "New Perspectives in Benzodiazepine Therapy—International Symposium. Heidelberg, 1979," *Arzeimittelforschung/Drug Research* 5a (1980): 898–901, quote 900.

122. John Marks, *The Benzodiazepines: Use, Overuse, Misuse, Abuse*, 2nd ed. (Lancaster: MTP Press, 1985), 6–7, 48.

123. See, for example, Peter Tyrcr, "Benzodiazepines on Trial," *BMJ* 288 (Apr. 14, 1984): 1101–1102, who began his editorial with, "Anyone who believes that a drug treatment can combine sound efficacy with no adverse effects whatsoever must be due for a nasty fall." Anthony W. Clare, "Benzodiazepines, Alcohol or Nicotine?" in *Benzodiazepines Divided: A Multidisciplinary Review*, ed. Michael R. Trimble, 1–13 (Chichester: Wiley, 1983).

124. Kevin Power, "Some Characteristics Contributing to Benzodiazepine Dependence," in *Benzodiazepines: The Basis for Controversy: Proceedings of an Extended Panel Discussion Held in London on 15 July 1988*, ed. Hugh Freeman, 39–43 (London: Royal Society of Medicine, 1988), quote 42.

125. On annual prescribing see David Taylor, "Current Usage of Benzodiazepines in Britain," in *The Benzodiazepines in Current Clinical Practice* ed. Hugh Freeman et al., 13–18 (London: Royal Society of Medicine Services, 1987). For a comment on the CRM guidelines, see Robert G. Priest, letter, *BMJ* 280 (Apr. 19, 1980): 1085.

126. Ian Hindmarch, "A Measured Performance: Psychometrics in Psychopharmacology," in *From Psychopharmacology to Neuropsychopharmacology in the 1980s*, ed. Thomas Ban et al., 201–205 (Budapest: Animula, 2002), quote 203. The list was of drug preparations that would no longer be paid for by the NHS.

127. "Benzodiazepines," in Great Britain. Committee on Safety of Medicines, *Current Problems*, no. 21 (Jan. 1988): 1–2. In the United Kingdom 66 percent of benzos were given without a co-prescription, as opposed to 51 percent of prescriptions for imipramine and 47 percent for chlorpromazine. But this is

normally seen as a psychopharmacologic plus: Benzos had such activity or so few side effects that a co-prescription was not required. See John Marks, "Interactions Involving Drugs Used in Psychiatry," in *The Scientific Basis of Drug Therapy in Psychiatry*, ed. John Marks et al., 191–201 (Oxford: Pergamon, 1965), see 192, table 1.

128. "Significant Decline," *Scrip*, June 11, 2003, 6.

129. David Sheehan interview, "Angles on Panic," in *The Psychopharmacologists*, ed. David Healy, 3: 479–503 (London: Arnold, 2000), quote 488.

130. Paul Leber, discussion, FDA, Psychopharmacologic Drugs Advisory Committee, 31st Meeting, vol. II, Sept. 22, 1989 [triazolam]: 9–10; obtained from FDA through Freedom of Information Act.

131. Hollister, discussion, in Hollister, "Valium," 52.

132. Karl Rickels, discussion, in Hollister, "Valium," 49.

133. Karl Rickels, "Benzodiazepines: Use and Misuse," in *Anxiety: New Research and Changing Concepts*, ed. Donald F. Klein and Judith G. Rabkin, 1–26 (New York: Raven, 1981), quote 8. Rickels, discussion, in Freeman, *Benzodiazepines in Current Clinical Practice*, 12.

134. National Institute on Drug Abuse, *Statistical Series: A Decade of DAWN: Benzodiazepine-Related Cases, 1976–1985*, Series H, No. 4 (Rockville, MD: NIDA, Division of Epidemiology and Statistical Analysis, 1988), 8, table 4. These data concern total number of benzo-related visits. The trend for some benzodiazepines more recently released on the market, such as Xanax (alprazolam) and Ativan (lorazepam), was up. Yet the huge declines in numbers for Valium (diazepam) and Librium (chlordiazepoxide) swamped these less commonly used substances.

135. Michael Weintraub et al., "Consequences of the 1989 New York State Triplicate Benzodiazepine Prescription Regulations," *JAMA* 266 (1991): 2392–2397, on the basis of IMS America data.

136. Elavil advertisement, *JAMA* 206 (Dec. 2, 1968): 2193.

137. American Psychiatric Association, *Benzodiazepine Dependence, Toxicity, and Abuse: A Task Force Report* (Washington, DC: APA, 1990), 56–58.

138. Cheryl Nelson, *Drug Utilization in Office Practice, National Ambulatory Medical Care Survey, 1990*. Advance Data from Vital and Health Statistics, no. 232 (Hyattsville, MD: National Center for Health Statistics, Mar. 25, 1993), 4, table 2.

139. I am anonymizing the members of the listserv psycho-pharm@psychom. net, as they did not necessarily realize they were posting for publication. Post of Feb. 13, 2007.

140. In Hindmarch, *Benzodiazepines*, 112.

141. Thomas Ban, interview, Dec. 5, 2005.

NOTES TO CHAPTER 6

1. FDA Oral History Program, Interview with J. Richard Crout, Nov. 12, 1997, part I: 3 of 3; http://www.fda.gov/oc/history/oralhistories/crout (accessed June 25, 2002).

2. To be exact, the NAS/NRC contract was renewed in July 1969 for one more year to tie up loose ends. Yet the bulk of the work at NAS/NRC had

finished at that point. See "NAS/NRC Efficacy Contract Extended One Year," *F-D-C Reports/Pink Sheet*, July 7, 1969, T&G2.

3. The Drug Amendments of 1962 are quoted in Division of Medical Sciences, National Research Council, *Drug Efficacy Study: Final Report to the Commissioner of Food and Drugs, Food and Drug Administration* (Washington, DC: National Academy of Sciences, 1969), 1.

4. On this conflict, see "Grandfather Clause," *F-D-C Reports/Pink Sheet*, Sept. 17, 1962, 4–5.

5. Paul De Haen, "Quarterly Review of Drugs: Medicinal Chemistry and Synthetic Drugs," *New York State Journal of Medicine* 69 (Dec. 15, 1969): 3157–3162, see 3159.

6. *Hearings Before the Subcommittee on Reorganization and International Organizations of the Committee on Government Operations, United States Senate, 88th Congress, First Session, Agency Coordination Study, Part 4, Mar. 21, 1963* (Washington, DC: GPO, 1964), 1327.

7. Ibid., part 5, session of June 19, 1963: 2182–2183.

8. Ibid., part 5, reprints letter from Humphrey to Larrick, Feb. 21, 1964: 2384.

9. Ibid., Larrick to Humphrey, Mar. 20, 1964, 2384–2385.

10. "FDA Reversed Position," *F-D-C Reports/Pink Sheet*, Mar. 22, 1971. 12.

11. "Memorandum of Meetings, Office of Commissioner," Jan. 31, 1964, NARA RG 88, General Subject Files, 1964, UD-WW, E35, file 505.

12. Arthur Egelman to Ralph G. Smith, Feb. 5, 1964, file 505, as above.

13. *Federal Register*, Feb. 28, 1964; 21 CFR Part 130, reprinted in *Hearings Subcommittee on Reorganization*, part 5: 2370–2373.

14. *Hearings Subcommittee on Reorganizations*, part 5, "Summary Memorandum of Comments by Senator Hubert H. Humphrey," June 1964: 2832–2843, quote 2842.

15. R. Keith Cannan, "NAS-NRC Background," part of a larger article, "The Washington Briefing on FDA's Drug Efficacy Review," *FDA Papers*, 2 (Mar., 1968): quote 10.

16. Information in this section is largely based on Division of Medical Sciences, National Research Council, *Drug Efficacy Study*, 1–8.

17. Statistic from the *New York Times*, Dec. 31, 1967.

18. *Drug Efficacy Study*, 7.

19. Abuse of Depressant and Stimulant Drugs Advisory Committee, Minutes of the Seventh Committee Meeting, Sept. 19, 1967: 4, NARA, RG 88, UD-WW, E9, 88–79–49.

20. "PMA [Pharmaceutical Manufacturers Association] Charges . . .," *F-D-C Reports/Pink Sheet*, Jan. 29, 1968, 17.

21. Louis Lasagna to Duke Trexler, June 21, 1971, FDA, DESI papers, "NAS-NRC Reviews," correspondence; obtained through the Freedom of Information Act (FOIA).

22. Smith, Kline & French Laboratories, *A Chronology and Review of the National Academy of Sciences/National Research Council Drug Efficacy Study* (Philadelphia: SKF, 1971), 15.

23. "FDA Makes First Real Departure . . .," *F-D-C Reports/Pink Sheet* May 5, 1969, 22.

24. Joseph D. Cooper, discussion, in Cooper, ed., *Quality of Advice* (Washington, DC: Interdisciplinary Communication Associates, 1971), 132.

25. William M. Wardell, "Regulatory Assessment Model Reassessed," in *Regulation, Economics, and Pharmaceutical Innovation*, ed. Joseph D. Cooper ed., 235–267 (Washington, DC: American University, 1973), quote 242.

26. Louis Lasagna, "Consensus Among Experts: The Unholy Grail," *Perspectives in Biology and Medicine* 19 (1976): 537–548, quote 540.

27. Louis Lasagna, discussion, in Joseph D. Cooper, ed., *Decision-Making on the Efficacy and Safety of Drugs* (Washington, DC: Interdisciplinary Communication Associates, 1971), quote 41.

28. "Critical Review of NAS/NRC Drug Efficacy Study," *F-D-C Reports/Pink Sheet* Oct. 26, 1970, TG-1.

29. "Edwards' New Thinking . . .," *F-D-C Reports/Pink Sheet* May 10, 1971, 28.

30. Telephone interview with Sidney Merlis, July 19, 2002.

31. The psychiatry panel did not necessarily evaluate all drugs used in psychiatry, even though as a rule drugs used across specialties were considered by the various specialty panels; the anesthesia panel, for example, evaluated the hypnotic methyprylon (Noludar) as an anesthetic agent. The psychiatry panel did not judge it. FDA, DESI papers, NAS/NRC reports, box 6, no. 1778 (methyprylon); obtained through FOIA.

32. Jonathan Cole interview, July 17, 2002.

33. Yet there clearly was some overall suspiciousness of combination drugs, either at NAS/NRC or FDA, for the DES final report inveighed against them, *Drug Efficacy Study*, 8, 72–76.

34. R. Craigin Lewis, "Drug Efficacy Ratings: Will They Box You In?" *Medical Economics* June 19, 1972: 27–32, quote 30. Italics in original.

35. "Nelson Witnesses Hit Ads," *F-D-C Reports/Pink Sheet* Aug. 4, 1969, 10.

36. Daniel Freedman, discussion, in Cooper, ed., *Decision-Making*, 42.

37. "Nelson Witnesses Hit Ads," *F-D-C Reports/Pink Sheet* Aug. 4, 1969, 10. Parentheses in original.

38. For details on the antineurotics, see Edward Shorter, "Looking Backwards: A Possible New Path for Drug Discovery in Psychopharmacology," *Nature Reviews Drug Discovery* 1 (2002): 1003–1006. The full list of antineurotics considered by the panel that ultimately were withdrawn: mephenesin, phenaglycodol, aspartate salts, mephenoxalone, emylcamate, meparfynol (methylparafynol), ectylurea, hydroxyphenamate, oxanamide, captodiame, benactyzine, and deanol.

39. Donald Klein, "Reaction Patterns to Psychotropic Drugs," interview, in *The Psychopharmacologists*, ed. David Healy, 1: 347 (London: Chapman and Hall, 1996).

40. William Karliner, "Use of Psychopharmacological Agents," *American Practitioner* 11 (1960): 278–281, quote 280.

41. See, for example, the psychiatry panel's report on chlorpromazine, FDA, DESI papers, NAS/NRC, box 2, no. 1330 tablets (liquid) and no. 1344 (injectable); obtained through FOIA.

42. Jonathan Cole, interview, July 17, 2002.

43. Smith, Kline & French continued to fight for expanding the chlorpromazine label, and in 1980 the FDA accepted several additional

indications, including "severe behavioral problems in children" and the "short-term treatment of hyperactive children." *Federal Register* 45 (June 17, 1980): 41070–41074, esp. 41073.

44. Cole interview.

45. The eight stimulants remaining on the market were: mephentermine, methamphetamine, phentermine, phenmetrazine, methylphenidate, diethylpropion, and benzphetamine.

46. "Over half": see Robert J. Bazell, "Drug Efficacy Study: FDA Yields on Fixed Combinations," *Science* 172 (June 4, 1971): 1013–1015.

47. See FDA, Advisory Committee on Abuse of Depressant and Stimulant Drugs, Summary of Proceedings, Second Meeting, April 25–26, 1966: 7, NARA, RG 88, UD-WW, E9, 88–79–49.

48. FDA, NAS/NRC, box 3, no. 2147.

49. FDA archives, NAS/NRC, box 8, no. 1729.

50. Karl Rickels et al., "Combination of Meprobamate and Benactyzine (Deprol) and Constituents in Neurotic Depressed Outpatients," *Diseases of the Nervous System* 32 (1971): 457–467.

51. FDA, NAS/NRC, box 2, no. 1308. The combo product was evidently saved by trial data resuscitated from NDA 12–042, showing Eskatrol "to be an effective anorectic agent while producing a minimum of side effects. In addition, 'Eskatrol' has been shown to be efficacious for the relief of the anxieties and tensions seen in the obese patient."

52. Louis Lasagna, discussion, in Cooper, *Quality of Advice*, 213.

53. Herbert Ley, discussion, in Cooper, *Quality of Advice*, 155.

54. See "Combination Drugs for Human Use . . . [21 CFR Part 3]," *Federal Register* 36 (Feb. 18, 1971): 3126–3127.

55. See Paul A. Bryan and Lawrence H. Stern, "The Drug Efficacy Study, 1962–1970," *FDA Papers*, 4 (Oct. 1970): 14–17. The authors were director and assistant director of DESI, respectively.

56. Herbert Ley, Louis Lasagna, discussion, in Cooper, *Quality of Advice*, 156.

57. "FDA Plans to Revoke 1938–62 'Not New' Letters . . ." *F-D-C Reports/Pink Sheet* Feb. 5, 1968, 12–13. In this arcane FDA terminology, "not new" was not the same as "old," the latter having been launched before 1938.

58. At a meeting at the FDA on Jan. 23, 1968, Chester Williams of the Department of Justice asked FDA counsel Goodrich "whether it is possible that withdrawal of an NDA for a useful drug which has some unsupported claims 'could be used as a club to prevent a mfr. from litigating claims which he believes in, which would ordinarily be handled by seizure action and litigation in the courts?'" "PMA Charges . . .," *F-D-C Reports/Pink Sheet* Jan. 29, 1968, 14.

59. "Antibiotic Drugs," *Federal Register* 35 (May 8, 1970): 7250–7253.

60. Robert Temple's paper, "Reevaluation of Marketed Drugs: the DESI Program," presented at the Third International Conference of Drug Regulatory Agencies in Stockholm, Sweden, June 11–14, 1984, p. 21. ". . . We have from time to time found that the published results did not in fact reflect the data collected by the investigator," a reason for demanding two controlled trials. FDA, NAS/NRC.

61. It was also widely held among insiders that the courts never reversed FDA decisions; hence, struggle was pointless. See the remarks of Vincent Kleinfeld, a Washington regulatory lawyer in Cooper, *Decision-Making*, 28–29.

62. Temple, "Reevaluation of Marketed Drugs," 15.

63. William W. Goodrich, "Legislative Background," in "The Washington Briefing on FDA's Drug Efficacy Review," *FDA Papers* 2 (Mar. 1968): 12–15.

64. See "Summary Authority to Suspend Drug Marketing," attached to Linda Horton (chief, Legislative Services Staff) to Morton Fromer (consumer safety officer), Dec. 3, 1974; this document was, in turn, attached to acting director, Bureau of Drugs to Morton Fromer, Dec. 19, 1977, in NARA, RG 88, General Subject Files, box 5031, 505.

65. Louis Lasagna, "The Development and Regulation of New Medications," *Science* 200 (May 26, 1978): 871–873, quote 872. The actual DESI unit had been dismantled in 1972. See Marion Finkel to Director, Bureau of Drugs, Dec. 4, 1972, together with attached Position Paper, DESI Project Office, Dec. 1, 1972, RG 88, General Subject Files, box 4647, 505.52.

66. Bryan and Stern, "The Drug Efficacy Study," 15.

67. William M. Wardell, "The U.S. Drug Efficacy Study and Its Implication (DESI)," *Agents and Actions* 8 (1978): 421–422. On the administrative shuffling of the DESI Task Force within the FDA, see "FDA Concentrates Responsibility . . .," *F-D-C Reports/Pink Sheet* June 23, 1969, 20.

68. "New Procedure for Handling NAS/NRC Review," *F-D-C Reports/Pink Sheet* Jan. 18, 1971, TG7–TG8.

69. *Federal Register* 36 (Apr. 28, 1971): 7989.

70. Edwin Ortiz (director, Division of Metabolic and Endocrine Drug Products) to Hoffmann-La Roche, Dec. 8, 1972, FDA, NAS/NRC reports, NDA 12–750/S-010.

71. Jonathan Cole interview, July 17, 2002.

72. "Roche's Marplan . . .," *F-D-C Reports/Pink Sheet* Apr. 28, 1975, TG8.

73. *Federal Register* 41 (Oct. 5, 1976): 43938–43940.

74. Having too few subjects to show a result at a certain level of effect is called "type II" error and it was first described in 1933 by J. Neyman and E. S. Pearson; this classical essay is reprinted in Neyman and Pearson, *Joint Statistical Papers* (Cambridge: Cambridge University Press, 1967), 186–202, see 190, 201. But only in the 1970s did it start to become common coin within the trialist community.

75. *Federal Register* 44 (Aug. 28, 1979): 50409–50410.

76. *Physicians' Desk Reference*, 39th ed. (Oradell, NJ: Medical Economics Company, 1985), 1690.

77. Jonathan Cole, interview, July 17, 2002. Alertonic was NAS/NRC box 2, file no. 1322.

78. Temple, "Reevaluation of Marketed Drugs," statistics from table 3, quote 19.

79. Robert L. Dean, director of regulatory affairs, Smith Kline & French Laboratories, discussion, in Cooper, *Quality of Advice*, 176–177.

80. William C. Triplett to John Young, July 10, 1972, NARA, RG 88, General Subject Files, box 4647, 505.52. Italics in original.

81. Memorandum of Conference, Sept. 20, 1973, between Mr. Robert Tutag and Theodore E. Byers, Albert Lavender and Charles Mitchell (Office of Compliance). RG 88, General Subject Files, box 4866, 515. Shortly thereafter, Tutag learned that Zenith Labs were marketing generic chlorpromazine without an NDA. In a furious phone call to Lavender, he said, as the FDA memo preserved the gist, "industry will consider our [FDA] failure to follow-up on Zenith's chlorpromazine as a signal to ignore the conditions for marketing as stated in the DESI announcements." Memorandum of Telephone Conversation, Albert Lavender, Oct. 31, 1973. In above file. (It is of interest that on Dec. 12, 1973, Zenith agreed to recall its generic chlorpromazine.) In 1979 Ciba-Geigy acquired Tutag, its generics arm becoming "Geneva Generics."

82. Albert Lavender to Director, Office of Compliance, Jan. 17, 1973. NARA, RG 88, General Subject Files, box 4863, 505.52.

83. Durward G. Hall to Charles C. Edwards, Dec. 15, 1972. Edwards responded with a boilerplate letter on Dec. 29, 1972, to "Dear Mr. Hall." NARA RG 88, General Subject Files, box 4647, 505.52.

84. Alexander M. Schmidt, interview, FDA Oral History Program, Mar. 8–9, 1985; http://www.fda.gov/oc/history/oralhistories/schmidt/default/htm, part 3: 4 of 9 (accessed June 25, 2002).

85. Clark Havighurst, discussion, in Cooper, *Quality of Advice*, 167. Italics in original.

86. FDA, Goodwin interview, part 2: 10 of 12.

87. "Havoc in Administering . . .," *F-D-C Reports/Pink Sheet* June 22, 1970. 21.

88. Paul J. Quirk, "Food and Drug Administration," in *The Politics of Regulation*, ed. James Q. Wilson, 191–235 (New York: Basic Books, 1980), quote 210–211.

89. FDA, NAS/NRC, box 8, file no. 1760. A notice in the *Federal Register* of June 25, 1970, on "Oxanamide and Certain Other Drugs," declared it lacking in efficacy (see 10395).

90. FDA, NAS/NRC, box 8, file no. 1730, box 6, file no. 1744.

91. "Methylphendiate Hydrochloride for Oral Use," *Federal Register* 43 (Apr. 28, 1978): 18256–18257.

92. "Pfizer Laboratories," *Federal Register* 39 (June 5, 1974): 19973.

93. *Physicians' Desk Reference*, 29th ed. (Oradell, NJ: Medical Economics Co., 1975), 1571.

94. FDA, NAS/NRC, box 2, no. 1284; *Physicians' Desk Reference*, 57th ed. (Montvale, NJ: Thomson, 2003), 1602.

95. FDA, NAS/NRC, box 2, no. 1330.

96. *Federal Register* 35 (Aug. 26, 1970): 13608–13609.

97. Cole interview, July 17, 2002, 25.

NOTES TO CHAPTER 7

1. Frank Berger interview by Leo Hollister, December 1995, 16, American College of Neuropsychopharmacology (ACNP), Oral History Project; I am grateful to Thomas Ban for sharing this transcript with me.

2. This paragraph is based on Michael Alan Taylor and Max Fink, *Melancholia: The Diagnosis, Pathophysiology, and Treatment of Depressive Illness* (New York: Cambridge University Press, 2006); Tom G. Bolwig and Edward Shorter, eds., *Melancholia: Beyond DSM, Beyond Neurotransmitters, Acta Psychiatrica Scandinavica* 115, no. 433 (Copenhagen: Blackwell/Munksgaard, 2007); Conrad M. Swartz and Edward Shorter, *Psychotic Depression* (New York: Cambridge University Press., 2007).

3. Henry M. Wetherill, Jr., "The Modern Hypnotics," *American Journal of Insanity* 46 (1889): 28–47, quote 28.

4. Donald W. Goodwin and Samuel B. Guze, *Psychiatric Diagnosis*, 4th ed. (1974; New York: Oxford University Press, 1989), vii.

5. Daniel Greenwald to Robert Spitzer, undated (sometime in 1978, on the basis of internal evidence), Janet Williams Papers, DSM-III-R, box 1, DSM-III files, "Affective comments in notebook," American Psychiatric Association Archives, Arlington, VA. (Hereafter cited as APA Archives.) Dr. Greenwald's note was apparently preserved for reconsideration in the drafting of the revised edition of the manual, *DSM-III-R*, which began soon after *DSM-III* appeared in 1980.

6. Robert Spitzer interview by Max Fink and Edward Shorter, Mar. 14, 2007, at Irvington, New York, 7.

7. Walter E. Barton (medical director) to Sidney Malitz (chair, APA Council on Research and Development), Mar. 20, 1973, APA Archives, Professional Affairs, box 17, folder 188, "Origins of the Task Force on Nomenclature and Statistics." Spitzer at this point had not yet been appointed.

8. Spitzer interview, 22.

9. J[ulius] Hoenig, "Nosology and Statistical Classification," *Canadian Journal of Psychiatry* 26 (1981): 240–243, quote 240.

10. Spitzer interview, 7.

11. Spitzer interview, 7.

12. Spitzer interview, 21.

13. Eli Robins and Samuel B. Guze, "Establishment of Diagnostic Validity in Psychiatric Illness: Its Application to Schizophrenia," *AJP* 126 (1970): 983–987.

14. John P. Feighner, Eli Robins, Samuel B. Guze, Robert A. Woodruff, Jr., George Winokur, and Rodrigo Muñoz, "Diagnostic Criteria for Use in Psychiatric Research," *Archives of General Psychiatry* 26 (1972): 57–63.

15. Robert Spitzer, Jean Endicott, and Eli Robins, "Research Diagnostic Criteria," *Archives of General Psychiatry* 35 (1978): 773–782.

16. Spitzer to "Fellow Deans of the Invisible College," May 10, 1979; APA Archives, Williams Papers, Research DSM-III-R, box 3, misc. DSM-III files.

17. Paula Clayton interview, by Max Fink and Edward Shorter, Hollywood, FL, Dec. 4, 2006.

18. APA Task Force on Nomenclature and Statistics, meeting of Sept. 4–5, 1974, New York; APA Archives, Professional Affairs, box 17, folder 188.

19. Spitzer interview, 8.

20. [Robert Spitzer], "Progress Report on the Preparation of DSM-III," 10–11, APA Archives, Professional Affairs, box 17, folder 193 (70, no. 3).

21. World Health Organization, *International Classification of Diseases: Manual of the International Statistical Classification of Diseases, Injuries, and Causes of Death, Based on the Recommendations of the Ninth Revision Conference, 1975, and Adopted by the Twenty-ninth World Health Assembly* (Geneva: WHO, 1977), 1: 191–193.

22. Committee on Nomenclature and Statistics of the American Psychiatric Association, *DSM-II: Diagnostic and Statistical Manual of Mental Disorders*, 2nd ed. (Washington, DC: APA, 1968), 8.

23. Spitzer interview, 34.

24. The phrase "Chinese menu" for the lists of diagnostic criteria was Gerald Klerman's. See Samuel Guze, "The Neo-Kraepelinian Revolution," interview, in *The Psychopharmacologists*, ed. David Healy, 3: 395–414 (London: Arnold, 2000), see 408.

25. Robert L. Spitzer, Jean Endicott, Eli Robins, Judith Kuriansky, and Barry Gurland, "Preliminary Report of the Reliability of Research Diagnostic Criteria Applied to Psychiatric Case Records," in *Predictability in Psychopharmacology: Preclinical and Clinical Correlations*, ed. Abraham Sudilovsky et al., 1–47 (New York: Raven, 1975), see 23–29.

26. "Initial Draft Version of DSM-III Classification of Aug. 1, 1975," attached to Bernard Stotsky to Lissy F. Jarvik, Nov. 8, 1976, Paula Clayton Papers, box 30, folder 13, International Neuropsychopharmacology Archives, Eskind Biomedical Library, Vanderbilt University Medical Center, Nashville, TN.

27. Karl Leonhard, *Die Aufteilung der endogenen Psychosen* (Berlin: Akademie-Verlag, 1957).

28. See "Final General Session [of meeting in St. Louis]," June 10, 1976, Donald Klein remarks, 1, APA Archives, Medical Director's Office, Range 37, box C-1, "Summary of Conference . . . DSM-III in Mid-stream, 1976." On the history of "endogenous" depression, see Shorter, *Historical Dictionary of Psychiatry* (New York: Oxford University Press, 2005), 83.

29. Spitzer interview, 36.

30. Later evidence suggests that Spitzer disliked "minor" because of the problem of insurance reimbursement for clinicians. Yet he may be just accommodating others' opinions, without himself, a researcher, fearing this problem. See Rachel Gittelman to Robert Spitzer, Feb. 18, 1976: "I am not too clear what would replace the major/minor heading," APA Archives, Williams Papers, DSM-III-R, box 1, DSM-III files, major depressive disorder. The March 1976 draft was attached to Task Force on Nomenclature and Statistics, "Progress Report on the Preparation of DSM-III," March 1976, APA Archives, Professional Affairs, box 17, folder 193 (70, no. 3). This draft also made mention of demoralization disorder, the only point in the *DSM-III* process at which this interesting diagnosis seems to have been officially considered.

31. The draft of Aug. 19, 1976, was attached to Spitzer to Organic Mental Disorders Subcommittee, Sept. 23, 1976; Clayton Papers, box 30, folder 13.

32. Robert Spitzer to Task Force, Nov. 5, 1976, Clayton Papers, box 30, folder 13.

33. See APA [Board of Trustees], re "Task Force on Nomenclature & Statistics," minutes of meeting of May 1, 1977, Toronto.

34. "Draft of Axes I and II of DSM-III Classification," Jan. 16, 1978, Clayton Papers, box 30, folder 15.

35. DSM-III draft text, "Comparative Listing of DSM-II and DSM-III, undated [c. August 1979]. "Appendix C: Annotated Comparative Listing of DSM-II and DSM-III"; APA Archives, Williams Papers, Research—DSM-III-R, box 3. The sentence about chronic equaling neurasthenia was edited out of the published version, which stated simply of neurasthenia, "This DSM-II category was rarely used." APA, *DSM-III* (Washington, DC: APA, 1980), 377.

36. Robert Spitzer to Task Force, June 6, 1977, Clayton Papers, box 30, folder 12.

37. "Draft of Axes I and II . . ." Jan. 16, 1978, Clayton Papers, box 30, folder 15.

38. Spitzer interview, 34.

39. "Draft of Axes I and II of DSM-III Classification," Mar. 30, 1977, attached to "DSM-III Draft, Table of Contents," Apr. 15, 1977, APA Archives, Professional Affairs, box 16, folder 176, DSM-III draft (1).

40. John Racy to Robert Spitzer, Mar. 21, 1978, APA Archives, Williams Papers, Research—DSM-III-R, box 1, DSM-III files, folder "misc. affective."

41. Robert Spitzer to John Racy, Mar. 31, 1978, Williams Papers, Research—DSM-III-R, box 1, DSM-III files, folder "misc. affective."

42. Robert Spitzer to "Affective Disorder Mavens," July 10, 1978, APA Archives, Williams Papers, Research—DSM-III-R, DSM-III files, "misc. affective."

43. This point was brought out even before the renaming occurred. At a meeting of the task force on May 7, 1978, in Atlanta, the minutes note, "In the Affective Disorders section, consideration is being given to renaming the Chronic Affective Disorders, Chronic *Minor* Affective Disorders. The Episodic Disorders, then, would become the Major Affective Disorders." Janet B. W. Forman to Members of the Task Force, May 25, 1978, Clayton Papers, box 31.

44. Spitzer to "Dear Colleagues," Apr. 30, 1979, Williams Papers, DSM-III-R, loose DSM-III files, "neurosis" folder.

45. See John J. McGrath (Legislative Representative of Area III) to Alex H. Kaplan (president, American Psychoanalytic Association), Mar. 12, 1979, Williams Papers, Research—DSM-III-R, loose DSM-III files.

46. Spitzer interview, 20.

47. Spitzer to task force members, memo entitled "Neurotic Depression Once Again," Apr. 27, 1979, Clayton Papers, box 31.

48. Donald F. Klein to Task Force, Mar. 30, 1979, Clayton Papers, box 31.

49. *DSM-III*, 214, 223. The diagnostic criteria for a major depressive episode specified that "At least four of the following symptoms have each been present nearly every day for a period of at least two weeks" (p. 213). The symptoms include poor appetite; insomnia or hypersomnia; psychomotor agitation or retardation; loss of interest or pleasure in usual activities; loss of energy or fatigue; feelings of worthlessness, self-reproach, or excessive or inappropriate guilt; diminished ability to think or concentrate; and recurrent thoughts of death or suicidal ideation, desire, or attempts (p. 214). For dysthymic disorder, "During the past two years . . . the individual has been bothered most or all of the time by symptoms characteristic of the depressive syndrome . . . (although a major depressive episode may be superimposed on Dysthymic Disorder)" (p. 222). The specific *DSM-III* symptoms of dysthymic disorder, of which

three must be present for the diagnosis, include insomnia or hypersomnia; low energy level or chronic tiredness; feelings of inadequacy; decreased productivity; decreased attention, concentration, or ability to think clearly; social withdrawal; loss of interest in or enjoyment of pleasurable activities; irritability or excessive anger; inability to respond to praise or rewards; less active or talkative than usual; pessimistic attitude toward the future, brooding about past events, or feeling sorry for oneself; tearfulness or crying; and recurrent thoughts of death or suicide (p. 223). If a patient could have both disorders at once, there was little difference between them aside from episodic versus chronic—and episodes that repeated became "chronic" by definition. See also the following note.

50. Herman van Praag, past chair of psychiatry at Albert Einstein College of Medicine, writes of *DSM-III*, "Major depression and dysthymia are introduced as discrete syndromal entities, but for the greater part they overlap and the major criterion that seems to properly differentiate them is *severity*." He said "differentiability" of major depression and dysthymia was even less in *DSM-III-R*, published in 1987. Herman van Praag, *"Make-Believes" in Psychiatry or The Perils of Progress* (New York: Brunner, 1993), 53, 57.

51. In 2005, 90.1 percent of all visits to psychiatrists ended with a prescription, making psychiatry the highest-prescribing specialty. (For internal medicine, by contrast, it was 82.3 percent; the average for all specialties was 70.5 percent.) D. K. Cherry et al., *National Ambulatory Medical Care Survey: 2005 Summary*, Advance Data from Vital and Health Statistics 387 (Hyattsville, MD: National Center for Health Statistics, 2007), 33, table 24.

52. Arthur Rifkin to Robert Spitzer, Mar. 30, 1978, Williams Papers, Research—DSM-III-R, box 2; "DSM-III- unfiled."

53. Martin B. Keller and Diane L. Hanks, "The Natural History and Heterogeneity of Depressive Disorders: Implications for Rational Antidepressant Therapy," *Journal of Clinical Psychiatry* 55, suppl. A (1994): 25–33.

54. Bernard J. Carroll to Robert Spitzer, Feb. 19, 1979, Williams papers, DSM-III-R, box 1, DSM-III files, major depressive disorder.

55. Donald Klein to Robert Spitzer, Mar. 6, 1979, Clayton Papers, box 31.

56. Donald Klein to Robert Spitzer, Aug. 31, 1984; Williams Papers, Research, DSM-III-R, box 2, loose DSM-III-R papers.

57. Wilson M. Compton et al., "Changes in the Prevalence of Major Depression and Comorbid Substance Use Disorders in the United States Between 1991–1992 and 2001–2002," *AJP* 163 (2006): 2141–2147.

58. Gavin Andrews et al., "Lifetime Risk of Depression: Restricted to a Minority or Waiting for Most?" *BJP* 187 (2005): 495–496.

59. Gordon Parker, "Editorial: Commentary on Diagnosing Major Depressive Disorder," *Journal of Nervous and Mental Disease* 194 (2006): 155–157, quote 156.

60. Donald Klein to Robert Spitzer, Apr. 24, 1978, Williams Papers, Research, DSM-III-R, box 1, DSM-III files, folder "Misc. Affective."

61. Spitzer interview, 36–37.

62. Mark Olfson and Gerald L. Klerman, "Trends in the Prescription of Antidepressants by Office-Based Psychiatrists," *AJP*, 150 (1993): 571–577, table 1, p. 572.

63. Ross Baldessarini interview with Max Fink and Edward Shorter, Feb. 17, 2006, Belmont, MA.

64. Gordon Parker, "Beyond Major Depression," *Psychological Medicine* 35 (2005): 467–474, quote 471.

65. According to an ABC News Report, http://abcnews.go.com/GMA/OnCall/story?id=2640591&page=1 (accessed May 15, 2007).

66. Fred A. Bernstein, "The New Kitchen Is Done," *New York Times*, Feb. 22, 2007, D7.

67. Spitzer interview, 48.

NOTES TO CHAPTER 8

1. S. Raofi et al., *Medication Therapy in Ambulatory Medical Care: United States, 2003–04*. National Center for Health Statistics, *Vital Health Statistics* 13, no. 163 (2006), 27, table 10. In 2005, antidepressants led drugs in all other therapeutic classes in percent of mentions in office visits: Antidepressants constituted 5.3 percent of all drug mentions, antihypertensive agents 5.2 percent, and so on down the list. D. K. Cherry et al., *National Ambulatory Medical Care Survey: 2005 Summary*, Advance Data from Vital and Health Statistics, no. 387 (Hyattsville, MD: National Center for Health Statistics, 2007), 34, table 25.

2. Arvid Carlsson interview by David Healy and Edward Shorter, part II, Gothenburg, Sweden, Feb. 28, 2007, 25–26.

3. On the repositioning of phenyltoloxamine, see "Bristol Lab Tranquilizer," *F-T-C Reports/Pink Sheet*, June 24, 1957, 17.

4. Einar Hellbom, "Chlorpheniramine, Selective Serotonin-Reuptake Inhibitors (SSRIs) and Over-the-Counter Treatment," *Medical Hypotheses* 66 (2006): 689–690.

5. Robert L. Bowman et al., "Spectrophotofluormetric Assay in the Visible and Ultraviolet," *Science* 122 (July 1, 1955): 32–33; Solomon H. Snyder, Julius Axelrod et al., "A Sensitive and Specific Fluorescence Assay for Tissue Serotonin," *Biochemical Pharmacology* 14 (1965): 831–835.

6. Arvid Carlsson tells this story in his Nobel Lecture, Dec. 8, 1999, "A Half-Century of Neurotransmitter Research: Impact on Neurology and Psychiatry," *Bioscience Reports* 21 (Dec. 2001): 691–710. For the 1960 paper and the conference, see Arvid Carlsson et al., "On the Biochemistry and Possible Functions of Dopamine and Noradrenaline in Brain," in *Ciba Foundation Symposium Jointly With Committee for Symposia on Drug Action on Adrenergic Mechanisms*, ed. J. R. Vane et al., 432–439 (Boston: Little and Brown, 1960).

7. Alec Coppen et al., "Potentiation of the Antidepressive Effect of a Monoamine-Oxidase Inhibitor by Tryptophan," *Lancet* 1 (Jan. 12, 1963): 79–81.

8. The seminal contribution is B. Falck, N.-A. Hillarp, G. Thieme and A. Torp, "Fluorescence of Catechol Amines and Related Compounds Condensed with Formaldehyde," *Journal of Histochemistry and Cytochemistry* 10 (1962): 348–354.

9. P[aul] Kielholz and W[alther] Pöldinger, "Die Behandlung endogener Depressionen mit Psychopharmaka," *Deutsche Medizinische Wochenschrift* 93 (Apr. 5, 1968): 701–704.

10. In his published work, Carlsson makes virtually no reference to this Kielholz article. Yet he told David Healy in 1996 that Kielholz's data were the reason that he, Carlsson, did the experiment. Arvid Carlsson, "Rise of Neuropsychopharmacology" (interview), in *Psychopharmacologists*, ed. David Healy, 1: 51–80 (London: Chapman and Hall, 1996), see 60. Carlsson reinforced the importance of the Kielholz article in the Healy–Shorter interview, Feb. 27, 2007: 72.

11. Arvid Carlsson, Hans Corrodi, Kjell Fuxe, and Tomas Hökfelt, "Effect of Antidepressant Drugs on the Depletion of Intraneuronal Brain 5-Hydroxytryptamine Stores Caused by 4-Methyl-alpha-Ethyl-Meta-Tyramine," *European Journal of Pharmacology* 5 (1969): 357–366.

12. Arvid Carlsson, Hans Corrodi, Kjell Fuxe, and Tomas Hökfelt, "Effect of Antidepressant Drugs on the Depletion of Intraneuronal Brain Catecholamine Stores Caused by 4, alpha- Dimethyl-Meta-Tyramine," *European Journal of Pharmacology* 5 (1969): 367–373.

13. Arvid Carlsson and Margit Lindqvist, "Central and Peripheral Monoaminergic Membrane-Pump Blockage by Some Addictive Analgesics and Antihistamines," *Journal of Pharmacy and Pharmacology* 21 (1969): 460–464.

14. For a fluent overview of these events, see David Healy, *Let Them Eat Prozac: The Unhealthy Relationship Between the Pharmaceutical Industry and Depression* (New York: New York University Press, 2004). Some observers consider early research on clomipramine as touching off the SSRI era. Yet clomipramine metabolizes in the body to a norepinephrine reuptake inhibitor.

15. Swedish patent no. 361 663, published Nov. 12, 1973.

16. These details are mainly from Ivan Oestholm [Ostholm], *Drug Discovery: A Pharmacist's Story* (Stockholm: Swedish Pharmaceutical Press, 1995), 101–110.

17. Zelmid advertisement, *BJP* 140 (March 1982).

18. See the two big symposia: Arvid Carlsson et al., eds., *Recent Advances in the Treatment of Depression: Proceedings of an International Symposium, Corfu, Greece, April 16–18, 1980, Acta Psychiatrica Scandinavica* 63, no. 290 (Copenhagen: Munksgaard, 1981); Carl-Gerhard Gottfries, ed., "Recent Advances with Zimeldine, the 5-HT Reuptake Blocker," in *The Treatment of Depression: Proceedings of a Symposium in Laxenburg, Austria, July 9, 1983, Acta Psychiatrica Scandinavica* 68, no. 308 (Copenhagen: Munksgaard, 1983).

19. FDA, Psychopharmacologic Drugs Advisory Committee, vol. 2, Dec. 4, 1981 [dothiepin], II-164.

20. Arvid Carlsson interview, Feb. 27, 2007, 69.

21. Leslie Iversen, "Neuroscience and Drug Development" (interview), in *The Psychopharmacologists*, ed. David Healy, 2: 325–350 (London: Altman, 1998): 325–350, quote 343.

22. Robert Temple to Director, Division of Neuropharmacological Drug Products [Paul Leber], Sept. 15, 1983, NARA, RG 88, UD-04W, E3, 88–89–16, box 28.

23. R. Langlois et al., "High Incidence of Multisystemic Reactions to Zimeldine," *European Journal of Clinical Pharmacology* 28 (1985): 67–71.

24. Carlsson interview, 69.

25. P[er] Bech, "A Review of the Antidepressant Properties of Serotonin Reuptake Inhibitors," *Advances in Biological Psychiatry* 17 (1988): 58–69, see 64.

26. For a comprehensive list of SSRIs in development in the late 1980s, see Scrip's *Serotonin Report* (Richmond, Surrey: PJB Publications, 1988), 109–120.

27. V. Claassen et al., "Fluvoxamine, a Specific 5-Hydroxytryptamine Uptake Inhibitor," *British Journal of Pharmacology* 60 (1977): 505–516.

28. Gérard Le Fur et al., "On the Regional and Specific Serotonin Uptake Inhibition by LM 5008," *Life Sciences* 23 (1978): 1959–1966; Claude Gueremy et al., "3-(4-iperidinylalkyl)indoles, Selective Inhibitors of Neuronal 5-Hydroxytryptamine Uptake," *Journal of Medicinal Chemistry* 23 (1980): 1306–1310.

29. See Klaus Bogeso's account "Drug Hunting" (interview), in Healy, *Psychopharmacologists*, 2: 561–579, esp. 569.

30. "Citalopram Launched," *Scrip*, Feb. 13, 1991, p. 22.

31. Date given in *Eli Lilly and Company* v. *Barr Laboratories et al.*, IP 96–0491-C-B/S, United States District Court for the Southern District of Indiana, Indianapolis Division, 100 F. Supp. 2d 917; 1999 U. S. Dist. LEXIS 21852; decided Jan. 12, 1999, 2. On Benadryl, see the testimony of Lilly scientist Louis Lemberger, who explained that to get nisoxetine, a norepinephrine-reuptake-inhibitor, Lilly reversed the oxygen and the carbon on the Benadryl side chain; they then tweaked nisoxetine to get fluoxetine. FDA, Psychopharmacologic Drugs Advisory Committee, 28th Meeting, Oct. 10, 1985 [fluoxetine]: 140–141; obtained through the Freedom of Information Act (FOIA).

32. See Iversen interview, in Healy, *Psychopharmacologists*, 2: 344.

33. One study with a database of over 172,000 patients on antidepressants found that fluoxetine had an unusually high suicide rate per 10,000 person years of use; the classic tricyclic antidepressants by contrast had suicide rates rather lower than average (taking dothiepin as the "average"). Susan S. Jick et al., "Antidepressants and Suicide," *BMJ* 310 (Jan. 28, 1995): 215–218. For data indicting the tricyclics as highly dangerous to suicidal patients, see John A. Henry, "A Fatal Toxicity Index for Antidepressant Poisoning," *Acta Psychiatrica Scandinavica* 80, no. 354 (1989): 37–45. All such studies are bedeviled by not knowing the actual cause of death, as opposed to the coincidental presence of a given drug.

34. A[ndré] Uzan, discussion, in "Colloque international sur 'Approches biologiques de l'anxiété et des troubles de l'humeur,' Sousse (Tunisie), 16–17 Oct. 1981," *L'Encéphale*, n.s., 8 (1982): 324–325. Uzan was an industry scientist associated with the discovery of indalpine (Upstène).

35. This list of side effects is from FDA, "Summary Basis of Approval: Fluoxetine Hydrochloride," NDA 18–936, Oct. 3, 1988, 33. FDA Archives.

36. Carlsson interview, 73.

37. For a list of co-prescribed drugs, see Dorothy S. Dobbs to FDA, Dec. 17, 1984, http://www.healyprozac.com/trials/criticaldocs/dobbsexhibits.pdf (accessed June 22, 2006).

38. Lilly's Gary Tollefson waffled in answering a question about this but made it clear that a certain number were indeed recruited in advertisements. FDA, Psychopharmacologic Drugs Advisory Committee, Sept. 20, 1991 [antidepressants and suicide], 251–253 http://www.fda.gov/ohrms/dockets/ac/prozac/2443T1.pdf (accessed Oct. 23, 2006).

39. The main published trials were quite opaque from the viewpoint of recruitment and psychopathology. We learn mainly that fluoxetine beat placebo, not difficult in a large trial, and that fluoxetine lacked the anticholinergic side effects characteristic of the tricyclic antidepressants. Nothing was said about impotence. John Feighner et al., "Double-Blind Comparative Trials of Fluoxetine and Doxepin in Geriatric Patients with Major Depressive Disorder," *Journal of Clinical Psychiatry* 46 (1985): 20–25; J. B. Cohn et al., "A Comparison of Fluoxetine, Imipramine, and Placebo in Patients with Major Depressive Disorder," *Journal of Clinical Psychiatry* 46 (1985): 26–31; Paul Stark et al., "A Review of Multicenter Controlled Studies of Fluoxetine vs. Imipramine and Placebo in Outpatients with Major Depressive Disorder," *Journal of Clinical Psychiatry* 46 (1985): 53–58.

40. Prozac advertisement, *JAMA* 259 (June 3, 1988): 309a–c.

41. See Elora Weringer, "The History of Psychotropic Drugs at Pfizer," in *Reflections on Twentieth-Century Psychopharmacology.* ed. Thomas Ban et al., 58–64 (Budapest: Animula, 2004).

42. Willard M. Welch, "Discovery and Preclinical Development of the Serotonin Reuptake Inhibitor Sertraline," *Advances in Medicinal Chemistry* 3 (1995): 113–148.

43. See FDA, Psychopharmacologic Drugs Advisory Committee (PDAC), 33rd Meeting, Nov. 19, 1990 [sertraline], 83–86, 93, obtained through FOIA.

44. Jorgen Buus Lassen et al., "Comparative Studies of a New 5HT-Uptake Inhibitor and Some Tricyclic Thymoleptics," *European Journal of Pharmacology* 32 (1975): 108–115; Buus Lassen, "Potent and Long-Lasting Potentiation of Two 5-Hydroxytryptophan-Induced Effects in Mice by Three Selective 5-HT Uptake Inhibitors," *European Journal of Pharmacology* 47 (1978): 351–358. Arvid Carlsson remembers that Buus Lassen prompted the synthesis after a conversation with Carlsson. Carlsson interview, Feb. 27, 2007, 74.

45. For the facts in this paragraph, see *SmithKline Beecham* v. *Apotex Corp.*, 98 C 3952, United States District Court for the Northern District of Illinois, Eastern Division, 286 F. Supp. 2d 925; 2001 U.S. Dist. LEXIS 19766; decided Nov. 30, 2001.

46. Paxil advertisement, *AJP* 150 (March 1993), advertisement section.

47. FDA, PDAC, Feb. 2, 2004 [adolescent suicide and antidepressants], 171; http://www.fda.gov./ohrms/dockets/ac/04/transcripts/4006T1.pdf (accessed March 12, 2004).

48. Jonathan Cole interview by Edward Shorter, July 17, 2002, 15.

49. Leber, FDA, PDAC, Apr. 26, 1994 [fluoxetine for treatment of bulimia], 284, obtained through FOIA.

50. For Detre and Leber, see FDA, PDAC, 23rd Meeting, Feb. 24, 1983, 1: 165–166; obtained through FOIA.

51. FDA, PDAC, 18th Meeting, Nov. 6, 1980 [antidepressant guidelines], 192; obtained through FOIA.

52. FDA, PDAC, 38th Meeting, Apr. 30, 1993 [venlafaxine], 207; obtained through FOIA.

53. FDA, PDAC, Feb. 25, 1983 [nomifensine], 2: 141; obtained through FOIA.

54. FDA, PDAC, June 10, 1982 [alprazolam], 1: 135; obtained through FOIA.

55. FDA, PDAC, Apr. 26, 1994 [fluoxetine for treatment of bulimia], 284; obtained through FOIA.

56. FDA, PDAC, Dec. 4, 1981 [dothiepin], 2: 168–169; obtained through FOIA. The day previously nomifensine had been under discussion.

57. FDA, PDAC, 32nd Meeting, Dec. 1, 1989, 131 [clomipramine in OCD]; obtained through FOIA.

58. On the subject of possibly carcinogenic elevations of prolactin in the drug risperidone, Leber said, do we just communicate to physicians and public the facts,

> Or do you think we have an added responsibility to also interpret them in light of what current judgment among experts is about them. I mean, what is the purpose of this. Is it to put on record that we know these things happen, because, believe me, every day there will be reports in the literature, in SCIENCE or NATURE or somewhere else about some other phenomena that has been described in relationship to a drug class. And if all you want to do is inform people, the list will grow and grow. The question is the difference between information and knowledge in these areas.

Robert Temple added,

> So, there is more than usual skepticism about what these findings mean. And I guess I would echo what Paul said. I mean, we have a fairly hard time knowing what this means. The best people in the business have grappled with it for decades, and they don't know what it means. So, what would you be telling a patient if you told them that these tumors are there in a very conspicuous way, like in a patient insert. It is not that anybody wants to hide it, but when you bring it out and put it in there, why did you pick that. That is my question. That is a real problem.

Temple said later in the session, "If you write something down as if it means something, but it doesn't, you shape what people use, and this might not be the best basis . . . for making a choice of antipsychotic drugs. . . . It is doubly hard for a lay audience to make much sense out of animal tumorigenicity studies." FDA, PDAC, 39th Meeting, July 19, 1993 [nefazodone, risperidone], 242–244, 260; obtained through FOIA.

59. FDA, PDAC, June 10, 1982 [alprazolam, bupropion], 1: 141; obtained through FOIA.

60. Ibid., 271.

61. FDA, PDAC, 23rd Meeting, Feb. 24, 1983 [antidepressant labeling], 1: 137, obtained through FOIA. Donald Klein coined the term "endogenomorphic depression," by which he meant any depression with the features of retardation, agitation, and dysphoria, regardless of whether precipitated or not; he saw such depressions as eminently drug responsive. Klein, "Endogenomorphic Depression," *Archives of General Psychiatry* 31 (1974): 447–454.

62. "PMA [Pharmaceutical Manufacturers Association] Charges FDA 'Numbers Game' in Efficacy Review," *F-D-C Reports/Pink Sheet* Jan 29, 1968, 14.

63. Peter Barton Hutt (general counsel) to Charles C. Edwards (commissioner), Oct. 24, 1972, NARA, RG 88, General Subject Files, box 4647, 505.52.

64. Charles C. Edwards (commissioner) to Richard J. Pierce, Aug. 18, 1972, NARA, RG 88, General Subject Files, box 4647.

65. Joseph Sadusk to J. B. Roerig and Company, July 27, 1965, NARA, RG 88, General Subject Files, box 3751, 505.2.

66. Louis Lasagna, discussion, in *Decision-Making on the Efficacy and Safety of Drugs* [1970 conference], ed. Joseph D. Cooper (Washington, DC: Interdisciplinary Communication Associates, 1971), 180.

67. "PMA Tries Again for FDA Reply on Relative Effectiveness Policy," *Washington Drug and Devices Newsletter*, July 14, 1972, copy in NARA, RG 88, General Subject Files, box 4647.

68. "Memo of OSE Rounds," Aug. 8, 1974, NARA, RG 88, General Subject Files, UD-04W, E3, 88–89–16, box 27.

69. FDA, PDAC, 23rd Meeting, Feb. 24, 1983 [antidepressant labeling], 1: 143–144; obtained through FOIA.

70. FDA, PDAC, vol. 2, Dec. 4, 1981 [dothiepin], 59–61; obtained through FOIA.

71. FDA, PDAC, 28th Meeting, Oct. 11, 1985 [haloperidol decanoate], 2: 62; obtained through FOIA.

72. FDA, PDAC, 30th Meeting, Apr. 26, 1989 [clozapine], 17, obtained through FOIA.

73. Leber said of this design, "The reason for looking at three doses is to try to find out where the fair and comparable comparisons are. It is by no means the standard thing we do. We do it often or recommend it when people really have an interest in saying, 'I am better than another drug.' We say, 'All right, prove that you are in the right operating range to make this comparison.'" PDAC, "Workshop on Antipsychotic Drug Development (Open Public Hearing)," July 25, 1995, 131; obtained through FOIA.

74. Leber occasionally cited Walter Modell and Raymond W. Houde, "Factors Influencing Clinical Evaluation of Drugs," *JAMA* 167 (Aug. 30, 1958): 2190 2199, who made a strong case for placebo controls. The authors wrote, "It is suggested that in clinical evaluations another demonstrably effective drug always be used in addition to the placebo control to indicate this essential competence [being 'sensitive'] of the method" (2198).

75. FDA, PDAC, 39th Meeting, July 19, 1993 [nefazodone], 184; obtained through FOIA.

76. T[homas] P. Laughren, "The Scientific and Ethical Basis for Placebo-Controlled Trials in Depression and Schizophrenia: An FDA Perspective," *European Psychiatry* 16 (2001): 418–423, quote 419.

77. FDA, PDAC, Feb. 14, 2001 [olanzapine IM], 207; obtained through FOIA.

78. FDA, PDAC, 41st Meeting, Oct. 18, 1993 [fluvoxamine], 92; obtained through FOIA.

79. Ibid., 106.

80. *FDA's Role in Protecting the Public Health: Examining FDA's Review of Safety and Efficacy Concerns in Antidepressant Use By Children. Hearing Before the Subcommittee on Oversight and Investigations of the Committee on Energy and Commerce, House of Representatives*, 108th Congress, 2nd Session, Sept. 23, 2004, serial no. 108–125, 58–61, http://www.access.gpo.gov/congress/house (accessed Feb. 10, 2006).

81. Dorothy S. Dobbs (Medical Adviser, Lilly Regulatory Affairs), to FDA, June 16, 1982, http://www.healyprozac.com/trials/criticaldocs/dobbsexhibits. pdf (accessed June 22, 2006).

82. FDA, PDAC, Oct. 10, 1985 [fluoxetine], 39–40; obtained through FOIA.

83. Ibid., 127–128.

84. In the meeting on sertraline, see Thomas Laughren's comment that Prozac as well lacked effectiveness in inpatients. FDA, PDAC, 33rd Meeting, Nov. 19, 1990 [sertraline], 73; obtained through FOIA.

85. PDAC, Oct. 10, 1985, 118.

86. Ibid., 129.

87. Ibid., 87.

88. Ibid., 133–134.

89. PDAC, Nov. 19, 1990, 97.

90. FDA, "Summary Basis of Approval, NDA 18–936, Drug Generic Name: fluoxetine hydrochloride," Oct. 3, 1988, p. 48; FDA Archives.

91. D[avid] Healy et al., "Suicide in the Course of the Treatment of Depression," *Journal of Psychopharmacology*, 13 (1999), 94–99.

92. Healy, *Let Them Eat Prozac*, 133.

93. See Jack Dolan and Dave Altimari, "Memos Display Drug Firms' Optimism," *Hartford Courant* Sept. 21, 2003; http://www.ctnow.com. There is, however, considerable evidence that Lilly suppressed negative trial data regarding Prozac. See *Susan K. Forsyth* v. *Eli Lilly and Company*, Civil No. 95–00185 ACK, United States District Court for the District of Hawaii, 1998 U.S. Dist. LEXIS 541, decided Jan. 5, 1998.

94. See Alexander Glassman interview by Edward Shorter in New York, Oct. 5, 2004, 23–25. Lilly ultimately did get its combo of Prozac and Zyprexa approved as Symbyax for "bipolar depression."

95. Arif Khan et al., "Are Placebo Controls Necessary to Test New Antidepressants and Anxiolytics?" *International Journal of Neuropsychopharmacology* 5 (2002): 193–197, see 194, table 1.

96. William Guy et al., "Double-Blind Dose Determination Study of a New Antidepressant—Sertraline," *Drug Development Research* 9 (1986): 267–272.

97. Michael Babyak et al., "Exercise Treatment for Major Depression: Maintenance of Therapeutic Benefit at 10 Months," *Psychosomatic Medicine* 62 (2000): 633–638.

98. Thomas E. Donnelly, Jr. (SKB Regulatory Affairs), memorandum, "FDA Conversation Record," Nov. 19, 1990. I am grateful to David Healy for sharing this document with me.

99. Quoted in a web communication by Karen Barth Menzies (a partner at Baum Hedlund, a law firm representing plaintiffs in drug litigation), Dec. 1, 2004; posted by Chris Gupta, Dec. 8, 2004, at http://www.newmediaexplorer. org/chris/2004/12/08 (accessed Mar. 5, 2007). The letter was presumably discovered in legal proceedings.

100. FDA, PDAC, 33rd Meeting, Nov. 19, 1990 [sertraline], 53; obtained through FOIA. (The version that I received from FDA was unpaginated; I paginated the copy I printed out; according to the table of contents, the official FDA transcript apparently had a different pagination.)

101. Ibid., 40.
102. Ibid., 54.
103. Ibid., 59.
104. Ibid., 54–55.
105. Ibid., 64.
106. Ibid., 66.
107. Ibid., 75–76.
108. Zoloft advertisement, *AJP* 149 (March 1992). This was the first Zoloft ad in that journal.
109. Khan, "Are Placebo Controls Necessary?" 194.
110. FDA, PDAC 36th Meeting, Oct. 5, 1992 [paroxetine], 38; obtained through FOIA.
111. Ibid., 127.
112. Danish University Antidepressant Group, "Paroxetine: A Selective Serotonin Reuptake Inhibitor Showing Better Tolerance, but Weaker Antidepressant Effect than Clomipramine in a Controlled Multicenter Study," *Journal of Affective Disorders* 18 (1990): 289–299, quote 297.
113. Paul Leber to Wyeth-Ayerst Laboratories, Aug. 26, 1996; FDA, Center for Drug Evaluation and Research, Approval package for Ativan (lorazepam), NDA 18-140/S-003; http://www.fda.gov/cder/foi/nda/97/018140ap_s003.pdf (accessed July 16, 2002).
114. Delia Gavrus, "The Gatekeepers of American Psychiatry: The FDA and the Approval of SSRIs for Depression, 1985–1992," in *Proceedings of the 15th Annual History of Medicine Days*, ed. W. A. Whitelaw, 138–156 (Calgary: University of Calgary Faculty of Medicine, 2006).
115. FDA, PDAC, 23rd Meeting, Feb. 24, 1983 [antidepressant labeling], 1: 158; obtained through FOIA.
116. PDAC, Nov. 19, 1990, 95–96.
117. Readers are reminded that the PDAC transcripts on which this chapter heavily relies were obtained through requests to the FDA on the basis of the Freedom of Information Act (FOIA). FDA document transfers to the National Archives and Records Administration of the federal government, as of this writing, go little beyond 1982. See Edward Shorter, "The Liberal State and the Rogue Agency: FDA's Regulation of Drugs for Mood Disorders, 1950s-1970s," *International Journal of Law and Psychiatry*, 31 (2008): 126-135.
118. PDAC, Nov. 19, 1990, 98.
119. Louis Lasagna, "Congress, the FDA, and New Drug Development: Before and After 1962," *Perspectives in Biology and Medicine* 32 (1989): 322–343, quote 337.
120. Paul J. Quirk, "Food and Drug Administration," in *The Politics of Regulation*, ed. James Q. Wilson, 191–235 (New York: Basic Books, 1980), quote 211.
121. For an update, see Gardiner Harris, "Potentially Incompatible Goals at F.D.A.," *New York Times*, June 11, 2007, A16.
122. Thomas Ban, personal communication, May 31, 2006.
123. David Sheehan, "Angles on Panic," interview, in *The Psychopharmacologists*, ed. David Healy, 3: 479–503 (London: Arnold, 2000), quote 487.
124. "The Promise of Prozac," *Newsweek*, Mar. 26, 1990, 39.

125. "Psychotropic Sales $7.6 Bill by 1996?" *Scrip*, May 22, 1992, 26.

126. "'Another Excellent Year' for Lilly," *Scrip*, Mar. 14, 1990, 14.

127. Editorial, "If at First You Do Succeed," *Lancet* 337 (Mar. 16, 1991): 650–651.

128. "US Oral Antidepressant Market," *Scrip*, Jan. 23, 1991, 30.

129. "SmithKline Beecham Stresses New Product Growth," *Scrip*, Mar. 2, 1993, 7.

130. "Pfizer's Jump in World Rankings," *Scrip*, Feb. 18, 1994, 10–11.

131. National Institute for Health Care Management data; see "Drug Spending Jumps 17%," *Wall Street Journal*, Mar. 29, 2002, A3.

132. Marie N. Stagnitti, *Trends in the Use and Expenditures for the Therapeutic Class Prescribed Psychotherapeutic Agents and All Subclasses, 1997 and 2004*, Statistical Brief 163. (Rockville, MD: Agency for Healthcare Research and Quality, Feb. 2007); http://www.meps.ahrq.gov/mepsweb/data_files/publications/st163/stat163.pdf (accessed March 13, 2007).

133. Decision Resources data, "Antidepressant Market to Decline Slightly," *Psychiatric News*, Jan. 3, 2003, 1.

134. Mark Olfson et al., "National Trends in the Outpatient Treatment of Depression," *JAMA* 287 (Jan. 9, 2002): 203–209, see 207, table 3.

135. K. M. Brett et al., *Utilization of Ambulatory Medical Care by Women: United States, 1997–98*, National Center for Health Statistics, *Vital Health Statistics* 13, no. 149, (2001): 38, table 14.

136. Heather Mallick, "As If," *Globe and Mail* [Toronto], Jan. 5, 2002, F7.

137. FDA, Psychopharmacologic Drugs Advisory Committee, Sept. 13, 2004 [antidepressants and pediatric suicide], 57–58.

138. FDA, Joint Meeting of the PDAC and the Pediatric Advisory Committee, Sept. 14, 2004 [day II], 338–339; http://www.fda.gov/ohrms/dockets/ac/04/transcripts/2004-4065T1.pdf (accessed March 30, 2005).

139. Michael E. Thase, "How Should Efficacy Be Evaluated in Randomized Clinical Trials of Treatments for Depression?" *Journal of Clinical Psychiatry* 60, no. 4 (1999): 23–31, quote 23.

140. "Relapse Prevention Trials for Long Term Depression Advocated in EU," *Pink Sheet*, Jan. 25, 1999, 17.

141. David Healy, personal communication, July 6, 2007. He based his calculation on data in Marc B. Stone and M. Lisa Jones, "Clinical Review: Relationship Between Antidepressant Drugs and Suicidality in Adults," Nov. 17, 2006, FDA internal document, attached to Thomas P. Laughren to Members of PDAC, Nov. 16, 2006, re "Overview for December 13 Meeting of Psychopharmacologic Drugs Advisory Committee"; www.fda.gov/ohrms/dockets/ac/06/briefing/2006-427261-01-FDA.pdf (accessed Jan. 20, 2007). The Stone and Jones data concerned all currently marketed antidepressant drugs, not just SSRIs.

142. Thomas Ban, personal communication, Feb. 25, 2003.

143. Irving Kirsch et al., "The Emperor's New Drugs: An Analysis of Antidepressant Medication Data Submitted to the U.S. Food and Drug Administration," *Prevention & Treatment* 5, article 23, posted July 15, 2002, http://journals.apa.org/prevention/volume5/pre0050023a.html (accessed Oct. 27, 2002).

144. FDA, Joint meeting of PDAC with the Pediatric Subcommittee of the Anti-Infective Drugs Advisory Committee, Feb. 2, 2004 [pediatric suicide], 173,

http://www.fda.gov/ohrms/dockets/ac/04/transcripts/4006T1.pdf (accessed Mar. 25, 2004).

145. In the dozens of trials comparing TCAs to SSRIs virtually no study has ever found the SSRIs superior to the TCAs from the viewpoint of efficacy, and the consensus is that the dropout rates and side effects of the two drug classes are virtually identical. For a definitive opinion, see J. R. Geddes et al., "Selective Serotonin Reuptake Inhibitors (SSRIs) for Depression (Cochrane Review)," *The Cochrane Library*, Issue 3 (Oxford: Update Software, 2002).

146. Lars F. Gram, "Fluoxetine," *NEJM* 331 (Nov. 17, 1994): 1354–1361, quote 1359.

147. Jan Fawcett et al., "Efficacy Issues with Antidepressants," *Journal of Clinical Psychiatry* 58, no. 6 (1997): 32–39, see 35, table 2.

148. Alan Schatzberg interview, Dec. 12, 2001, 11, ACNP, Oral History Project.

149. David Healy, "Some Continuities and Discontinuities in the Pharmacotherapy of Nervous Conditions Before and After Chlorpromazine and Imipramine," *History of Psychiatry* 11 (2000): 393–412, quote 398.

150. Steven Hollon, "The Emperor's New Drugs: Effect Size and Moderation Effects," *Prevention & Treatment* 5, article 28, posted July 15, 2002, http://journals.apa.org/prevention/volume5/pre0050028c.html.

151. P. K. Gillman places the supposed dangerousness of the tricyclics in some perspective. "The mortality from nortriptyline in overdose (5.5 deaths per million scripts is similar to that from SSRIs, and better than both dothiepin (53.3) and venlafaxine (13.2 deaths per million scripts.)" (Confidence intervals in the original have been omitted here.) Gillman, "Tricyclic Antidepressant Pharmacology and Therapeutic Drug Interactions Updated," *British Journal of Pharmacology* 151 (2007): 737–748, quote 739.

152. John Donoghue, "Selective Serotonin Reuptake Inhibitor Use in Primary Care: A 5-Year Naturalistic Study," *Clinical Drug Investigation* 16 (1998): 453–462.

153. Evelinda Trindade, et al., "Adverse Effects Associated with Selective Serotonin Reuptake Inhibitors and Tricyclic Antidepressants: A Meta-analysis," *Canadian Medical Association Journal* 159 (1998): 1245–1252.

154. Anita H. Clayton et al., "Prevalence of Sexual Dysfunction Among Newer Antidepressants," *Journal of Clinical Psychiatry* 63 (2002): 357–366, quote 363.

155. "Glaxo's Wellbutrin/Zyban U.S. Half-Year Sales More Than Double," *Pink Sheet* Aug. 3, 1998, 15.

156. FDA, PDAC, Dec. 4, 1997 [triazolam], 58; obtained through FOIA.

157. Roland Kuhn, "From Imipramine to Levoprotiline: The Discovery of Antidepressants," in Healy, *Psychopharmacologists*, 2: 93–118, 114. This is the only one of Healy's published interviews that I sat in on, simply because Kuhn wished to be interviewed in German, which I speak but David doesn't.

158. Desyrel advertisement, *AJP* 139 (April, 1982): A51–A58.

159. B[ernard] J. Carroll, "Neurobiologic Dimensions of Depression and Mania," in *The Origins of Depression: Current Concepts and Approaches*, ed. J[ules] Angst, 163–186 (Berlin: Springer, 1983), quote pp. 164–165; the conference occurred Oct. 31–Nov. 5, 1982.

160. Torgny Svensson, discussion, in Ruth Porter, ed., *Antidepressants and Receptor Function*, Ciba Foundation Symposium 123 (Chichester: Wiley, 1986), 275.

161. P. S. Whitton et al., "The Effect of the Novel Antidepressant Tianeptine on the Concentration of 5-Hydroxytryptamine in Rat Hippocampal Dialysates *in Vivo*," *Neuropharmacology* 30 (1991): 1–4.

162. For a summary of this research, see Fridolin Sulser, "My Becoming a Psychopharmacologist," in *Reflections on Twentieth-Century Psychopharmacology*, ed. Thomas Ban et al., 299–307 (Budapest: Animula, 2004), quote 304.

163. J[ohn] Evenden, S[tephen] J. Peroutka, discussion, in Merton Sandler et al., eds., *5-Hydroxytryptamine in Psychiatry: A Spectrum of Ideas* (Oxford: Oxford University Press, 1991), 20.

164. George Beaumont, discussion, in E. M. Tansey and D. A. Christie, eds., "Drugs in Psychiatric Practice: The Transcript of a Witness Seminar Held at the Wellcome Institute for the History of Medicine, London, on 11 March 1997," in *Wellcome Witnesses to Twentieth Century Medicine*, ed. Tansey et al., 2: 133–204, (London: Wellcome Trust, 1998), 196.

165. "CINP Meeting with the Nobels, Montreal, Canada, June 25, 2002: Speaker's Notes—Dr. Arvid Carlsson," *Collegium Internationale Neuro-Psychopharmacologicum Newsletter*, March 2003, 5.

166. See Jeffrey R. Lacasse and Jonathan Leo, "Serotonin and Depression: A Disconnect Between the Advertisements and the Scientific Literature," *PloS Medicine* 2, no. 12 (Dec. 2005): e392; doi:10.1371/journal.pmed.0020392.

167. Louis Lasagna, "Clinical Trials of Drugs from the Viewpoint of the Academic Investigator (A Satire)," *Clinical Pharmacology and Therapeutics* 18 (1975): 629–633, quote 632.

168. Jamie Reidy, *Hard Sell: The Evolution of a Viagra Salesman* (Kansas City: Andrews McMeel, 2005), 49–50.

169. Personal communication of a physician who wished to remain anonymous to Edward Shorter, July 27, 2005.

170. Melody Petersen, "Heartfelt Advice, Hefty Fees: Companies Pay Stars to Mention Prescription Drugs," *New York Times*, Aug. 11, 2002, 3.1, 14.

NOTES TO CHAPTER 9

1. See psycho-pharm@psycom.net, posts of May 17, 2007.

2. Bruce G. Charlton, "Editorial: Boom or Bubble? Is Medical Research Thriving or About to Crash?" *Medical Hypotheses* 65 (2006): 1–2.

3. J[ulius] Hoenig, "Psychiatric Nosology," *Canadian Journal of Psychiatry* 26 (1981): 85.

4. A. John Rush et al., "Bupropion-SR, Sertraline, or Venlafaxine-XR after Failure of SSRIs for Depression," *NEJM* 354 (Mar. 23, 2006): 1231–1242.

5. Ivan Feinstein, discussion, in Joseph D. Cooper, *The Efficacy of Self-Medication*, Philosophy and Technology of Drug Assessment, (Washington, DC: Interdisciplinary Communication Associates, 1973), 4: 146.

6. Roland Kuhn, "From Imipramine to Levoprotiline: The Discovery of Antidepressants," in *The Psychopharmacologists*, ed. David Healy, 2: 93–118 (London: Chapman & Hall, 1998), quote 99.

7. E. M. Tansey et al., eds., *Wellcome Witnesses to Twentieth Century Medicine* (London: Wellcome Trust, 1998), discussion, 171. The group discussion in which Sandler made the comment occurred in 1997.

8. Jonathan O. Cole, "The Future of Psychopharmacology," in *Depression in the 1970's: Modern Theory and Research*, ed. Ronald R. Fieve, 81–86 (Amsterdam: Excerpta Medica, 1971). The conference took place in 1970.

9. Mario Roy and Jacques Bernier, "A Rapid Response with Psychostimulants in the Treatment of Depressed Persons with Medical Illnesses," *Canadian Journal of Psychiatry* 44 (1999): 283–284, quote 283.

10. Fridolin Sulser, "From the Presynaptic Neurone to the Receptor to the Nucleus" (interview), in *The Psychopharmacologists*, ed. David Healy, 3: 239–258 (London: Arnold, 2000), quote 247.

11. I am anonymizing the author of this post of Mar. 25, 2007, to psycho-pharm@psycom.net, on the grounds that he did not realize he was speaking for publication.

12. See Peter Temin, *Taking Your Medicine: Drug Regulation in the United States* (Cambridge: Harvard University Press, 1980), 42–44.

Acknowledgment

I gratefully acknowledge financial support of this research from the Canadian Institutes of Health Research (CIHR), the Social Sciences and Humanities Council of Canada (SSHRC), and the Scion Natural Science Association.

Index

Abbott Laboratories, 26, 30
Abraham, Hilda, 62
Abraham, Karl, 62
Adair, James, 12
Addiction concerns, 16, 44, 75, 80, 81
   amphetamines, 31, 33, 75, 81, 138
   barbiturates, 22–23, 75, 80, 81
   benzodiazepines, 113–15, 122, 180
   downplayed by Leber, 182
   as hysteria and over-reaction, 74,
     103–4, 115–25
   as marketing ploy, 197
   meprobamate, 44, 74, 75, 77–92
   SSRIs, 197
   vs. "dependence," 23, 44, 80
   vs. "habituation," 75
Addiction Research Center. *See*
   National Institute of Mental
   Health (NIMH), Addiction
   Research Center
Adjustment disorder, 159
Adrenaline. *See* epinephrine
Affective disorders, 4, 15, 43, 158, 159.
   See also Mood disorders
Agnew, Spiro, 117
Akathisia, 190
Alexander, Leo, 18, 58, 87, 90
Alprazolam. *See* Xanax
American Medical Association, 42, 57,
   59, 98, 133
   conferences, 57, 59
   Council on Drugs, 42, 98

American Psychiatric Association
   (APA), 124, 155, 158, 205, 206
   DSM series, 4, 151, 154
   DSM-III process, 159, 160, 162, 165
Amine theory of depression. *See*
   Monoamine reuptake theory of
   depression
Amitriptyline (Elavil), 119, 137, 148,
   149, 198
   comparative studies, 173, 174, 186
   norepinephrine reuptake inhibition,
     172
Amphetamines, 24–33, 56, 64
   addiction concerns, 75, 80, 81
   as antidepressants, 24–25, 212
   combined with barbiturates, 31–33
   controlled-drug status, 84, 88
Amytal (amobarbital), 19–21, 30, 32, 33
Andreasen, Nancy, 156
Angst, Jules, 25
Anhedonia, 58
Annis, Edward, 87, 88
Anslinger, Harry, 75
Antianxiety drugs. *See* Anxiolytics
Antidepressants, 152, 180–81, 183,
   211. *See also* Monoamine oxidase
   inhibitors (MAOIs), Selective
   serotonin reuptake inhibitors
   (SSRIs), Tricyclic antidepressants
   (TCAs)
   amphetamines as, 24–30, 32–33, 212
   antipsychotics as, 46–52

291

Durham–Humphrey Act (1951), 91, 107
Dysthymia, 162, 163, 164

Ecstacy (hallucinogen), 26
ECT. *See* Electroconvulsive therapy
Eddy, Nathan, 75
Edeleano, Lazar, 25, 27
Edwards, Charles, 145, 184
Effexor (venlafaxine), 197, 199, 211
Efficacy, drug, 130, 132, 134, 140.
    See also Drug Efficacy Study
    (DES), Drug Efficacy Study
    Implementation (DESI)
  comparative studies rejected, 184–88
  decline in, 4, 39, 184, 194, 207
  disadvantages of mandating, 213
  drug removals, 142–43
  controlled-trial vs. clinical
      experience, 6–9, 130, 131, 135,
      139
  in inpatient vs. outpatient
      populations, 191–92, 193–94
  mandated by Kefauver–Harris Act
      (1962), 97, 127
  "possibly" effective ratings, 131,
      133, 135, 136, 137, 141, 143, 144
  "probably" effective ratings, 131,
      133, 135, 138, 143, 144, 148
Electroconvulsive therapy (ECT), 47,
    48, 50, 60, 66, 192
  in catatonia, 8
  in melancholia, 48, 64, 165
  vs. Marsilid, 54, 55, 56
Eli Lilly, 19, 187, 190–91
  Prozac, 176–77, 189, 190, 194,
      198, 202
Ellenhorn, Matthew, 104, 105
Ellis, Havelock, 26
Elsasser, Gunter, 16
Elvehjem, Conrad Arnold, 14
Endicott, Jean, 156, 158
Engelhardt, David, 134
Ephedrine, 25, 27, 28, 53
Epilepsy, 18, 24, 32
Energizers. *See* Monoamine oxidase
    inhibitors (MAOIs)
Epinephrine (adrenaline), 25, 26, 27,
    28, 53
Equanil. *See* Meprobamate
Escobar, Javier, 192

Essig, Carl, 75, 88, 89
Evenden, John , 204
Evidence-based medicine, 8
Ewing, John, 89
Extrapyramidal motor syndromes
    (EPS), 48, 96

Family medicine, 39, 134, 137, 138
  benzodiazepines in, 100–1, 124
Fawcett, Jan, 201
Feighner, John, 155
Feighner criteria (1972), 155, 156, 158
Feinstein, Alvan, 211
Feldman, Paul, 100
Felix, Robert, 76
Fieve, Ronald, 67
Fink, Max, 24, 50, 64, 165, 168
Finlator, John, 106, 107
Finney, Thomas, 108, 109
Fischer, Emil, 19
Fish, Frank, 35
5-HT. *See* Serotonin
Fluoxetine. *See* Prozac
Flurazepam (Dalmane), 99
Fluvoxamine (Luvox), 175, 188, 194
Food and Drugs Act (1906), 73
Food and Drug Administration (FDA),
    3, 5, 35, 38, 57, 96
  on comparative efficacy studies,
      184–87
  drug efficacy study. *See* Drug
      Efficacy Study Implementation
      (DESI)
  expansion of powers, 81–83, 92, 127,
      129, 130, 139, 140, 144–46
  growth of agency, 73, 74, 77, 81,
      140, 146
  impact on drug supply, 33, 207, 213
  interference in medicine, 88, 143–44,
      148–49, 212–13
  and Kefauver–Harris Amendments
      (1962), 8, 104, 127, 128, 140
  Librium and Valium, assault on, 10,
      95, 100, 103–12, 126
  lithium, 65, 67
  meprobamate, assault on, 10, 44,
      78–92, 95, 126
  relations with pharmaceutical
      industry, 77–78, 84, 92, 104–5,
      126, 130–31, 179, 194–96
  and SSRIs, 178–96

Monoamine neurotransmitters. *See*
    Neurotransmitters
Monoamine oxidase inhibitors
    (MAOIs), 52–59, 68, 167, 212
  in atypical depression, 165
  decline of, 64
  and DESI, 130, 137, 141, 147–148
  proposed withdrawal by FDA, 129
  reuptake inhibition and, 71
  tryptophan augmentation, 171
  vs. SSRIs, 195, 199
Monoamine reuptake theory of
    depression, 52, 54, 71
  dismissed by scientists, 203–5
Mood disorders, 3, 4, 10, 15,
    20, 158. *See also* Affective
    disorders
  current bankruptcy of concept, 168
  drug treatments, 43, 58, 61, 65, 101
  in *DSM-II*, 158
  in *DSM-III*, 160
  intermittent, 159
  melancholic vs. nonmelancholic, 14
  pre-psychopharmacologic remedies,
    12–13, 15–18
Morphine, 16
Mosholder, Andrew, 188
Moulton, Barbara, 77
Moxness, Bennie, 84
Murphy, Alfred, 85
Musto, David, 17
Myerson, Abraham, 29, 32

Nabenhauer, Fred, 27, 29
Nagai, Nagayoshi, 25
Narcolepsy, 25, 28, 147
Narcotics, 15–18, 73, 79
Nardil. *See* phenelzine
Natenshon, Adolph, 40
Nathanson, Morris, 29
National Academy of Sciences,
    National Research Council
    (NAS/NRC), 74, 75, 130,
    131, 133
  Drug Efficacy Study (DES), 127, 129,
    130–39, 140, 147, 184
  gastrointestinal panel, 137
  psychiatry panel, 134–39, 141, 148
National Archives and Records
    Administration, 110, 111
National Heart Institute, 54, 69, 170

National Institute of Mental Health
    (NIMH), 76, 210, 211
  Addiction Research Center,
    Lexington, Ky, 75, 88, 107
  Psychopharmacology Research
    Center (PSC), 63, 96, 114,
    134, 212
National Institutes of Health (NIH),
    69, 76, 170. *See also* National Heart
    Institute, National Institute of
    Mental Health
National Institute on Drug Abuse
    (NIDA), 113, 118–19
National Research Council (NRC). *See*
    National Academy of Sciences,
    National Research Council
Neuroleptics, 46, 50, 51. *See also*
    Antipsychotics
Neurosis, 49, 126, 157
  depressive, 158, 162, 163
Neurotransmitters, 13, 64, 69,
    171, 212. *See also* Dopamine,
    Norepinephrine, Serotonin
  dismissed as basis of depression,
    203–5
  reuptake inhibition, 52, 62, 70–71,
    172
New Drug Applications (NDAs), 35,
    57, 67, 74, 77, 184
  addition of efficacy provisions, 76,
    97, 128
  considered by PDAC, 180, 186
  extension to old drugs, 129, 140
  meprobamate, 78–79, 85
  SSRIs, 178, 188, 189, 191, 193
  withdrawal of, 139, 141
"New drug" status, 94, 130, 184
New York State Psychiatric Institute
    (PI), 36, 64, 154, 190
  and DSM-III, 155, 156, 162
Newman, Thomas, 199, 200
Nialamide (Niamid), 58
NIMH. *See* National Institute of
    Mental Health
Nixon, Richard, 79, 117
Nonmelancholia/Nonmelancholic
    depression, 10, 14, 158, 165, 183
  amphetamines in, 24–25, 28–29
  benzodiazepines in, 100, 101–2
  as comparable to "neuroses," 157
  heterogeneity of, 150, 152